THE OPEN FIELD / PENGUIN LIFE

THE NEW RULES OF WOMEN'S HEALTH

Meghan Rabbitt is an award-winning journalist covering health, nutrition, and psychology. She's currently an editor at Maria Shriver's *The Sunday Paper* and has written for *Prevention*, *Health*, *Women's Health*, and more. She's previously worked at *Parenting*, *Alternative Medicine*, *Natural Health*, and *Yoga Journal* magazines.

The
NEW RULES
of
WOMEN'S
HEALTH

Your Guide to Thriving at Every Age

Meghan Rabbitt

THE OPEN FIELD / PENGUIN LIFE

PENGUIN BOOKS

An imprint of Penguin Random House LLC
1745 Broadway, New York, NY 10019
penguinrandomhouse.com

The Open Field/A Penguin Life Book

THE OPEN FIELD is a registered trademark of MOS Enterprises, Inc.

Illustrations by Allan Santos

Set in FS Brabo
Designed by Sabrina Bowers

LIBRARY OF CONGRESS CONTROL NUMBER: 2025006010
ISBN 9780143137962 (paperback)
ISBN 9780593512050 (ebook)

Printed in the United States of America
1st Printing

The authorized representative in the EU for product safety and compliance is
Penguin Random House Ireland, Morrison Chambers, 32 Nassau Street,
Dublin D02 YH68, Ireland, https://eu-contact.penguin.ie.

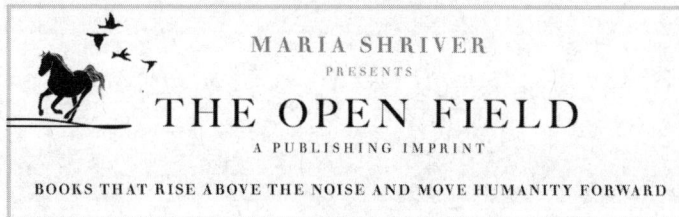

MARIA SHRIVER

PRESENTS

THE OPEN FIELD

A PUBLISHING IMPRINT

BOOKS THAT RISE ABOVE THE NOISE AND MOVE HUMANITY FORWARD

Dear Reader,

Years ago, these words attributed to Rumi found a place in my heart:

Out beyond ideas of
wrongdoing and rightdoing,
there is a field. I'll meet you there.

Ever since, I've cultivated an image of what I call "the Open Field"—a place out beyond fear and shame, beyond judgment, loneliness, and expectation. A place that hosts the reunion of all creation. It's the hope of my soul to find my way there—and whenever I hear an insight or a practice that helps me on the path, I love nothing more than to share it with others.

That's why I've created The Open Field. My hope is to publish books that honor the most unifying truth in human life: We are all seeking the same things. We're all seeking dignity. We're all seeking joy. We're all seeking love and acceptance, seeking to be seen, to be safe. And there is no competition for these things we seek—because they are not material goods; they are spiritual gifts!

We can all give each other these gifts if we share what we know—what has lifted us up and moved us forward. That is our duty to one another—to help each other toward acceptance, toward peace, toward happiness—and my promise to you is that the books published under this imprint will be maps to the Open Field, written by guides who know the path and want to share it.

Each title will offer insights, inspiration, and guidance for moving beyond the fears, the judgments, and the masks we all wear. And when we take off the masks, guess what? We will see that we are the opposite of what we thought—we are each other.

We are all on our way to the Open Field. We are all helping one another along the path. I'll meet you there.

Love, Maria S

For my nieces,
Maeve, McKenna, and Sydney

Contents

PART II

The Specialties: Staying Informed and Attuned

PART III

Optimize Your Health: The Road to Strength and Resilience

Foreword

I'm thrilled that you have picked up this book because every woman I know will benefit greatly from it. I wish this book had been around when I was young, or even when I was approaching midlife. That's why I commissioned the amazing health reporter Meghan Rabbitt to write it.

This book belongs in every woman's hands. It needs to go with you to every doctor's appointment. You need to share it with everyone in your life. Because the truth is that women's health has been misunderstood, overlooked, and underresearched for far too long. Women make up half the population, yet every single woman I talk to, no matter where in the country I'm visiting, tells me the same thing: "I can't get the healthcare answers I need to help myself, my mother, my grandmother, my sister, my daughter."

I imagine you have some version of that story, too—one where at some point in your life, you were left with more questions than answers about your body or about one of the many diseases that disproportionately impact women.

You're not alone. After all, even our healthcare providers admit to having more questions than answers about countless women's health topics. This is the state of women's healthcare due to our woeful lack of female-specific health research.

Why do women make up a staggering two-thirds of all Alzheimer's diagnoses? How does hormonal birth control impact the brain and body over time? Why do gynecologic conditions, such as endometriosis and polycystic ovary syndrome (PCOS), remain so poorly understood and so rarely discussed? Why don't we have more data on perimenopause—one of the most consequential hormonal transitions of a woman's life? Why are women the majority of those who develop autoimmune diseases, multiple sclerosis, and migraine headaches? Why is it that a staggering 80 percent of women aged fifty-five and older have at least one chronic condition, such as asthma, arthritis, cancer, or cardiovascular disease?

The sad truth is that we don't have definitive answers. We live in a country that prides itself on medical innovation, yet we are failing women—failing to study them, failing to listen to them, and failing to provide the much-needed explanations to their most important queries.

Women deserve better. We deserve answers. And the only path forward is research that recognizes women's health as the essential, urgent priority it is.

For decades now, I've been relentlessly asking for this research, and hearing the unsatisfying answer that it just doesn't exist. When my father was diagnosed with Alzheimer's disease in 2003, I couldn't fathom how this man who was the founding director of the Peace Corps and launched the War on Poverty could go from knowing so much about so many things to being unable to remember my name or his own. It sparked countless questions about the disease: When, why, and how does it start? What can one do to prevent it from developing? This led me to write a children's book, *What's Happening to Grandpa?*, and to produce an HBO documentary on the disease and its impact on kids and families. But it wasn't until I started hearing from women— stories from my peers—about the Alzheimer's diagnoses their grandmothers, mothers, sisters, and even they were dealing with themselves that I realized something was amiss. I started asking doctors if Alzheimer's disproportionately affected women's brains. I got a lot of non-answers that included information about plaques and tangles and the dismissive explanation that women simply lived longer. This didn't square with what I was seeing and hearing.

Driven by this disconnect, I partnered with the Alzheimer's Association to launch *The Shriver Report: A Woman's Nation Takes on Alzheimer's*. Our investigation revealed a startling truth that I reported to the country: A staggering two-thirds of those living with Alzheimer's are women. And even more concerning, nobody knows *why*. The realization—and frustration— that we hadn't adequately researched women's brains fired me up.

My drive for answers ultimately led me to launch the Women's Alzheimer's Movement (WAM), now part of the esteemed Cleveland Clinic, to raise awareness and fund research on Alzheimer's disease and particularly its impact on women. Why is it that two out of every three brains that are diagnosed with Alzheimer's disease belong to women? I founded WAM to answer that question, and we've since spent millions of dollars on research and given many grants to scientists who are passionate about answering that question as well. Thankfully, the narrative has changed, and we have more awareness and research than ever before about the cognitive changes that disproportionately impact women. But we are still decades behind, and not nearly enough has been done at the national level to make up for lost time.

I'm proud to say that WAM led to the first-ever Women's Alzheimer's Movement Prevention and Research Center at Cleveland Clinic, which in turn paved the way for the first of its kind Women's Comprehensive Health and Research Center at Cleveland Clinic, which opened in the spring of 2024 and has already cared for thousands of women facing the many conditions that disproportionately impact them. I serve as chief visionary and strategic advisor for this center, and we're on a mission to provide women— particularly those in midlife and beyond—with research-informed, comprehensive, and compassionate healthcare. It's a place for women at every stage of their lives to feel seen, to feel heard, and to get the care they deserve.

My twenty-plus years of work advocating for women's health led me to the White House, where I spoke to First Lady Jill Biden about the critical need for a more nuanced and comprehensive approach to studying women's health. Can you believe that it wasn't until 2024 and the leadership of President Biden and Dr. Jill Biden that we had a White House Initiative on Women's Health Research, a program aimed at funding and advancing women's health research and development?

These are all big advancements. And I believe there will be many more in the years to come, because women are advocating for change across the board. They're starting organizations to push for menopause legislation. They're demanding answers about conditions like PCOS, endometriosis, autoimmune diseases, and more. Clinicians are banding together to enact change as well, such as a group of menopause specialists urging the Food and Drug Administration to take black box warnings off menopause hormone therapy. A growing number of doctors are also speaking out about how shockingly little education focused on women's health they received in medical school, and they're trying to change that for future students.

Collectively, we must continue to fight for change. Every woman should have access to healthcare providers who understand that women aren't just small men and that our health needs are different and often more complex than our male counterparts. We deserve research that gives our clinicians robust evidence to inform how they care for us. But until this happens, we must be relentless. We must advocate for ourselves and for our loved ones, push through the current barriers, and refuse to stop until we have the answers we need. The days of neglecting ourselves are officially over. The days of accepting the old status quo are over. It's time to stop doubting ourselves and our symptoms. It's time to own our stories and share them. And it's time to demand that our healthcare providers believe us when we tell them how we feel.

We must become the CEOs of our own health. And I believe this book will help us do just that.

Journalist Meghan Rabbitt has spent the last twenty-five years on the women's health beat, reporting on what we know—and don't know—about the many conditions that disproportionately impact girls and women. Why is puberty happening earlier than ever before? Why are so many women underestimating their lifetime risk of breast cancer, and why are too many doctors not using the tools available to them to calculate this risk? Why do women make up a whopping 70 percent of chronic pain patients, yet we're more likely than men to have our pain dismissed by medical providers?

Meghan has tackled these questions and many more in articles for print magazines and digital media outlets. She also writes about these topics for Shriver Media's award-winning weekly digital newsmagazine *The Sunday Paper*. She has spent her career interviewing researchers, clinicians, and other leading experts in a range of fields to bring women the information they need to make actionable changes in their lives based on the evidence we *do* have. For this book, Meghan interviewed more than a hundred experts to bring you the critical knowledge you need about your body, provide you with the language to talk to your doctors about your health, and empower you to care for yourself and the ones you love in a way that helps you feel like you're thriving at every age and stage of your life.

Throughout my childhood, I watched my mother struggle with her health. She went from doctor to doctor to get answers for the health issues that plagued her. My mother was a force of nature and the sister of the president of the United States, and even *she* had to navigate a healthcare system that left her with more questions than answers. From a very early age, I realized that if my mom struggled, what were women without the same access to top-notch healthcare and the resources to pay for that care dealing with and feeling?

Women's health begins at birth, and it spans puberty, pregnancy, motherhood, menopause, and beyond. Yet at every stage of our lives, we are still faced with critical gaps in knowledge. Filling in those gaps by raising awareness and funding research has been a passion and mission of mine for the last several decades.

Even though too many of us aren't getting the care we deserve, and even though we *still* have far more questions than answers when it comes to women's health, I'm deeply optimistic about the future because I believe in the power of women. We have the power to educate ourselves about our health, to speak up for ourselves, to seek out better care, and to fight for better research and a more equitable healthcare system for all.

This book is a testament to that power. It is an invitation to become more informed and engaged so you can navigate your own health journey with confidence and clarity. It is a call to join the growing movement of women who are ready to demand the research they need and the care they deserve. It is the guide you need to become a fierce advocate for your own health, for the women and girls in your life, and for our sisters all around the world.

—MARIA SHRIVER

Introduction

It's Time to Own Your Health and Advocate for Yourself.

Here's Where to Start.

> Communities and countries and ultimately the world are only as strong as the health of their women.
>
> —Michelle Obama, address to students at the Elizabeth Garrett Anderson School, 2009

As women, we get a lot of confusing messages about our bodies starting at a young age—and not a lot of clear explanations about how they work.

If we're lucky, we spend our early years simply *being* in these sophisticated machines, getting acquainted with how they feel and what they can and can't do as we explore the world. There may be a sense of wonder and admiration for the running, jumping, and playing our bodies help us do. We feel powerful in our bodies—and either unaware of or indifferent about what anyone else might think about them.

Then the world gets to us. We hear a nasty comment from the elementary school bully and start to suspect that our bodies are for *looking at*, not *living in*. A well-meaning parent or caregiver gives us the general gist of where babies come from—some version of "You grew in Mommy's belly, and one day you'll grow a baby in your belly, too!"—and the follow-up questions this inevitably inspires are often met with vague, confusing answers. As puberty hits and everything starts changing in strange and oftentimes shocking ways, we become aware that our bodies are transforming but get little or no explanation about *why* these changes are taking place.

The closest most of us come to that kind of education happens in a middle or high school health class that typically covers some basic anatomy with a unit on sex ed that's almost always focused on what *not* to do. ("Don't have sex, and if you do, don't get pregnant or contract a sexually transmitted disease.") We pick up information and *misinformation* from social media and the internet.

As time goes on, it's no wonder so many of us lose our sense of wonder about our bodies and, worse, start to feel disempowered: We lack the information we need to take ownership of our health and become our own best advocates.

This book is here to empower you with that information. Because being able to truly care for yourself starts with an understanding of the body you're caring for.

You can think of this book as a user's manual for your female body—an easy-to-understand primer about how it works, what can go wrong, and the newest research on disease prevention, as well as how to heal and recover from health setbacks. The insights and advice you'll find in these pages have been culled from more than a hundred interviews with women's health researchers and clinicians who've made it their life's work to understand women's bodies and help you understand yours. Their mission—and mine—is to leave you feeling like you have what you need to take ownership of your health at every stage of life and restore the sense of wonder, awe, and admiration your body so deeply deserves.

Why I Wrote This Book

As a journalist who has spent the last twenty-five years talking to some of the world's leading health experts and learning everything I can about various health conditions, you'd think I'd have a deep knowledge of my body and the ability to detect when something was a sign of an underlying health issue.

Yet for years, I experienced debilitatingly heavy menstrual cycles, and I'd brush them off as no big deal. Every month, I'd joke about my week of "hemorrhaging," and as it got worse in my early forties, I blamed it on perimenopause.

I casually mentioned this to my gynecologist at my annual exam, joking with her that even the Costco-sized package of pads was now not enough to get me through one cycle. Next thing I knew, a vaginal ultrasound showed that my uterus was filled with fibroids—a veritable fruit basket of them. I choked back tears as I asked a slew of questions: *What does this mean? Why did they develop? What can I do about them?* I could only half listen to the responses due to the internal self-berating that quickly set in: *Why didn't I raise a flag about those heavy periods? Why didn't I have more conversations with my doctor about what I could do to prevent fibroids, given my mother's history of them?* Even now, five years after that initial diagnosis, I'm still trying to shake off that "if only" thinking.

Despite the many years I've spent writing about conditions that disproportionately impact women—interviewing patients struggling with disease, the doctors caring for them, and the researchers working passionately to find new treatments—there's still much more I'd like to understand about my body and my health. I suspect this is true for you, too. And in this time of the endless scroll—where countless articles, social media influencers, and other questionable sources hawk health advice and wellness hacks that are rarely evidence-based—it can be tricky to sort the legit from the ludicrous. Now more than ever, we need a trusted guide.

Years ago, that guide might've been a primary care physician (PCP). These days, one-fourth of adults and nearly half of those under age thirty don't have a PCP.[1] Even if you do have a go-to doctor, you're probably lucky if you can sneak in for an appointment when you're sick, let alone spend thirty minutes or more asking questions that would give you the foundation to be proactive about your health. And when you do bring up what's bothering you, there's a chance you'll get dismissed and be disbelieved. Most women can tell stories about their healthcare providers' shoulder shrugs and facial expressions that say, *I'm sorry you're dealing with this, but I don't know how to help you.* Too many of us have also had our ailments blamed on our diet, weight, age, or "lifestyle choices"—points that tend to prompt shame in even the most self-assured among us.

And so we shut down. We don't share the full story about how we're feeling and what we're experiencing. We don't feel like reliable storytellers of our own experiences because we fear we don't have our facts right. And the cycle of not talking can lead us into not advocating for the care we need and deserve.

Since that day when I found myself on the ultrasound tech's table, looking at an image of countless lumpy (though thankfully benign) growths in my uterus, I've had more experiences that have left me scared about my health and filled with questions. My annual mammograms usually require follow-up breast ultrasounds to make sure the cysts are just cysts. I make twice-yearly appointments with my dermatologist due to the number of precancerous moles I've had removed and biopsied. I've been lucky to have some incredible healthcare practitioners who've held my hand as I've looked at them wide-eyed and worried—kind clinicians who've walked me through their action plan for treatment and follow-up care. But I've also had plenty of experiences with less skillful practitioners—ones who've left me with more questions than answers and with that dreaded feeling of shame that I should know more about what's happening with my body than I do.

I'll never forget those helpful healthcare providers who treated me with care and respect. And one of the reasons I wrote this book is because I wish such a resource had been there for me to turn to after those not-so-great interactions with the less helpful clinicians. It's the book I want my nieces to be able to pick up when they have questions about what's happening to them—a source of information that'll encourage them to listen to their symptoms and give them the confidence to not take "I don't know" as an acceptable answer when they seek help.

My hope is that this book will help you do the same.

Some of the information you'll find here may feel like a refresher on what you already know. Some of it will feel brand-new and downright surprising. Some of it may quite possibly save your life—or the life of someone you love. While interviewing experts for this book, I lost track of the number of times I stared open-mouthed in surprise at the information I was learning. Some of the revelations were filling in holes in my education. Other pieces, however, felt shockingly new because the information itself *is* new. We've entered an era where women's bodies and health are beginning to be as rigorously studied as our male counterparts', and this new world of knowledge is teeing us up for better health than ever before.

Women's Health Is Having a Moment

For far too long, women were treated medically as if our bodies were the same as men's, just smaller and with a few different parts. The medical bias reflects a broader scientific one. Indeed, the movement to consider sex-specific differences in medical research didn't really begin in earnest until 1985. That's when a report from the U.S. Public Health Service Task Force on Women's Health Issues concluded that "research should emphasize disease unique to women or more prevalent in women."[2] Finally, an organization with the power to enact some change on this front was essentially saying that women are not small men, and that it would make sense to study how all kinds of diseases impact us—not just the ones that affect our reproductive organs.

Yet while that report got the ball rolling, it wasn't until 1993 that the U.S. National Institutes of Health (NIH) required women and minorities to be included in NIH-funded research.[3] Fast-forward to 2012, and the NIH finally started a gynecologic branch.[4] This represented some progress, but still, too few research dollars were dedicated to women's health issues. Finally, in 2024, the first-ever White House Initiative on Women's Health Research was established to accelerate research aimed at preventing, diagnosing, and treating conditions that affect women uniquely, disproportionately, or differently.

There is a long list of reasons why it's taken so long for scientists to study women. For starters, there's a real and serious sexism problem in science, with women largely excluded from the labs and research groups doing the studying. Think about it: Scientists are people, too, interested in studying what's on their radar. It's not so surprising, then, that men—who've never experienced the stabbing pelvic pain that comes with conditions like endometriosis or polycystic ovary syndrome or the years of angst and multiple doctor visits often involved in getting an autoimmune disease diagnosis—haven't exactly prioritized their attention or requests for funding toward these conditions.

For many years, there were also justifications for excluding females from experiments. One common one was that the male body was the "norm" and could adequately represent the entirety of the human species. Another was the idea that our fluctuating hormones make us more "variable" than males and too troublesome to research as a result. One of the more understandable rationales was the concern that testing new medical treatments on women of childbearing age might impact unborn children—yet this reasoning is why females make up only about 30 percent of the participants in drug trials[5] and why most drugs haven't actually been tested on pregnant women.

While we've made progress, women's health is still under-studied, and sex-specific research continues to be underfunded.[6] Too many of our medications and treatments are based on men's bodies. Even the medical school textbooks that educate the next generation of healthcare providers still contain little information or emphasis on important women's health topics. If you've ever been baffled about why your clinician couldn't answer questions about sexual dysfunction or menopause hormone therapy, there's a reason for those blank spots in their knowledge. We still have a lot of work to do to close the major gaps in our understanding of how and why so many conditions impact women differently from men.

Thankfully, women are taking matters into our own hands, and we're talking more openly and honestly than ever before on both the local and the national stage about the ways this lack of sex-specific research and lackluster understanding of women's health have real, life-threatening consequences.

Tennis great Serena Williams and Olympic track-and-field star Allyson Felix have been heartbreakingly honest about their potentially life-threatening experiences related to giving birth, helping shine a much-needed light on the obstacles Black women face in getting healthcare and why, as a result, they are disproportionately dying during childbirth.[7]

Comedian Amy Schumer has cracked jokes and earnestly shared details about her decades-long struggle with undiagnosed endometriosis, the debilitating pain that came along with it, and how not knowing what was wrong with her for so many years drastically impacted her life.

Actress Angelina Jolie was a trailblazer in her openness talking about her genetic risk of breast cancer and the preventive double mastectomy she chose to get. Olivia Munn told her story of how getting a breast MRI—which showed an aggressive cancer in both of her breasts—saved her life. And Halle Berry shouted, "I'm in menopause!" on Capitol Hill to help lift the stigma that still exists around this period of a woman's life and to lobby for millions more research dollars to be allocated to this pivotal health transition we still know far too little about.

The rest of us are choosing to be more open with one another about what's going on with our health, too. We're being more specific with our kids when we give them "the talk" about sex and pleasure. We're talking about our stabbing cramps, heavy periods, hot flashes, and countless other common symptoms that our mothers were taught to power through and stay quiet about. We're also demanding better care from our healthcare providers, and a new crop of (largely female) clinicians—many of whom you'll see quoted in the pages of this book—are committed to meeting our needs by giving themselves the women's health education they should've gotten in medical school but didn't. One group of these clinicians who care for women at midlife have even banded together and given themselves a name—"the Menoposse"—to amplify their efforts to educate themselves and the rest of us so we're able to get better quality menopause care.

The progress we've made has ignited a new conversation and a new way of talking about women's health. The science is catching up, too, with new research emerging and bringing with it new understandings of women's health in all its aspects. This book is an invitation for all of us to take steps to optimize our health, advocate for ourselves based on the research we do have, and jump on the momentum that's putting women's health at the center of our collective conversation.

Whom This Book Is For—and How to Use It

This book is for young women who are coming of age just as much as it's for those of us who know that as women, we are *always* coming of age. It's for those of us who believe that when we're going through massive changes like puberty and pregnancy, motherhood and midlife, knowledge is power.

You can read this book cover to cover for an in-depth education on your body and how to optimize your health. Or you can treat it more like an à la carte menu, flipping right to the chapters that are most relevant to you (or the people you love) right now.

It's important to note that I am a journalist, not a healthcare provider. I rigorously reported and fact-checked the information in this book, but it is not meant to be used to diagnose specific health concerns or replace essential conversations with your healthcare team. This book is meant to be used as a tool to inform you so that you can take that knowledge and talk to your clinicians about any health concerns you have, as well as the testing and treatment that's right for *you*.

The book is divided into three sections.

In part I, we'll talk about the women's health concerns and conditions that would prompt you to make an appointment with a gynecologist or other women's health specialist. In this section, we'll . . .

- **Give you a primer on female anatomy** that's so much more vast (and fascinating!) than that cartoon illustration of the uterus, uterine tubes, and ovaries most of us have seen.

- **Walk through the essential information you need about puberty,** why it's starting earlier in girls than ever before, and how understanding your own puberty transition—even if it was years ago—can help you show up for and support the young people in your life.

- **Outline what to know about your sexual and gynecologic health,** as well as fertility, pregnancy, childbirth, and hormones.

- **Explain what to expect during the menopause transition,** how to manage the symptoms, and the steps you can take to optimize your health through this period of life.

In part II, we'll dive into the major health specialties with an eye toward pinpointing the important differences in how various diseases develop in women versus men. In this section, we'll . . .

- **See how the female immune system works** and why nearly 80 percent of people with autoimmune disease are women.

- **Talk about why women make up just over 70 percent of chronic pain patients** and may feel pain more intensely than men, and why women and people of color are more likely to have symptoms dismissed by medical providers, even when facing life-threatening situations.

- **Look at the groundbreaking research that's transformed how we think of women's brain and heart health.** The research advances we've made in the last decade have shed light on why women make up two out of every three Alzheimer's diagnoses and why heart disease is the number one cause of death among women. And we finally have clear advice on the steps we can take to stay optimally healthy.

- **Unpack what "gut health" means**, how your gut microbiome works, and what you need to know to spot and treat the most common gastrointestinal disorders in women.

- **Dive into what you most need to know to keep your skin healthy** and looking great at every age.

In part III, we'll look at areas of our health that often get lumped into the vague category of "lifestyle"—things that affect our strength and resilience. In this section, you'll find information that'll help you . . .

- **Take care of your mental health**, including what we know about conditions like depression and anxiety that disproportionately impact women and the new thinking on the best ways to care for our emotional and spiritual selves.

- **Get better-quality sleep (and more of it!).** This is an especially important issue when you consider women are more likely than men to have insomnia and other sleep problems, thanks in part to our fluctuating hormones—especially during the "big P's": pregnancy, the postpartum period, and perimenopause.

- **Learn how to build an exercise routine that has the best shot at improving your health now *and* later on**, with information on the female-specific factors that influence exercise performance and research-backed advice on how your workouts need to change during big hormonal transitions.

- **Understand how food works in the body and how to use nutrition to fuel your body.** We'll work to stamp out diet-culture myths and replace them with expert-based advice on how best to eat to take care of yourself.

- **Stay informed in our ever-changing digital age.** None of us can avoid the steady flow of often contradictory new studies and facts doled out by our favorite news sites and social media feeds, but we can learn how to be more discerning when it comes to what information we pay attention to and what experts we trust.

We'll end with everything you need to create a playbook for optimizing your health, lining up the care you need, and managing disease if it strikes. We all want a game plan for how to stay healthy if we're feeling great. And when it comes to illness—whether it's the common cold or a chronic disease or a global pandemic—women often bear the brunt of the fallout. We're typically the ones scheduling the doctors' appointments and missing days of work to care for sick kids and aging parents. This makes it crucial to consider how we'll handle illness if it strikes and care for ourselves even when we're caring for others.

You'll finish this book feeling prepared to chart a path forward with the tools you need to get and stay optimally healthy and to face potential health scares when they happen to you or the people you love.

A Word About Language . . .

Words matter. This is especially true when it comes to talking about our physical and emotional health.

It is my intention to be inclusive to all in this book. I believe each of us should be able to be gendered in whatever way feels true to us, no matter what sex we were assigned at birth. I also believe it's up to all of us—you, me, the scientists who study us, and the clinicians who put those findings into practice—to make progress when it comes to creating a more inclusive world. Which is why I want to let you in on why you'll see the terms *female*, *woman*, and *women* in this book.

When you read these terms, think of them as shorthand for those born with two X chromosomes and female hormone ratios and body parts. While not all people with ovaries are women and not all people with testicles are men, being born with female genitals means you have specific health concerns that are important to keep in mind as you move through life. Whenever possible, I've included specific advice for those who don't fit the cisgender, heterosexual category.

It's also important to distinguish between *sex* and *gender*, two words that are often used interchangeably but have very different meanings—especially when you read these terms in the context of health research. *Sex* refers to the organs and ratio of hormones you were born with: female or male. When referring to sex-based research, it's an issue of biology: Researchers are studying and reporting the results on those with female genitals and hormone levels. *Gender* includes factors outside of our biology—things like social roles, expectations about those roles, and other social constructs that impact our health and well-being. Even though sex and gender impact each other, they can each have distinct roles in health outcomes.

At times, the words I use might not feel inclusive enough. I've tried hard to avoid using language that makes anyone feel less than, discriminated against, or left out. My goal is to provide information that makes all people feel informed and empowered.

Where We Go from Here

Our understanding of women's health has come a long way. Yes, there's still plenty of work to be done to further understand sex- and gender-based differences in medicine and how those findings can lead to better health for all of us who live in female bodies. But we have made a lot of progress.

Now it's up to us to take these findings and apply them to our own lives. It's time for us to run with what we've learned and share it with our sisters, daughters, mothers, aunts, friends, and other important women in our lives so they feel empowered and ready to advocate for themselves, too.

Optimizing our health and truly caring for ourselves requires facts. It requires learning the basics about our bodies from trusted sources so we're better able to know when something is wrong and seek help. Healing when we're sick also requires an ability to speak up for ourselves, and this is especially true for women, who are too often made to believe our symptoms are all in our heads.

When we have a basic understanding of how our bodies work—and the language needed to talk about our health with our partners, our kids, our friends, and our caregivers—we can truly care for ourselves and our communities. And that is power.

Part I

Women's Healthcare

What You Need to Know

Chapter 1

Essential Anatomy

Why Understanding the Basics
Sets You Up for Better Health

> *Women have been programmed to view our bodies only in terms of how they look and feel to others, rather than how they feel to our-selves, and how we wish to use them.*
>
> —Audre Lorde, *The Cancer Journals*

When you think about female anatomy, there's a good chance the image that comes to mind is the illustration most of us were first shown in middle school health class. You know the one. It looks vaguely like the head of a steer.

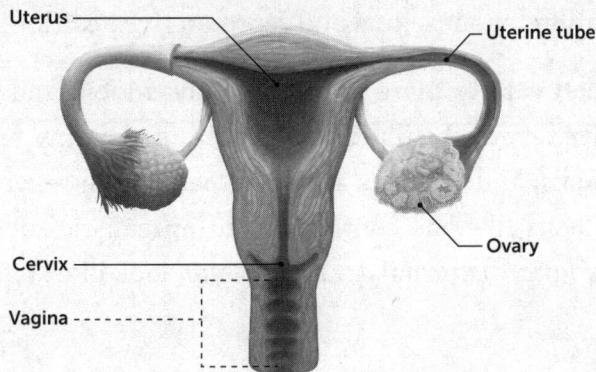

Uterus — Uterine tube — Ovary — Cervix — Vagina

And while, yes, what's depicted in this illustration and others like it are some of the key structures of the female reproductive system, it's missing some important details, like the clitoris, which is the female erectile body that's a lot more similar to the male penis than you might imagine—and is mostly *inside* your body.

It also should come with an asterisk that explains that this isn't actually how these important organs are situated inside your body. For example, your uterine tubes and ovaries sit behind the uterus, and they're quite close together. In fact, your ovaries are so close to each other that either tube can draw in an egg from either ovary. (This is one reason why, if you have one tube surgically removed for a medical reason like an ectopic pregnancy or an infection, your fertility won't change that much.) What's more, the uterine tubes open into the pelvic cavity—and are *not* connected to their corresponding ovary, as you might assume from looking at the illustration—which is why they have fimbriae ("little fingers") to sweep the egg into their openings. Illustrations like this also lack important facts and pieces of context, like how big the uterus is (about the size of your fist) or where it's located in your body (in most of us it's tipped forward and sits on top of the bladder).

In this chapter, we'll cover . . .

- **The external and internal organs and structures you have if you were assigned female at birth**. Many of us were taught that "girls have vaginas and boys have penises"—but our genitals involve a lot more than our vaginas. Understanding this anatomy (and using accurate terminology to describe it) has many benefits, including reducing the stigma and shame associated with these body parts, ensuring patients and clinicians are talking about the same body parts, and encouraging open conversations about sexual and reproductive health.

- **How much variety there is in how vulvas look**, and how the lack of vulva diversity in the illustrations used in anatomy textbooks, educational books, and websites aimed at teaching those of us with a vulva what it looks like has contributed to unrealistic social norms about what a woman's external genitalia *should* look like.

- **How sexism has existed in anatomy since the beginning of the field itself.** We'll hear from the new wave of anatomists who are committed to using anatomical terms for all of our parts rather than eponyms (names for our organs that come from the—usually white—men who claim to have discovered them).

- **Anatomy terms** that'll not only help you read and understand this chapter but also be useful as a cheat sheet to help you decode the medical jargon in those post-visit reports delivered on your healthcare provider's online portal.

Meet the Experts

Heather F. Smith, PhD, professor of anatomy at Midwestern University

Amanda J. Meyer, PhD, senior lecturer in anatomy and pathology at James Cook University

Carrie Pagliano, PT, DPT, doctor of physical therapy who specializes in women's pelvic floor health, spokesperson for the American Physical Therapy Association, and CEO of Carrie Pagliano Physical Therapy

Female Genitalia

Most of us are taught from an early age to think about our genitals in a binary way: Women have vaginas, men have penises. Yet this overly simplistic—and potentially harmful—way of thinking about our genitalia prevents us from knowing the full scope of our bodies and using accurate terminology to describe ourselves. Having a clearer picture of all of the external and internal organs and structures you have if you were assigned female at birth can go a long way toward encouraging healthy conversations about sexual and reproductive health and can help each of us discuss important issues related to our reproductive rights and gender equality. Here,

Dr. Heather Smith, professor of anatomy, walks us through what we need to know.

External Genitalia

Vulva: This is the term used for the mons pubis, labia majora, labia minora, clitoris, vestibular bulbs, vulva vestibule, greater vestibular glands (Bartholin's glands), lesser vestibular glands (Skene's glands), urethra, and vaginal orifice (opening). Many people use the term *vagina* when they mean *vulva*, or they use the terms interchangeably, but they aren't the same! Your vagina is a canal-like organ located *inside* your body that extends from your cervix to your vulva, ending as a hole outside your body called the vaginal opening.

Mons pubis: This is the round, fleshy area located over the pubic bone that becomes covered in pubic hair during puberty. It provides cushioning in some positions during sexual intercourse.

Prepuce and glans clitoris: The clitoris is an erectile organ analogous to the male penis, and its only known purpose is to provide sexual pleasure. It's the most sensitive erogenous zone of the female body, with the highest concentration of nerve endings. The visible parts of the clitoris are the *prepuce* (aka the clitoral hood) and the *glans*. But these are only part of a larger clitoral structure, most of which is inside the skin and not visible.

Labia majora: Also known as the outer lips, these are the large, fleshy folds of skin that extend down from the mons pubis and can vary in size, color, and shape from person to person. The labia majora protect the more delicate structures inside, help maintain moisture in the vulvar area, and play a role in sexual arousal. During puberty, the labia majora become covered in pubic hair.

Labia minora: Also known as the inner lips, these are the two smaller folds of skin enclosed by the labia majora that extend from the clitoral prepuce to the vaginal opening. The labia minora have many highly sensitive nerve endings and play a crucial role in sexual stimulation. They also serve a protective function for the clitoris, external urethral orifice, and entrance to the vagina.

External urethral orifice: This is the external opening of the urethra, the tube that carries urine from the bladder out of the body.

Vaginal orifice: Also known as the vaginal opening, this is the entryway to the vagina. Its size and shape can vary greatly from person to person and change in response to sexual arousal (becoming wider and more relaxed) or as a result of childbirth or, sadly, trauma.

Vulvar vestibule: This is the area beneath the glans clitoris and prepuce, between the labia minora. It's where the external urethral orifice and vaginal orifice are located; it also contains the (smaller) openings of the greater vestibular glands and lesser vestibular glands.

Perineum: The region between the vagina and the anus.

Perineal body: This is a fibromuscular structure located in the perineum that's a critical point of attachment for several muscles that are part of the pelvic floor and perineum. During childbirth, the perineal body stretches and sometimes it can tear. In some cases, an episiotomy—a surgical cut in the perineal body that's done to enlarge the vaginal opening during childbirth—is necessary.

Anus: This is the opening through which waste from the digestive tract is expelled from the body.

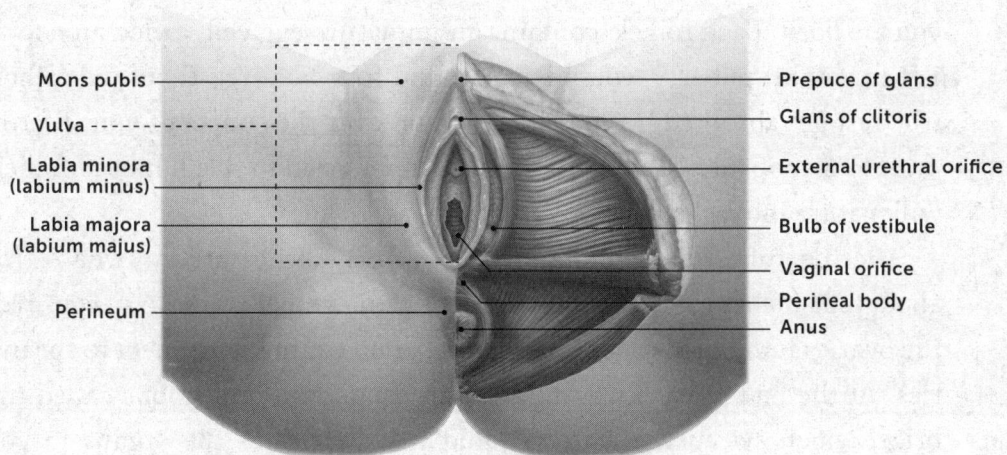

Mons pubis

Vulva

Labia minora
(labium minus)

Labia majora
(labium majus)

Perineum

Prepuce of glans

Glans of clitoris

External urethral orifice

Bulb of vestibule

Vaginal orifice

Perineal body

Anus

Internal Genitalia

Vestibular glands: These are two sets of glands located near the vaginal opening that aren't typically able to be seen or felt by touch. (They can enlarge as a result of infection or vulvar cancer. If they are enlarged, seek medical care.)

Lesser vestibular glands (aka Skene's glands): These are located on either side of the urethra and secrete a fluid that helps lubricate the urethral opening and is also believed to have antimicrobial properties to help prevent urinary tract infections (UTIs). They're involved in producing a fluid that's sometimes released during sexual arousal or orgasm (often referred to as female ejaculation).

Greater vestibular glands (aka Bartholin's glands): These are located to the left and right of the opening of the vagina and secrete a mucus-like lubricant during sexual arousal.

Vestibular bulbs: These are two structures located on either side of the vaginal opening. They are composed of erectile tissue. When you are sexually aroused, these bulbs become engorged with blood, causing them to swell and expand the vagina in preparation for sexual intercourse.

Ovaries: These primary reproductive organs in female bodies are about the size of an almond and contain about one to two million follicles when you are born. Each follicle contains an immature egg cell, called an oocyte. When you hit puberty, you'll have around four hundred thousand follicles (the rest get absorbed by your body)—and over the course of your lifetime prior to menopause, anywhere from three hundred to five hundred follicles will mature into eggs.

Uterine tubes (aka Fallopian tubes): These tubes are anywhere from about four inches to five and a half inches long and exist to carry eggs from the ovaries into the uterus. Note that they don't actually connect to the ovaries. At the end of each uterine tube are fingerlike projections called fimbriae, which sweep the watery liquid that lubricates the organs in your abdominal cavity (called peritoneal fluid) to make currents that push the immature egg cell (oocyte) into the uterine tube opening.

Uterus: This muscular organ sits on top of the bladder and is typically shaped like an upside-down pear. It's about the size of a fist in a nonpregnant woman. The uterus is composed of a number of different parts: the *fundus* (upper domed part of uterus), the *body* (large, central portion of the uterus), and the *cervix* (lower end of the uterus). In most women, the uterus is anteverted, which means it's tipped forward at your cervix, pointing toward your mons pubis. In approximately 25 percent of women, the uterus tips backward (which is referred to as retroverted or tilted uterus).

The uterus is made of three layers of tissue:

1. *Serosa*: the smooth outer layer that covers the uterus

2. *Myometrium*: the bulky middle layer that's composed of thick muscles and expands during pregnancy to hold a growing baby, contracts during labor to push the baby out, and also contracts during menstruation to expel blood (and is the source of "period cramps")

3. *Endometrium*: the innermost layer, also referred to as the uterine lining, which is shed during menstruation

Vagina: This stretchy, muscular canal is about 3.5 inches deep and sits between your urethra (at the front) and your anal canal (at the back). It has three main functions: It enables sexual pleasure via penetration, whether from a penis, fingers, vibrators, or other sex toys; it channels menstrual blood out of the body; and it dilates to form a passage from uterus to the external world during childbirth.

Cervix: This tunnellike organ is made of dense, fibrous tissue. It's about an inch long and is located anywhere from three to six inches inside your vaginal canal. It connects your uterus and your vagina and allows fluids to pass between the two. It's a powerful gatekeeper, as it can open and close in ways that make pregnancy and childbirth possible. And it also changes position during the menstrual cycle and can feel different depending on where you are in your cycle, too. Spermatozoa (aka sperm) have to travel through your cervix to fertilize an egg, and cervical mucus plays a role in how easy or difficult it is for sperm to pass through. During pregnancy, your cervix secretes a mucus plug that seals entry to your uterus, which prevents your baby from slipping out. This plug dissolves or becomes loose and falls out when it's time to give birth. Your cervix also prevents objects inserted into your vagina—like tampons, menstrual cups, or diaphragms—from slipping inside your uterus.

Clitoral complex: While the glans clitoris and clitoral prepuce are considered part of the external genitalia, the *clitoral body* (or shaft), *crura* (which comes from Latin and means "legs"), and *vestibular bulbs* are inside the skin and not visible. (For a more detailed look at the clitoris, see page 53 in chapter 3.)

Hymen: This is the thin mucous membrane that usually surrounds or partially covers your vaginal opening. At puberty, estrogen stimulates the hymen to become more elastic. It can be stretched during sex, masturbation, trauma, or exercise, or even when you're inserting a tampon, which can be painful (or not). It's a myth that you can tell if someone is a virgin or not by looking at their hymen.

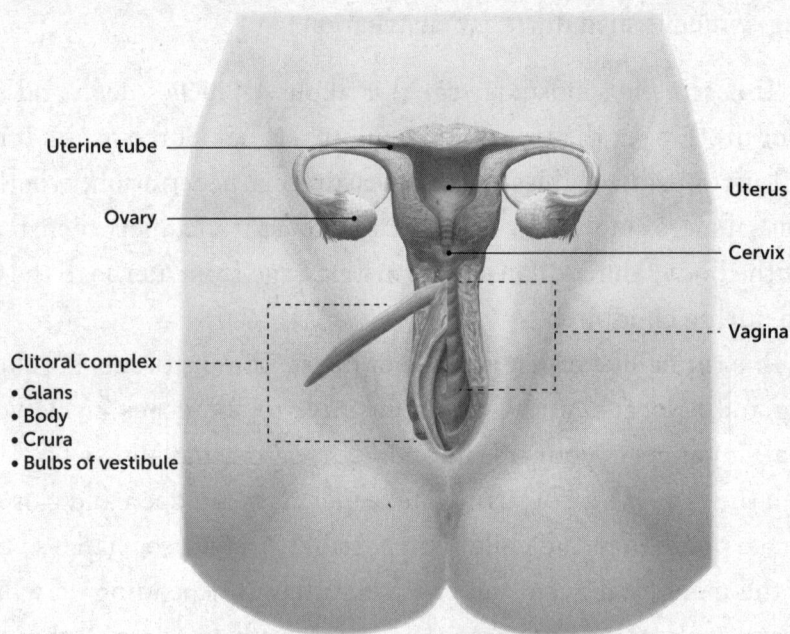

Uterine tube

Ovary

Uterus

Cervix

Vagina

Clitoral complex
- Glans
- Body
- Crura
- Bulbs of vestibule

There are three essential holes in your vulva area . . .

- *The external urethral orifice*: This tiny hole is located between your clitoris and vaginal opening and allows you to pee. Your urethra (the tube that carries urine from your bladder) empties at this opening.

- *The vaginal orifice*: This is where period blood flows during menstruation and where a baby exits your body during vaginal childbirth. It's also the opening where a finger, sex toy (such as a vibrator or dildo), penis, tampon, or menstrual cup can be inserted.

- *The anus*: This is the opening that allows feces (aka poop) to exit your body after it has traveled from your colon and through your rectum. It's also an opening where a finger, sex toy, or penis can be inserted.

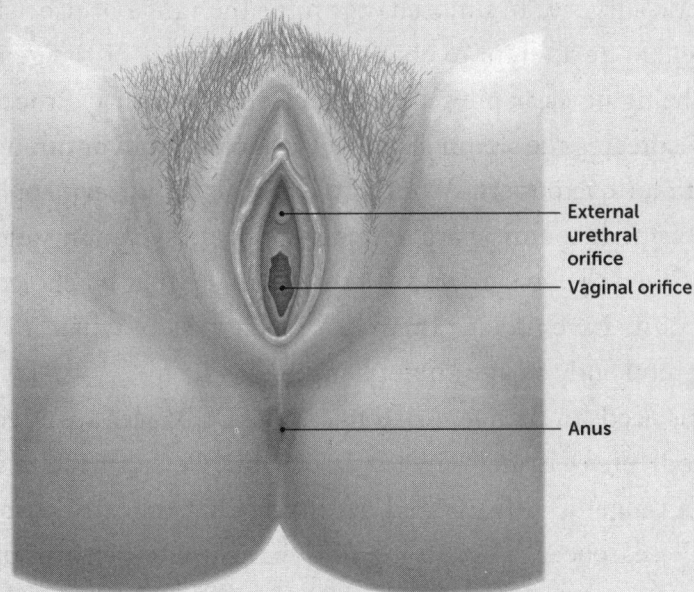

External urethral orifice

Vaginal orifice

Anus

Vulva Diversity:
Why Knowing Our Differences Matters

When anatomist Amanda J. Meyer, PhD, teaches the female genitalia section of gross anatomy, she asks her students to look around and notice how nobody in the room looks exactly alike. Sure, you could draw a picture of what a human face looks like: two eyes, a nose, a mouth, and so forth. But no two faces are exactly alike, right? Then she asks those students to look at the images of vulvas in their textbooks and points out the lack of vulvar diversity that's represented in even the most up-to-date, contemporary materials. "Given how we all look completely different on the outside, why would we think that what's inside our underwear would be any less variable?" she asks her students.

In fact, Dr. Meyer says a lack of vulvar diversity shown everywhere—from anatomy textbooks to the layperson's books and websites those with a vulva use to learn about their bodies to the media—is contributing to unrealistic social norms of what a vulva should look like. This affects all of us. Have you ever thought your vulva was "ugly" or looked "weird" or "too big," or been embarrassed to be seen naked by a partner?

This may be one reason for the recent increase in elective female genital cosmetic surgery, an umbrella term for the range of procedures performed in a deliberate attempt to change the appearance of the genital area despite there being no clear physical or functional necessity. Procedures like labiaplasty (altering the size or shape of the labia majora or minora), clitoral hood reduction (to expose the glans of the clitoris), and perineoplasty (tightening of the vaginal opening) are on the rise, including among adolescents.[1] That's right: Given the images we are exposed to—either by choice or by chance—many of us have no idea there's so much variety when it comes to vulvas, and genital body-image anxiety ensues.

This needs to change. Anatomists like Dr. Meyer are advocating for more vulvar diversity in anatomy textbooks, but we also need to start by normalizing a range of vulvas—and accepting that the way ours looks is totally okay. Researchers are studying how exposure to pictures of natural vulvas influences young women's genital self-image.[2] Not-so-surprising spoiler: It has a positive effect!

The Pelvic Floor

When you hear the term *pelvic floor*, there's a good chance you think about pregnancy and childbirth—and the resulting problems that can happen in this area, particularly as women age. However, this group of muscles, ligaments, connective tissues, and nerves that are woven together at the base of the pelvis plays a crucial role in several aspects of your health. Your pelvic floor muscles support:

- **Your bladder and urethra**, helping control the release of urine

- **Your rectum**, helping to maintain bowel control

- **Your sexual function and satisfaction**, with a well-functioning pelvic floor contributing to sexual pleasure and enhanced orgasms

- **Your growing uterus if you get pregnant**, helping to hold its increased weight and pressure

You can think of the pelvic floor kind of like a basket of intertwined muscles at the base of the pelvis that spans front to back—from the pubic bone at the front to the base of the sacrum, called the coccyx, at the back—and to the right and left sides of your pelvis.

There are two main pelvic floor muscles that intertwine to form the pelvic floor:

1. The levator ani, which consists of three separate muscle components:

- Iliococcygeus (from the ilium to the coccyx)

- Pubococcygeus (from the pubic bone to the coccyx)

- Puborectalis (forms a U-shaped sling from the pubic bone around the rectum and back to the pubic bone)

2. The coccygeus, which is located toward the back of your pelvis and is the smaller muscle component in your pelvic floor.

Your pelvic floor muscles intertwine to form a single sheet of layered muscle with openings for the anus, urethra, and vagina. You'll likely be able to feel where your pelvic floor muscles are by squeezing these openings.

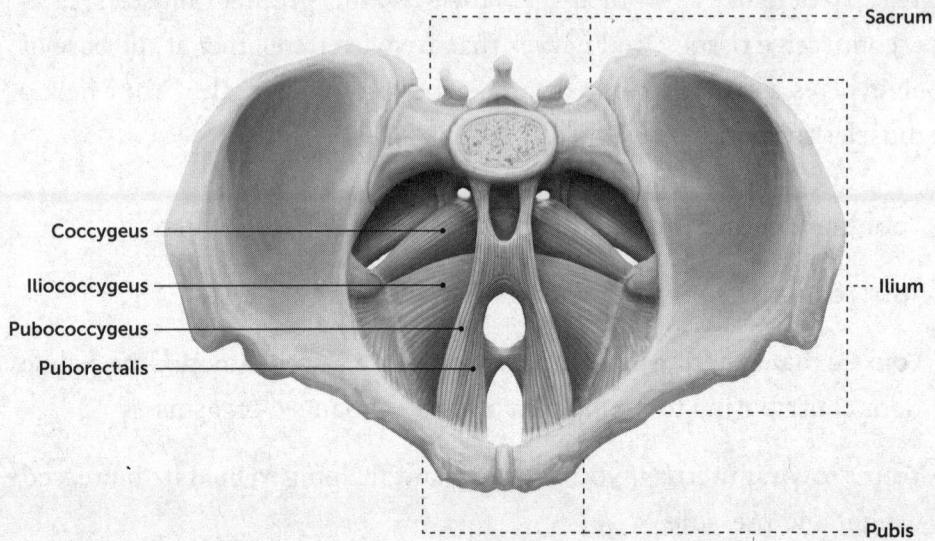

Sacrum

Coccygeus

Iliococcygeus

Pubococcygeus

Puborectalis

Ilium

Pubis

*Top-down
(aka superior) View*

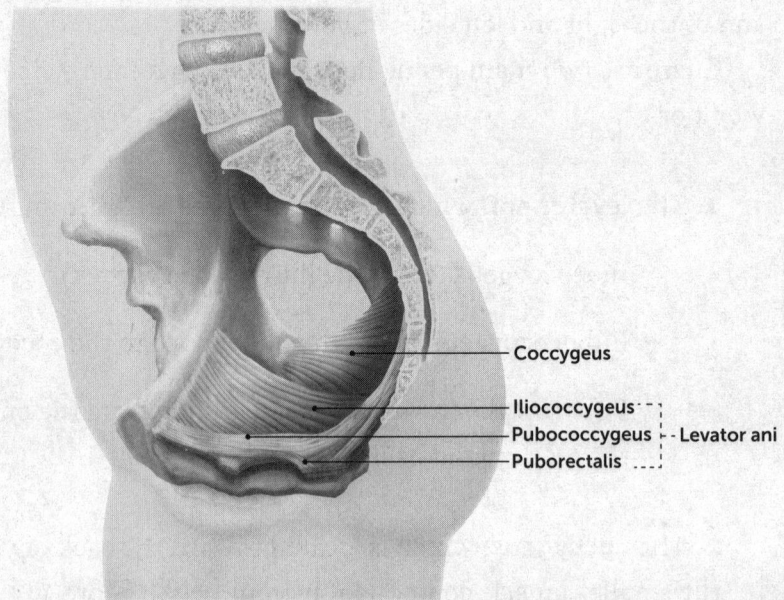

Coccygeus

Iliococcygeus
Pubococcygeus — Levator ani
Puborectalis

Side View

Source: Carrie Pagliano, PT, DPT

How Women and Men Are More Alike
Than We Are Different

When you consider female and male anatomy, it's easy to focus on our differences. Yet here's a fact that may feel surprising: All human embryos start with the same basic structures. Even though our genetic blueprint is fixed at conception (typically forty-six XX chromosomes in females and forty-six XY chromosomes in males), the structures that will develop into genitals aren't clearly "female" or "male" until around the fifth week of gestation.

In other words, our very different physical features can actually be traced back to the same structure. Anatomists call these "homologous structures," and knowing them just might open your mind to the ways we are more similar than different, which can help us claim sexual pleasure in new and more equal ways.

XX (FEMALE) ANATOMY	XY (MALE) ANATOMY	SAME, SAME—BUT DIFFERENT
Ovaries	Testes	Both the ovaries and the testes develop from the same embryonic gonads—and even after sexual maturation, both of these organs retain almost the same egg-like shape and function (the ovaries contain about one to two million egg cells, and testes produce about 1,500 sperm per second).
Clitoris	Penis	In utero, we all have genital tubercles that are pretty much identical until an embryo reaches about eight weeks. Genital tubercles in females and males both have a glans area, which develops into a clitoris or a penis. Both are what anatomists call "richly innervated" (translation: they have a ton of nerves!) and are the genitalia that are primarily responsible for orgasms. In fact, the same muscles control the erectile tissue in males and females, and in both sexes erection is required for orgasm.
Lesser Vestibular Glands (aka Skene's glands)	Prostate Gland	In women, these glands produce a watery substance that may help explain female ejaculation. The tissue surrounding these glands (including the part of the clitoris that reaches up inside the vagina) swells with blood during sexual arousal. In men, the prostate (along with the seminal vesicles) produces the watery component of semen.
Greater Vestibular Glands (aka Bartholin's glands)	Bulbourethral Glands (aka Cowper's glands)	In women, these pea-sized glands are situated under the skin on either side of the vaginal orifice, close to the anus, and secrete mucus, mostly for lubrication. In men, these glands are on either side of the urethra and produce an alkaline mucus that flushes out the male urethra and is commonly called preejaculate because it comes a short time before ejaculation.

How Our Genital Organs Develop

FROM CONCEPTION TO 10 WEEKS

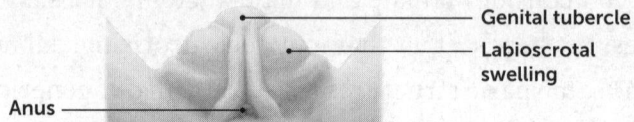

Genital tubercle

Labioscrotal swelling

Anus

FEMALE

MALE

AT ABOUT 10 WEEKS

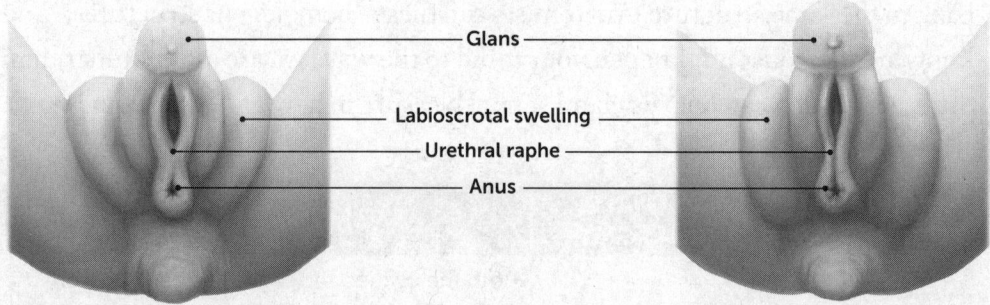

Glans

Labioscrotal swelling

Urethral raphe

Anus

FULLY DEVELOPED

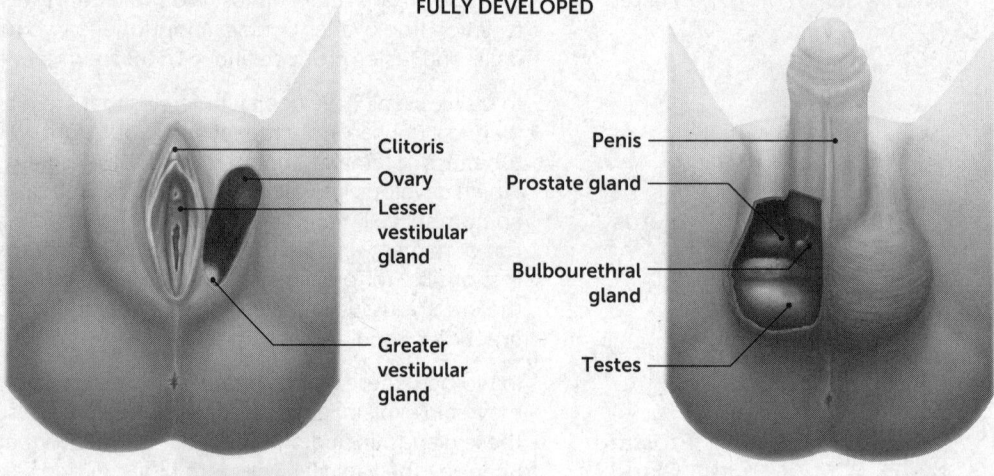

Clitoris

Ovary

Lesser vestibular gland

Greater vestibular gland

Penis

Prostate gland

Bulbourethral gland

Testes

Anatomy Terms 101

Consider this a cheat sheet to help you decipher anatomical words you'll frequently see.

Anterior: front, or in front of

Posterior: behind

Ventral: toward the front of the body

Dorsal: toward the back of the body

Distal: away from, farther from the origin

Proximal: near, closer to the origin

Median: midline of the body

Medial: toward the median

Lateral: away from the median

Superior: toward the top of the head

Inferior: toward the feet

External (aka superficial): toward the surface

Internal: away from the surface, deep

Why So Many Female Structures Are Named After Men: Eponyms and Why We Should Stop Using Them

Take a virtual tour inside the human body and you'll encounter a number of organs with a man's last name attached to them. Think *Fallopian tubes*, named after the Italian priest and anatomist Gabriele Fallopio, or *Bartholin's glands*, named after Caspar Bartholin, a Danish professor of medicine. These names are known as eponyms and were used to honor the people (mainly men) who first "discovered" or described the anatomical structure—or sometimes even had nothing to do with discovering the structure but simply wanted their names in an anatomy book!

Thankfully, there's a new wave of anatomists, scientists, and healthcare professionals who are pushing to use the official anatomical terminology— more descriptive terms that relate to the placement, function, size, shape, or color of a body part and reverse a stale view of anatomy as a field practiced exclusively by white, male scientists who got to name other people's body parts after themselves (like having an explorer march into your reproductive system and claim it for himself).

"Eponyms don't give any descriptive significance apart from the first white guy who was able to get his name published in a book," says Dr. Meyer, "which makes it more difficult for all of us—even those who are studying to become healthcare professionals—to learn and remember anatomy."

Toponyms—like the term *uterine tubes* instead of *Fallopian tubes* and *greater vestibular glands* instead of *Bartholin's glands*—are easier to learn. In fact, many anatomists argue that memorizing eponyms leads to more "cognitive load" that makes it tougher for students to learn them.[3] While toponyms are endorsed by the International Federation of Associations of Anatomists, they haven't been widely adopted—yet.

So throughout this book you'll see the descriptive terms used for anatomical structures, with eponyms in parentheses. There's been resistance, largely because eponyms are what have historically been taught. But the increasing focus on teaching anatomically descriptive terms rather than eponyms means the new generation of healthcare professionals are learning a more progressive and inclusive language for our bodies. And we can all do our part to use *that* language until eponyms are phased out.

• • • • •

Truly caring for ourselves requires an accurate understanding of what we're caring for. With this knowledge of female anatomy, you'll be better able to take charge of your health with confidence. It also has the potential to change and evolve the way we think about all bodies, so *everyone's* body is appreciated, understood, and respected.

Chapter 2

Puberty

A Guide to Helping Girls (and Their Caregivers)
Thrive Throughout This Major Transition

> *Forget (almost) everything you thought you knew about puberty, because modern puberty is more complex, more fascinating, and more demanding of our understanding than the version that we lived through.*
>
> —Cara Natterson, MD, *This Is So Awkward: Modern Puberty Explained*

D o you remember stammering your way through puberty feeling lost, confused, and even a little (or a lot) terrified about the changes that were happening to you? If the answer is yes, you're not alone. Too few of us received a clear explanation about what's involved in this major hormonal transition, why it was happening, and what all of these changes meant.

Sure, there was sex ed at school, filled with cringe-inducing videos meant to teach us about our reproductive organs. There may have also been a well-meaning parent or older sibling who supplemented what we learned in school with the old birds-and-the-bees talk. And while these lessons and discussions were a start, they probably didn't really involve the kind of detailed but easy-to-understand information kids actually need. The result? Most of us found ourselves navigating the grab bag of symptoms puberty presents largely on our own—and now we don't know how to help the next generation avoid the same fate.

In this chapter, we'll learn . . .

- **The typical timeline of puberty in girls** to understand what's happening to prompt the physical and emotional changes that take place. We'll also hear from the U.S.'s leading experts on why puberty is happening earlier and lasting longer these days, and what caregivers need to know about gauging where their daughters are in the transition.

- **What's a normal period symptom—and what's not.** You'll learn what to expect and when it's time to talk to the pediatrician about abnormal symptoms.

- **What it takes to foster a healthy body image in young girls.** With so many physical changes happening during puberty, this is prime time for body image issues to surface. But there are steps you can take to bolster a young person's confidence in their body and early signs of eating disorders that are important to be on the lookout for.

- **The information and language you need to support a child who may be questioning their gender identity.** Those who identify as lesbian, gay, bisexual, transgender, queer, intersex, asexual, questioning, or more (LGBTQ+) might struggle more during puberty. If we want to start helping our teens feel better, we have to understand the issues that are driving their increasing mental health challenges.

- **A better way to talk to kids about sex.** While puberty isn't just about reproduction, the end result of this transition *is* sexual maturity, which makes it essential to have "the talk" about sex—one that provides young people with the accurate, anatomically correct information they'll need to have safe, pleasurable sex.

Meet the Experts

Cara Natterson, MD, pediatrician, founder of Less Awkward, and author of *This Is So Awkward: Modern Puberty Explained*

Louise Greenspan, MD, pediatric endocrinologist, the Permanente Medical Group, and coauthor of *The New Puberty: How to Navigate Early Development in Today's Girls*

Julianna Deardorff, PhD, professor and head of the Maternal, Child and Adolescent Health program in the School of Public Health at UC Berkeley and coauthor of *The New Puberty: How to Navigate Early Development in Today's Girls*

Robbi K. Alexander, PhD, former administrative director of psychiatric services and director of the Princeton Center for Eating Disorders and the assistant vice president of behavioral health nursing at Penn Medicine in Princeton

Kelsie T. Forbush, PhD, clinical child psychology professor and director of the Center for the Advancement of Research on Eating Behaviors at the University of Kansas

Amy Lang, MA, sex educator and author of *Sex Talks with Tweens: What to Say & How to Say It*

Angela Dallara, spokesperson for GLAAD, the world's leading LGBTQ media advocacy organization

Peggy Orenstein, author of *Girls & Sex* and *Boys & Sex*

The Real Puberty Timeline: From Hormonal Changes to Periods

Too many of us still think the onset of puberty in a girl is marked by her first period. However, puberty actually starts a few years *before* menstruation—and even before there are any of the other outward signs most of us call to mind when we think about this transition.

Here's what's happening hormonally:

* The hypothalamus begins producing a hormone called gonadotropin-releasing hormone (GnRH), which gets sent to the pituitary gland.

- GnRH stimulates the pituitary gland to release luteinizing hormone (LH) and follicle-stimulating hormone (FSH).

- LH and FSH travel to the gonads—the ovaries in girls and the testes in boys.

- In girls, LH and FSH prompt the ovaries to produce estrogen and progesterone, which are responsible for breast development (medically referred to as thelarche). In boys, these hormones tell the testicles to produce testosterone, which is responsible for male sexual characteristics, like larger testes and penis.

- The adrenal glands start to secrete hormones, including small amounts of testosterone and estrogen, and dehydroepiandrosterone (or DHEA, which is used to make estrogen and testosterone). It's DHEA that's responsible for hair growth as well as oilier sweat, which can lead to acne and body odor.

- As all of these hormones are coming online, kids are forced to ride the feelings that come along with these big hormonal shifts—what we might consider "mood swings." This is why your once even-keeled daughter might start seeming more like a drama queen. As physician and puberty expert Cara Natterson, MD, describes it: "Those emotional ups and downs are a sign she's learning how to modulate these new hormones floating through her body and brain."

- The onset of menstruation. This can happen anywhere from age ten to sixteen, but that first period usually happens around age twelve.

So Why Are Girls Entering Puberty Earlier?

Experts still don't have a lot of definitive answers as to why many girls are at increased risk for going through puberty early, but they do have some theories. Here, Louise Greenspan, MD, and Julianna Deardorff, PhD—coauthors of multiple studies on early puberty as well as the book *The New Puberty: How to Navigate Early Development in Today's Girls*—explain three culprits widely believed to be affecting the pubertal process:

Suspect No. 1: Excess fat. Extra body fat has consistently been correlated to early breast development, which may be due to estrogen that's made and stored in fat tissue. (That's right, fat tissue produces and stores hormones!) Another hormone secreted by fat tissue is leptin, the appetite suppressant that rises before puberty. The thinking is that more fat cells lead to more leptin secretion, which in turn prompts puberty to start sooner. In both animal and human research, study subjects born without the ability to produce leptin become obese but do not go through puberty, proving the connection between leptin levels and the pubertal transition.

Suspect No. 2: Exposure to chemicals. It's impossible to accurately assess just how many chemicals the average person is exposed to, given how many of them are present in the air we breathe, the food we eat, the water we drink, the products we use, and practically everything we touch. In fact, our exposure starts before we're even born; studies have found toxic perfluoroalkyl and polyfluoroalkyl substances (aka PFAS or "forever chemicals" because they don't naturally break down and they accumulate both in the environment and in our bodies) in newborns.[1] Experts believe these chemicals lock onto estrogen receptors in the body, producing an estrogen-mimicking effect that prompts puberty to begin. What's worse, these chemicals are also thought to lead to more fat tissue, which in turn releases more hormones—creating a vicious cycle and double whammy for early puberty potential.

Suspect No. 3: Social and psychological stressors. A growing body of research shows that excessive stress and/or certain types of stressors early in life can correlate with early puberty, as stress can trigger hormonal responses that cue puberty. From an evolutionary perspective, this makes sense: In tough times, the survival of a species is best served if offspring mature and reproduce as soon as possible.

The Sexual Maturity Rating (SMR)

Mention the word *puberty* these days, and there's a good chance the first thing you'll hear about is how it's happening earlier in girls, which in turn may prompt you to wonder if your daughter is part of this growing trend.

If you have questions about this, schedule an appointment with your child's pediatrician. The doctor will probably use the Sexual Maturity Rating

(SMR) to gauge where they are in the pubertal transition. Having a basic understanding of the SMR can be helpful as a jumping-off point for conversations with your child's healthcare provider.

However, it's important to leave the examinations and official designations to a healthcare professional. They're the only ones who should be doing a medical evaluation and who can determine if your child is developing on track.

THE SEXUAL MATURITY RATING IN GIRLS[2]

STAGE	SIGNS
Stage 1	No changes since birth (no pubic hair, no breast buds)
Stage 2	Some pubic hair on the labia only and breast budding
Stage 3	Further enlargement of breast tissue; progression in the distribution and color of pubic hair
Stage 4	Increased breast size and elevation of the nipple area; pubic hair that's adultlike but doesn't reach the inner thighs
Stage 5	Mature female breasts; adultlike pubic hair that extends onto the thighs

Is It Breast Development—or Baby Fat?

Breast development is one clinical sign doctors will look for to diagnose the onset of puberty. One study showed that the average age of breast development is 8.8 years old for Black girls, 9.3 years old for Hispanic girls, 9.7 years old for white girls, and 9.7 years old for Asian Americans.[3]

How can you tell if a girl has true breast development or if it's simply fat accumulation? The short answer: *You* can't! Leave this discernment to your child's doctor, who'll be able to tell the difference by feel.

Your First Period: What's Normal—and What's Not

Yes, it's important to know the basics—like what the menstrual cycle is, why it happens, and practical things like how to track your cycle and use a tampon. For more details on the menstrual cycle, flip to page 82. But when it comes to puberty, there are a few specific things to keep in mind about what's normal (and not) when it comes to your cycle.

- **Vaginal discharge may increase in the months before your first period.** It can look like a raw egg white (clear and mucus-y) or feel sticky, thick, or gooey. If the color is deep yellow, green, or white, and/or if the texture is curdled (like cottage cheese), see a healthcare pro to make sure you're not dealing with an infection.

- **Your periods will probably be irregular at first.** This is because ovulation usually doesn't start happening regularly for a few years after your first period. If you're still experiencing irregular periods three years after your first menstrual cycle, talk to your doctor to rule out any potential health problems.

- **A "normal" period looks different for everyone.** After one to three years, your periods will likely start to settle into a pattern, with an average cycle length of twenty-eight days and bleeding lasting five to seven days. But keep in mind your cycle is considered "normal" if it's anywhere between twenty-four and thirty-eight days.[4] What's most important is to track your period so you find out what's "normal" for *you*.

- **Painful periods and losing lots of blood aren't normal.** Far too many women deal with pain and heavy bleeding during their cycles, writing it off as the downside of having a uterus and not seeking help because family members and friends have told them it's "just the way it is." However, debilitating pain in your pelvis, abdomen, or low back is not par for the course. Same goes for heavy menstrual bleeding, which is diagnosed if bleeding lasts more than seven days, if you need to change your tampon or pad every hour for several hours in a row, if your cycle stops you from your normal activities, or if you pass clots the size of a quarter or larger several times a day. It's important to talk to your healthcare provider if you're experiencing any of these symptoms or others that make your monthly cycle especially awful.

- **Your period is a sign of your overall health.** In fact, many clinicians think of the menstrual cycle as a vital sign, along with body temperature, blood pressure, heart rate, and respiratory rate. Paying attention to your period can be a way of tracking what's going on in your body, and it's a skill that's great to start cultivating when you're young.

Ask an Expert

When should I make that first ob-gyn appointment for my daughter?

The most recent evidence-based recommendations suggest a first gynecology exam take place when someone is planning to become or newly sexually active. However, this presumes there is another healthcare provider—like a pediatrician—doing all of the anticipatory guidance around relationships and everything-just-before-sex. It also presumes a teen isn't experiencing any issues separate from sex requiring a gynecology specialist. Consider making that first appointment if your teen hasn't gotten her first period by age fifteen or her periods are painful, very heavy, or persistently irregular. You can also talk it through with your pediatrician, who can help you figure out the right timing for that first visit.

—Cara Natterson, MD, pediatrician, founder of Less Awkward, and author of *This Is So Awkward: Modern Puberty Explained*

Changing Bodies: How to Raise a Teen with a Healthy Relationship to Her Body

All of us want to feel good about who we are and how we look. Yet this can become an uphill battle starting at a very young age. About two-thirds of parents of eight- to eighteen-year-olds say their child is self-conscious about some aspect of their appearance.[5]

Social media isn't helping, and research shows it's impacting girls' body images more negatively than boys'. In one study, adolescent girls using social media platforms experienced greater levels of body-related pressure, dissatisfaction, and self-criticism than boys. The researchers reported appearance comparisons, with peers, social media influencers, and celebrities as the main sources of body dissatisfaction.[6]

If you're a parent, it's easy to get discouraged, and many of us can probably relate to feeling uncomfortable in or dissatisfied with our bodies. Thankfully, you play a crucial role in shaping how your child sees themselves. Here are a few key things you can do to try to combat the increasing number of issues our young people are up against today:

- **Focus on function over appearance**. "We've gone from being revered for what our bodies can do—nurture and sustain life—to revered for what our bodies *look* like," says Dr. Robbi K. Alexander. To counter this, make statements that highlight what your child's body can do versus how it looks. For example, you might focus on how fast your child ran or how happy she seemed while playing her favorite sport instead of telling her how great she looked on the field or court; you could focus on how graceful and strong she was in her dance performance versus how beautiful she looked onstage. "Avoid starting sentences with 'You look . . . ,'" suggests Dr. Alexander.

- **Avoid comparisons**. It's so easy to make statements of comparison in a way that feels harmless. Maybe you describe another child as "taller" or "smaller" or even throw out a compliment, saying someone "always dresses so nicely." The implied difference can prompt a child to wonder how *she* stacks up, instilling a habit of comparison.

- **Watch how you talk about yourself.** The best thing you can do for a young girl is to be a role model for how you want her to talk about herself. If you don't want your kids placing too much emphasis on appearance or obsessing about what foods they eat, try not to do that yourself.

Spotting the Early Signs of Eating Disorders

Signs of eating disorders tend to fall into three categories: behavioral, psychological, and physical. Early intervention can help the treatment of an eating disorder begin before it becomes entrenched, so understanding the early warning signs is key. It will also help you make sure your child is at her ideal body weight, which is essential for normal brain development and bone growth. Talk to your child's pediatrician if you start to notice any of the following.

BEHAVIORAL SIGNS

- New food habits or "rituals," like having to cut food into tiny pieces before eating
- Food avoidance, including cutting out entire food groups (gluten, meat, anything that has white sugar) or making blanket statements, like "I don't like pizza"
- Little interest in food, extreme picky eating, or fear of the consequences of eating (signs that point to avoidant/restrictive food intake disorder, or ARFID)
- Preoccupation with the nutritional content of food; counting calories or carbohydrate content
- Not wanting to come to the table to eat with the family and choosing instead to eat alone
- Sudden or unexpected clothing changes, like wanting to wear only baggy clothes
- Changes in exercise habits
- Extreme anxiety if certain behaviors and routines are interrupted

PSYCHOLOGICAL SIGNS

- Increased anxiety

- Social withdrawal

- Preoccupation with body shape and size; a change in body image

- Big mood fluctuations, particularly if this feels new, as well as irritability

- Flat mood or lack of emotions

- Intense fear of gaining weight, or little concern over extreme weight loss

PHYSICAL SIGNS

- Changes in weight (both up and down)

- Gastrointestinal complaints, such as stomach cramps, constipation, or acid reflux

- Missed periods or other menstrual irregularities

- Dizziness or fainting

- Feeling cold all the time

- Sleep problems

- Dental problems, such as enamel erosion, tooth sensitivity, and cavities

- Dry skin, dry hair, brittle nails, and possibly cuts or calluses across the tops of finger joints (which can result from inducing vomiting)

- Fine hair on body or thinning of hair on head

- Abnormal lab results, including anemia, low thyroid and other hormone levels, low potassium, low blood cell counts

- Slow heart rate

This isn't an exhaustive list, and it's important to understand that some of these symptoms can happen in kids who aren't necessarily struggling with disordered eating. For example, a teen might express wanting to avoid processed, sugar-filled snacks and opt for healthier, whole-foods options instead. This is fine, says Dr. Alexander. Because that line between "normal" and extreme can be tough to gauge, talk to your child's doctor about the behaviors you're noticing. They can help you decide if consulting with a dietitian, psychiatrist, or eating disorder specialist is the next right move.

If you bring up these signs to your child's healthcare provider and feel like you're getting the brush-off, look for a practitioner with specific training in eating disorders. There's also a free eating disorder screening online through the National Eating Disorder Association, which is a great step to take before a doctor visit, especially if that healthcare provider isn't an eating disorder specialist.

Ask an Expert

I see the signs of an eating disorder in my child, and it's triggering because I've dealt with an eating disorder, too. What should I do?

This is a tricky situation that can bring up a lot of old memories for you. It's important to know that it's okay to focus on your mental health first. If you haven't achieved full recovery from your eating disorder, know that it's possible to get help now—no matter how old you are or how many years you've been struggling. Find a provider who offers evidence-based interventions for eating disorders so you can manage your condition while also getting help for your child. If you have made a full recovery, it's a good idea to talk to a mental health practitioner about what your child's behavior is bringing up for you, and to support you in figuring out the next steps.

—Kelsie T. Forbush, PhD, clinical child psychology professor and director of the Center for the Advancement of Research on Eating Behaviors at the University of Kansas

Navigating Gender Exploration: How to Arm Yourself with Facts for Supportive Conversations with Your Child

While only about 5 percent of young adults in the U.S. say their gender is different from their sex assigned at birth,[7] a growing number of kids are embracing a diversity of gender identities and exploring how they feel. Young people today have both the language and the social acceptance to question their gender identities, which can be challenging for older generations, who weren't exposed to the same kind of openness.

To support a child who may be exploring their gender identity, stay calm and open to having conversations about it, says sex educator Amy Lang, MA. You can start by sharing your understanding of gender. For example, you might say that you feel like a girl on the inside in addition to looking like a girl—and explain that this means you're cisgender. (For a cheat sheet on the terms all of us need to know to talk about gender identity in a supportive way, see the glossary on page 32.) Then you might ask how your child feels—without expecting or demanding a response. There are excellent online resources to help you navigate these talks, and Lang's book even includes scripts you can use if you're struggling.

If your kid is distressed about their gender and/or insistent that they are transgender, try to find a gender-competent therapist—someone who has focused training in gender identity development in childhood and adolescence. If your child is ultimately diagnosed with gender dysphoria (something a healthcare provider will do if certain criteria are met), there are several treatment options to address the distress and negative emotions kids may go through when their gender doesn't align with their sex at birth. A gender dysphoria specialist can tell you more about these options and what's age appropriate when considering how to support your child.

LGBTQ+ kids are at a considerably higher risk of mental health issues, including suicide, so it's essential to provide a safe and supportive space to discuss this topic. Most important, stay curious and open-minded as you have these conversations.

Sexual Orientation and Gender Identity Terms: A Cheat Sheet

Proper use of sexual orientation and gender identity terms and pronouns is an important way to show that you care about how someone identifies. When young people hear themselves being affirmed by the people who care for them—parents, teachers, healthcare providers, other adults—it helps them understand who they are and have language to best articulate what they're going through, says GLAAD spokesperson Angela Dallara.

Here are the GLAAD-approved definitions of a number of terms related to sexual orientation:

Asexual (aka ace): A term used to describe someone who has little or no sexual attraction to others. *Asexual* is an umbrella term that can also include people who are demisexual, meaning they do experience some sexual attraction but only in certain situations (for example, after they have formed a strong emotional or romantic connection with a partner).

Bisexual (aka bi or bi+): A term used to describe a person who has the potential to be physically, romantically, and/or emotionally attracted to people of more than one gender—though not necessarily at the same time, in the same way, or to the same degree.

Cisgender (aka cis): An adjective used to describe people who are not transgender.

Deadnaming: When someone refers to a trans, nonbinary, genderqueer, or gender-diverse person by their birth name without their permission or consent. A transgender person's chosen name is their real name, whether or not they are able to obtain a court-ordered name change (which can be expensive and involve complex bureaucratic obstacles). Transgender people should be referred to only by the name they use every day as their authentic selves, unless they have indicated otherwise.

Gender dysphoria: A concept designated in the *Diagnostic and Statistical Manual of Mental Disorders* (DSM) that refers to psychological distress resulting from an incongruence between one's sex assigned at birth and one's gender identity. The necessity of a psychiatric diagnosis for transgender people remains controversial, as both psychiatric and medical authorities recommend individualized medical treatment, considering every transgender person is different.

Gender identity: A person's internal, deeply held knowledge of their own gender. Everyone has a gender identity, including cisgender (aka nontransgender) people. For most people, their gender identity matches the sex they were assigned at birth. For transgender people, their identity does not align with the sex they were assigned at birth.

Gender nonconforming: A term used to describe people whose gender expression differs from conventional expectations of masculinity and femininity. Note that having nonconforming gender expression does not make someone trans or nonbinary.

Heterosexual (aka straight): A term used to describe a person whose enduring physical, romantic, and/or emotional attraction is to people of a sex different from their own.

LGBTQ+: An acronym for *lesbian*, *gay*, *bisexual*, *transgender*, *and queer*; the + is in recognition of all nonstraight, noncisgender identities.

Nonbinary (aka enby): An adjective used to describe people who experience their gender identity and/or gender expression as falling outside the binary gender categories of "man" and "woman." This is an umbrella term that encompasses many different ways to understand one's gender; some nonbinary people may also use words like *agender*, *bigender*, *demigender*, or *pangender* to describe the specific way in which they are nonbinary. Some nonbinary people identify as transgender, and some do not.

Pansexual: A term used to describe a person who has the capacity to form enduring physical, romantic, and/or emotional attractions to any person, regardless of gender identity. This is one of several terms under the bi+ umbrella.

Pronouns (she/her; he/him; they/them): These are the words we use to identify ourselves apart from our name. Using the correct pronouns for trans and nonbinary youth is a way to let them know you see them and accept their identity. *They* and *them* are used as singular pronouns when someone would like to remove gendered language in reference to themselves.

Sex at birth: This is the sex ("male" or "female") assigned at birth, usually by doctors and usually based on the appearance of external anatomy.

Sexual orientation: The term used for a person's enduring physical, romantic, and/or emotional attraction to another person. Sexual orientations can include heterosexual (straight), lesbian, gay, bisexual, queer, asexual, and other orientations.

Transgender (aka trans): An adjective used to describe people whose gender identity differs from the sex they were assigned at birth. Being transgender is not dependent upon physical appearance or medical procedures.

Transition: This is the process a person may undertake to bring their gender expression and/or their physical body into alignment with their gender identity. It can include:

Social transition: Coming out to family, friends, peers, and colleagues; using a different name; using different pronouns; dressing differently or wearing a different hairstyle

Legal transition: Changing your name and/or sex marker on identification documents like a birth certificate, driver's license, passport, Social Security record, bank accounts, and more

Medical transition: May involve puberty blockers, hormone replacement therapy, and/or one or more surgical procedures

It's important to note that many transgender people do not have the desire or financial means to legally or medically transition.

Queer: This is an adjective used by some people, particularly younger people, whose sexual orientation is not exclusively heterosexual. For those who identify as queer, the terms *lesbian*, *gay*, and *bisexual* may seem too limiting and/or fraught with cultural connotations they feel do not apply to them.

Here are a handful of outdated terms that should be avoided:

"Born a man/woman," "biologically male/boy or female/girl," "genetically male/female": These phrases were coined by anti-transgender extremists to imply that people who are transgender aren't who they say they are. A person's sex or gender is determined by a number of factors, and a person's biology does not determine a person's gender identity.

"Female-to-male" or "male-to-female": This implies someone is changing their gender from one binary gender to the other binary gender, when a person's gender is an innate sense of self that has not changed. Instead, use *transgender man*, *transgender woman*, or *transgender person*.

"Gender ideology" or "transgenderism": These are often used by antitransgender activists to dehumanize transgender people and reduce who they are to a dangerous "condition" or "political construct." These are not terms that transgender people use to describe themselves. The growing visibility of transgender and nonbinary people is not an ideology; being transgender is an authentic aspect of someone's personhood, and their existence is not up for debate.

"Homosexual": This is an outdated term that is often now used by anti-LGBTQ+ activists to suggest that people attracted to the same sex are somehow diseased or psychologically/emotionally disordered. Instead, use *gay*, *lesbian*, or, when appropriate, *bisexual*, *pansexual*, or *queer* to describe people attracted to people of the same gender or more than one gender. It's best to ask a person which term they use.

"Identifies as": This implies that gender identity is a choice.

"Lifestyle": An inaccurate term often used to denigrate LGBTQ+ people and inaccurately imply that being LGBTQ+ is voluntary or a "choice." Just as there is no one straight lifestyle, there is no one LGBTQ+ lifestyle.

"Sex change": This implies a person must have surgery in order to transition. Instead, use the word *transition*. Avoid overemphasizing surgery or transgender people's physical bodies when discussing transgender people or the transition process.

Sex Talks:
How to Have Healthy Conversations About Sex

Considering that the end result of puberty is sexual maturity, having sex talks with your child during this time—however uncomfortable or awkward you may feel—is key. Ideally, you'll want to start the conversation *before* puberty. After all, you want your child to learn about how sex works in a healthy way, which means learning about it from you, not from their friends or, worse, from porn. Your child should have healthy future sexual relationships and understand that pleasure is a must for everyone involved, including themselves.

Amy Lang is an expert at helping parents navigate these conversations. Here's her best advice about when, how, and why you need to have these talks:

- **Start laying the groundwork ASAP.** Far too many parents put off bringing up anything related to sexuality until it's time for the birds-and-bees talk. Lang recommends starting to talk to kids about sex when they're in preschool, or around age five. This doesn't mean going into detail, per se, but focusing on naming body parts—a topic preschoolers are naturally curious about—is a great place to start.

- **Be specific when talking about private parts, starting at birth.** This is especially important for girls, who often aren't given any terms for their private parts (unlike boys, who at least understand where their "pee-pee" is). Use the terms *vulva*, *vagina*, *clitoris*, *breasts*, and *anus* when talking about these body parts. (For a refresher on female anatomy, flip back to chapter 1.)

- **Talk about body safety.** Be specific about a child's private parts being private—and explain that kids can get hurt if someone touches them in a private area or puts anything (a toy, a shoe, a part of their body) in their vulva, anus, or mouth.

- **Explain that you want to know if anyone talks about or touches your child's private parts (and emphasize that you won't be mad!).** This is a crucial part of the body safety conversation that many of us ignore because we assume nothing bad will happen. Yet it's important to tell your child that if anyone ever talks to them about or touches their private parts, you want to know about it. Emphasize that you won't be upset at them; in fact, you'll be very proud of them for telling you. If your child does talk to you about inappropriate behavior, try to stay calm. Thank them for sharing it with you and tell them that you'll make sure the person who talked about or touched their private parts doesn't do it again.

- **Teach consent in a nonsexual way first.** At its core, "consent" means to agree, which is a word that makes sense to kids. Too often, we think about consent just in the context of sex. While having that conversation is crucial, it's also important to teach your child they have the right to say no to *any* kind of touch. Make setting these boundaries the norm at home. You might ask your spouse for a hug in front of your kid and agree beforehand that they'll say something like "No thanks, I'm not in the mood." You can also start asking your child if they want a hug or a high five rather than automatically going in for one. As your child builds up this boundary muscle, they become better prepared to say no when the stakes are higher.

- **Include all different types of sex when you talk about sex.** How detailed you get will depend on your kid's age, but overall, it's important to talk about sex as a way people share their bodies—and that a lot of different body parts are used.

- **Talk about the emotional aspects of sex in addition to the risks.** It can be easy to focus on the risks and dangers, like unintended pregnancy, sexually transmitted diseases, and sexual assault, when talking to your child about sex. While these are important safety issues to discuss, it's also important to emphasize that sex should feel good and be fun. Don't be afraid to talk about your values and beliefs. Maybe you hope your kid waits until she's in a relationship to have sex because you know being in a loving, committed relationship makes sex feel better. If that's how you feel, say it! "When you express your values, you develop some roots that'll keep *you* more settled when you talk about the tough stuff later on," adds Lang.

- **Bring up porn, even if you *really* don't want to.** Exposure to porn is a fact of childhood, whether you want to believe it or not. (The average age of porn exposure is about twelve years old.) Therefore, it's crucial to assume your kids will see it, to use monitoring and filtering on every device your kid uses, and to talk about what to do if it pops onto one of their screens.

  If your kid is eight years old or younger, talk about porn in general terms. You might say something like "Hey, when you're on your tablet, you might see videos of naked people. That's adult stuff and not safe for you to look at. If you see it, turn off the device and tell me what you saw—you won't be in trouble." You don't even have to say it's called porn at this stage, but you do have to give your kid a heads-up that it exists—and that you want to know right away if she sees it.

  After your kid is eight, you might add a bit more detail, explaining that it's called porn, that it's not safe for kids to see, and that while it can be fascinating to look at, it can hurt kids' hearts and minds. Given that kids this age are still very rule oriented, repeat the rules you've set earlier on—if you see porn, stop watching it right away and let me know you saw it—and emphasize that your child won't be in trouble.

  As kids get older, you can—and should—continue to address it. Your kid needs to understand that this is a topic you'll talk about, whether she wants to or not, and that it's always okay to ask questions.

  "Then stay super chill if she responds," says Lang, "and just do your best when it comes to answering."

If you're struggling to have "the talk," or your kid looks like she wants to run away from you:

- **Name your discomfort**. Is a conversation making you sweat, start to ramble, or even say things you wish you could take back? You're allowed to say outright, "I'm uncomfortable!" And if your kid starts squirming, name that too, says Lang: "You might say, 'I know it's uncomfortable to talk about this stuff. I'm uncomfortable. Life's uncomfortable. But here we go.'" You might also tell your kid she doesn't have to say a word; you just want her to listen and ask any questions if she has them. It's also okay to put off a conversation if your kid asks you something and you're not sure how to answer. You can reply, "You know what? I want to talk to you about this but I'm going to get back to you."

- **Revisit any topic you (or your kid) put off**. Let's say you have no idea how to answer a question your kid has, so you say something like "That's a grown-up thing. Can you finish unloading the dishwasher?" That's fine in the moment—but it's also important to circle back when you *do* know how to answer. You could say, "You know what? I messed that up. I was uncomfortable, but now I know how to answer your question."

  The beauty about this approach is twofold, says Lang: "You're buying time to craft an answer you feel good about, and you're showing your kid the human side of you that makes mistakes and knows how to go back and fix them. That's just all-around good parenting."

- **Give your kid a say when it comes to timing**. There are topics you simply have to talk about (read: porn) that your kid will likely try to push off. In those instances, give them a choice about when you talk. You might say something like "Hey, I want to talk to you about a sex thing. We can talk about it now or later." If "later" is the choice, that's fine—just make sure you bring it back up within forty-eight hours.

- **Have talks about sex stuff while you're on the move**. If you or your kid are a little uncomfortable about having these talks, being on the move can help things feel less formal. Bring things up while driving, biking, walking the dog, even folding the laundry.

"Plus," says Lang, "if you can have these conversations while you're doing other stuff, it starts to feel like a normal part of family life and reinforces to kids that you're going to bring up these conversations, and that they should expect them to happen."

- **Talk in the third person.** Consider for a moment how saying something like "I know you've seen porn" will land with your teenager versus something like "Hey, I know kids your age have seen porn." The latter is less accusatory—and more likely to keep a kid open to further discussion.

- **Enlist support (or a stand-in, if you really must).** Oftentimes, to avoid awkwardness or discomfort, kids will confide in another trustworthy adult what they might not share with a parent. It's okay to have another adult in your kid's life who talks to them about sex stuff, whether that's an aunt, grandparent, or family friend they're close with. Just make sure the person's okay with fulfilling that role before you tell your kid to go to them. Also, make sure your kid knows that if there's a safety issue, this person will talk to you about what's going on.

- **Remember, it's your job to have these chats about sex.** There's a myth that our kids will ask us about sex when they're ready. But it's not their job to ask; it's our job to give them the information they need. This is part of a parent's overarching role of keeping kids safe and healthy.

"Kids don't know what they need to know and when," says Lang. "Their caregivers do. And that makes it *our* responsibility to give kids consistent information throughout their childhood and into adolescence."

Talking to kids about sex doesn't have to be scary or weird. Think about what you want to say and how you want to say it—you can even find a script if needed, like the ones you'll find in Lang's excellent book *Sex Talks with Tweens: What to Say & How to Say It*—and then say those things. Your kids may confide in you or they may not. These conversations about sex may go smoothly or feel torturous. What you need to do is bring up these important topics, have the talks, and do the best you can. You'll feel good knowing you prepared your kids for this huge, important, sometimes crazy, and hope-fully happy-making part of life.

Helping Girls Feel Satisfied in Their Sexual Relationships

When it comes to young women and sex, Peggy Orenstein, author of *Girls & Sex* and *Boys & Sex*, has found that while they feel empow-ered to engage in sexual behavior, they don't necessarily feel enti-tled to *enjoy* it. In fact, from sexting to oral sex, girls often focus more on boys' enjoyment than on their own. While young men are more likely than their female partners to measure their satisfaction by their own orgasm, young women are more likely to measure it by their partner's pleasure.

How do we raise our young girls to not only think about their own pleasure when they have sex but even prioritize it? How do we help them see sex not as performative but rather as something they can (and should!) do for *their* enjoyment, too? Orenstein shares her thoughts.

Help girls understand that sex is about balancing responsi-bility (pregnancy prevention, safety) *and* joy. Rather than frame "the talk" about sex exclusively in terms of risk and danger or even consent, make it inclusive of the love, connection, mutuality, and pleasure that also come along with a healthy sexual encounter. There's great evidence that doing this leads to fewer negative con-sequences, like disease, pregnancy, regret, and even assault. It also leads to more positives, like being able to communicate with a part-ner and actually enjoying oneself.

Talk about the importance of asserting your own needs and desires. If you look at the media environment girls are up against—whether it's porn or mainstream media—the focus is largely on women being desirable rather than understanding their desire. Girls often described their sexual experiences to Orenstein as a one-way street.

"I heard so many stories of nonreciprocal blow jobs from girls who'd never had an orgasm with a partner," she says. "I asked them why that was okay, and they were confused. I started using an analogy about water, saying to them, 'If you always got your boyfriend a glass of water, but he never got you one—and if you asked for one, he sighed or grumbled—would you be okay with that?' That really got them! They'd laugh and say, 'Well, when you put it that way!'"

Teach girls to love living in their bodies. We can do this by helping them have a better understanding of all kinds of pleasure—not just sexual but also pleasure in food, music, art, dance, and in how their bodies *work* as opposed to how they *look*. Helping girls relate to their bodies doesn't always have to involve a big talk; it can be more about helping them become aware of how strong they feel when they're running down the soccer field or how much satisfaction they feel when eating their favorite fruit.

As kids get older, keep emphasizing that one's body is for living in, not just looking at. Orenstein remembers talking to a group of high school seniors where one girl asked a boy, "What do you do to express your sexuality?" The boy stared at her blankly. The girl then explained, "You know, we put on a sexy dress, do our makeup and hair . . . ," and the boy said, "I have sex."

"That's it in a nutshell," says Orenstein. "Girls think expressing sexuality is about an outfit or selfie. For boys, it's about the experience and sensations of the body—it's about sex."

Your Game Plan: How to Be a Supportive Adult During the Puberty Transition (and Stay Sane While You're At It)

This time in a kid's life is a wild ride, filled with all kinds of physical, emotional, and social changes. Given that, it's no surprise parents and caregivers will be impacted, too. How can you best navigate this big transition in a way that helps you show up for your kid—*and* yourself?

Educate yourself about all the ways puberty has changed since you went through it. From the earlier timing and longer time frame of hormonal surges before girls get their first period to navigating the social and emotional issues that come up due to the prevalence of social media and so much more happening in their world, all aspects of puberty have likely changed *a lot* since you were a kid. Understanding the new landscape will help you figure out what information to get your kids and at what age.

"You help your kids by knowing when they need your help, and the only way to know that is to educate yourself," says Dr. Natterson.

Make your puberty talks about *them*, not you. It can be tempting to tell your own stories about what happened to you during puberty in an attempt to be helpful. However, most of the time what kids really crave is for you to listen to what's happening in their world. Given that the experience of puberty has likely changed so much since you were a kid, try to stay more curious than all-knowing about what your child is going through.

"Remember, it's their puberty—not your puberty," says Dr. Natterson. "Plus, puberty—and the world—has changed so much since you were a kid. For instance, we have period underwear, so your story of leaking through white shorts isn't going to land the same way." An exception, says Dr. Natterson, is poking fun at yourself. Otherwise, less about you, more about your kid.

Help your kid understand what boys are going through, too. A growing number of experts on puberty (Dr. Natterson included) are on a mission to give puberty a new, less gender-focused image.

"Puberty tends to be all about periods and boobs and moods," says Dr. Natterson. Yet when we focus only on what a girl's body is going through without giving our daughters a sense of what their male peers are experiencing, we do kids a disservice. When we universalize the fact that everyone goes through puberty at a different time, in a different order, and probably feels a little shame *and* a little bit psyched about different parts of it, it helps all kids—girls, boys, and nonbinary kids—feel supported and seen.

"Your daughter should know that a sixth- or seventh-grade guy might get a spontaneous erection when he's standing in the front of the classroom," says Dr. Natterson. "If she knows this, she can have his back and not mock him, in the same way you'd hope a group of guys would throw her a sweatshirt to wrap around her waist if she gets her period for the first time at school."

Find yourself some support. There will be times you feel like you're losing your mind, don't know how to help your kid, or can't get over just how different life is for tweens and teens these days. There will be times you'll react to it all in ways that don't make you feel proud. You're not alone. Finding someone (or better yet, multiple people) to vent to, lean on, and share your own tried-and-true advice with is key. If you don't, you'll be more likely to mix up your own baggage from adolescence with what your kid is actually going through, which can lead to an unhealthy dynamic, says Dr. Natterson.

"Almost every parent I've talked to can remember some cringey or traumatic experience from their childhood, and every one of them is determined to spare their child from that experience," she says. "Having your own community to support you through this transition makes it more likely that you'll leave your own baggage at the door—or dump it on someone else—so you can be there for your kid when she comes to you with questions or concerns."

• • • • •

The beauty of all of us arming ourselves with this information *now*—whether we've already gone through puberty or not—is that it can help us understand our bodies and ourselves in new ways. And if we're mothers, grandmothers, aunts, or caregivers of young kids, we have an opportunity to help the young ones among us emerge from puberty feeling informed and empowered.

Chapter 3

Sexual Health

What We Really Need to Talk About When We Talk About Sex

> We did get a sex education. We got taught by our parents, religion, society, and all the movies that told us spontaneous desire is what everyone should have. We got sex education—we just didn't get accurate sex education. That's why everybody feels broken.
>
> —Kelly Casperson, MD, board-certified urologist, sexual medicine specialist, and author of *You Are Not Broken: Stop "Should-ing" All Over Your Sex Life*

For something that humans have been doing for as long as our species has existed, sex sure can feel *complicated*.

There are so many factors that play a role in what turns us on and gets our bodies physically ready for a sexual encounter. There's also so much variation—from person to person and even in ourselves from one point in time to another—in what feels good or not when we're physically intimate. And each of us have vastly different beliefs and expectations about sex based on the kind of education we received, our cultural and religious upbringing, and so much more.

In short, sex is a complex, multifaceted aspect of life—and therefore an area where accurate, fact-based information is crucial if we want to engage with it in a healthy, fun, and *pleasurable* way.

If you're one of the rare, magical unicorns who received a thorough, progressive education about sex, what you'll find in this chapter may feel like a refresher. For the rest of us, who got sex ed that resembled Coach Carr's approach in the movie *Mean Girls*—"Don't have sex, because you will get pregnant and die! . . . Okay, now everybody take some rubbers!"—the information here may feel new and revelatory.

In this chapter, we'll learn . . .

- **Why sexual health requires a biopsychosocial framework.** Exploring the underlying physical (bio), mental (psycho), and societal and interpersonal (social) factors that play into our sex lives can help us unpack the various aspects that often make sex feel less than stellar, and home in on areas that might be holding us back from having more *wow*-worthy sexual experiences.

- **The difference between sexual desire (often referred to as libido or sex drive) and arousal,** and the different ways they tend to show up in women versus men.

- **The physiology of female arousal and orgasm**, including the anatomy of the clitoris, known as the only human organ that exists strictly for the purpose of pleasure.

- **Which hormones are most closely tied to various aspects of our sexual health** and how changes in the levels of these hormones can impact our sexual function.

- **How to prevent and treat sexually transmitted infections (STIs)** and what precautions you can take to protect your health.

- **Why it's possible to have a healthy sex life after sexual abuse or trauma.** A good place to start is with the science-backed steps outlined on page 70.

Meet the Experts

Kelly Casperson, MD, board-certified urologist, sexual medicine specialist, and author of *You Are Not Broken: Stop "Should-ing" All Over Your Sex Life*

Emily Nagoski, PhD, sex educator and bestselling author of *Come as You Are: The Surprising New Science That Will Transform Your Sex Life* and *Come Together: The Science (and Art!) of Creating Lasting Sexual Connections*

Maria Uloko, MD, urologist, researcher, and comprehensive sexual medicine surgeon

Emily Morse, founder and CEO of *Sex with Emily* and author of *Smart Sex: How to Boost Your Sex IQ and Own Your Pleasure*

Sarah Cigna, MD, assistant professor of obstetrics and gynecology at The George Washington University and director of the first sexual medicine fellowship in the U.S. for ob-gyn physicians

Pelin Batur, MD, professor of ob-gyn and reproductive biology at Cleveland Clinic Lerner College of Medicine of Case Western Reserve University and physician lead of the Cleveland Clinic Women's Comprehensive Health and Research Center

Shannon Dowler, MD, family physician and author of *Never Too Late: Your Guide to Safer Sex After 60*

Wendy Maltz, LCSW, sex therapist who specializes in helping people heal after sexual abuse or trauma

Sex Is Biopsychosocial: Understanding All the Influences That Shape Our Sexual Health

While many of us think about sex as something that's solely driven by our hormones, most sex researchers, clinicians, and experts say it's way more helpful to think of it in terms of *all* the underlying factors that affect our sex lives, specifically the biological, psychological, and social processes. This is known as the biopsychosocial approach.

"As a physician, people come to me thinking their lack of sexual desire is due to hormones—they say, 'My hormones need adjusting so I have desire,'" says Dr. Kelly Casperson. "But hormones are only one piece of the picture. You also have to ask, 'How do I feel about sex? What does sex mean to me? What does it mean to my partner? What are my biases? How's my relationship? Am I having sex worth desiring?'" In other words, it's not just your hormones that play a role in your sex life.

Here Dr. Casperson walks us through what the *bio, psycho,* and *social* aspects of the *biopsychosocial* approach entail and how human sexuality exists within these three containers.

- **Biology** includes what's going on in your body. It entails your physical health, your hormones, and also things like how well you're sleeping, how fit you are (sex is a physical activity, after all), and any chronic diseases or chronic pain you may have. For example, if you're not sleeping well or you're dealing with back pain that won't go away, your body is unlikely to prioritize sex.

- **Psychology** includes what's going on in your mind. It encompasses your mental health, including conditions like depression, anxiety, and stress; sexual identity and orientation; body image and self-esteem; past sexual experiences (including sexual trauma); as well as expectations and attitudes about sex. For example, if you're having performative sex and are focused on what your partner(s) think about how you look or what you're doing, it'll impact your sex life.

- **Sociology** involves the sociocultural context in which we grew up and now live. It includes factors like the taboos around sex we learned growing up, what religion we practice, performance expectations we pick up due to fictionalized ideals we see in porn and movies, cultural norms or expectations, and access to sex education and information. For example, if you were taught that sex before marriage was a sin or you watched a lot of porn before having partnered sex, those early impressions can impact your sex life even after you've changed your beliefs and perceptions.

"Intimacy is created in talking about all of these things," says Dr. Casperson. "So many of us think sex is the intimate part when really, these are the conversations that help us feel more connected to our partners."

Demystifying Desire and Arousal

There are two processes that make us want and enjoy sex: desire and arousal. It might be tempting to think that desire is a necessary precursor to arousal. However, while desire and arousal are closely related to each other, they are decidedly not the same. Here are the basics about how they work.

Desire Versus Arousal

Desire is all about wanting sex. It's what we're talking about when we use the word *libido*, which is often described as a biological drive for sex. And as we just learned, while our biology does play a role in how much we want sex, it's also true that our desire is shaped by our minds, as well as what's happening in our lives and the world around us. After all, even when the hormones and neurotransmitters that regulate our sex drive (like testosterone, estrogen, and dopamine) start to surge, the stuff of life (like a sick child or stressful work deadline) can override the "I want sex" message our body is trying to send us.

Dr. Casperson also encourages asking yourself the following questions: *When I'm having sex, is it a good time? Am I having sex worth desiring?*

"If you don't like sex, or it's painful, or if you're just doing it because you think you should, it's like mushy broccoli," she says. "I can't make you desire mushy broccoli. You have to have sex worth desiring to have desire."

Arousal is the body's physiological response to sexual stimulation. This can include brain arousal (you see something sexy, you have a sexy thought or fantasy, or something you're doing is turning you on) and pelvic arousal (you experience an increase in blood flow, muscles relax, and the vagina lengthens and tilts back to expand and accommodate penetration).

"Erection is the classic sign of arousal in men, and it's important to know that female bodies do the exact same thing—we're just not told that," says Dr. Casperson. (For everything you were never taught about the clitoris—how it has erectile tissue, needs blood flow to get aroused, and even looks like its male equivalent, the penis—skip ahead to page 53.)

Spontaneous Desire Versus Responsive Desire

Once upon a time not so long ago, the consensus was that desire must come before arousal. It's a logical assumption, and sometimes it does work this way: You have a sexy thought, and it makes you want to have sex, which then prompts you to seek it out—whether partnered or solo. This is called spontaneous desire. Yet while this is one way the sequence of events can play out, it doesn't always go down like that. Some people experience arousal *first*, which can then trigger desire—and this is known as responsive desire.

Many people mistakenly believe that sex should happen only when spontaneous desire strikes. But for a lot of us, desire doesn't always come before sex. It can surface during or after intimacy and can emerge through connection, touch, or creating the right mood and environment. Ever find yourself saying, "Wow, that was amazing, I really enjoyed that!" after sex? That's responsive desire.

Now, this doesn't ever mean you should have sex when you don't want to, says Dr. Casperson. "But it's important to remember that when you pursue sexual experiences worth desiring, the desire can flow in during or after—and that is a very normal human experience, too."

Because we're not taught about these different types of desire or the fact that a desire discrepancy is common, we tend to make spontaneous desire the default—and in heterosexual relationships, we tend to compare female desire with the male normative experience. "The woman is broken because she wants sex more, or she's broken because she wants sex less," says Dr. Casperson. "She's always the broken one. But that's so much pressure on the woman! She shouldn't have to be the one who has to match her partner's desire."

If you're partnered with someone, you *will* have different desires—and that's okay. Sexual desire discrepancy is just like any other discrepancy you might have. Maybe you like different foods, different types of exercise, different movies. And just like any difference of opinion among two people trying to live together, it's important to talk about it and land on a compromise. "We think desire discrepancy is a big problem when really, we should normalize it," says Dr. Casperson.

I rarely experience spontaneous desire. What's wrong with me?

Nothing is wrong with you! Not experiencing spontaneous desire is 100 percent normal, and it's important to remind yourself that you likely experience responsive desire. Instead of desire just appearing—like kaboom!—because you had a stray thought or saw a sexy person, responsive desire emerges when you're like, *Okay, Saturday at eight o'clock, you, me, and the red underwear.* You put the last of the dishes away, you carry the last of the laundry upstairs, and you take off your clothes and get into bed and say, *Let's see what happens.* You put your body in the bed, you let your skin touch your partner's skin, and chances are, you're going to have fun.

Christine Hyde, a sex therapist in New Jersey, talks about responsive desire using the analogy of a party. If your best friend invites you to a party, you're probably going to say yes—because it's your best friend and it's a party. But then as the date starts to approach, you think, *I'm going to have to find childcare. There's going to be so much traffic on Saturday night. Am I going to want to put on my party clothes at the end of a long week?* But you said you would go—so you put on some dance music, put on your party clothes, arrange childcare, and show up to the party. And what usually happens? You have fun at the party. If the "party" is sex, this scenario is responsive desire.

If you're having fun at the party, you are doing it right. But here's the thing: There is no amount of spontaneously craving a party that will make that party worth going to if you don't feel good about your relationship with the people at the party, or if they're not serving the kind of food that you enjoy, or if you don't feel comfortable enough in your body to dance. Sex worth desiring is sex you like—it's sex that brings you pleasure.

In the end, it's not the desire that matters. It is the pleasure that you experience—or the obstacles that prevent you from accessing pleasure—that are the important targets of creating a more buoyant sexual experience.

—Emily Nagoski, PhD, sex educator and bestselling author of *Come as You Are: The Surprising New Science That Will Transform Your Sex Life* and *Come Together: The Science (and Art!) of Creating Lasting Sexual Connections*

The Female Orgasm: Why Understanding Our Anatomy Can Help Us Own Our Pleasure

There's an orgasm gap among women and men, and women are on the losing side of the divide—especially women in heterosexual relationships. According to one study, heterosexual women orgasm 65 percent of the time, compared with heterosexual men, who orgasm 95 percent of the time.[1]

First things first, and it's important to say this up front: Orgasm isn't necessarily the goal of sex. You don't have to have an orgasm to have a satisfying sexual experience. That said, orgasm *is* a marker for pleasure, which is why researchers look at who is having them.

So why is there a pleasure gap? There are many possible explanations, most of which point to sociocultural factors. Women are often more likely than men to be "in our heads" during sex, for example, thinking about how we look, how our partners are feeling, or how much we have to do when the sex is finished—a surefire pleasure killer. If we're not focused on our own pleasure, it can be tougher to have an orgasm.

Another big barrier to women reliably having an orgasm is that many of us don't understand the anatomy of our pleasure organ: the clitoris. There's a good chance more women would have more orgasms if more of us knew exactly how the female erectile network works. So let's geek out on this for a moment, shall we?

A Closer Look at the Clitoris

For such an important organ that's homologous to the extensively studied penis and widely known as *the* organ of pleasure for those who have one, the clitoris has historically been woefully under-studied. In fact, it was only in 2022 that urologist Maria Uloko, MD, and two colleagues discovered the mean number of nerve fibers in the structure: 10,281 (not 8,000, the oft-cited number that's based on a decades-old study on cows—yes, *cows*).[2]

Thankfully, we know more now. The first piece of information that blows many people's minds is this: The clitoris includes a lot more than that little spot at the top of the vulva (the glans clitoris). In fact, the majority of the clitoris is under the skin and becomes erect and spasms during orgasm, just like the penis. When you see the clitoris in its entirety, its similarities to the male pleasure organ, the penis, become a lot more apparent.

So let's take a closer look at what the clitoris actually looks like:

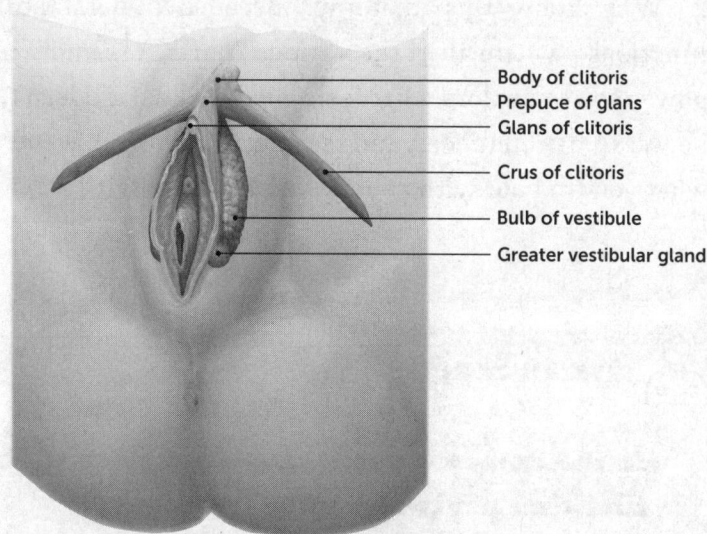

Body of clitoris
Prepuce of glans
Glans of clitoris
Crus of clitoris
Bulb of vestibule
Greater vestibular gland

Clitoral hood (aka prepuce): This is the movable skin over the glans clitoris (male equivalent: foreskin at the tip of the penis), but it's important to note that it's a different size in different bodies. Some hoods cover the glans; others don't.

Glans clitoris: This is the external part of the clitoris—what most people think of as the entirety of the clitoris but is really just the "tip of the iceberg."

Body or shaft of the clitoris: This runs along the pubic bone (below the mons) and splits into two parts that curve underneath the labia and both sides of the pelvic bone.

Crus (or crura, which is the plural): There are two crura or "legs" (*crus* is a Latin word that means "leg") of the body of the clitoris, which extend under the surface of the labia minora. The crura are made of erectile tissue (they become engorged with blood during arousal) and are about five to nine centimeters long.

Bulbs of the vestibule: These are located at the bottom of the crura and hug the urethra and vagina. They're made of spongy tissue that fills up with blood when you're aroused and may help compress the greater vestibular glands to release their secretions.

Greater vestibular glands: These are located on either side of the vaginal opening and secrete a mucus that lubricates the vulva during arousal.

Why know this anatomy? Because understanding how your body functions—where all of the various "parts" are and what they do—can empower you to explore what feels good and what doesn't, lead you to discover new sexual preferences, and feel more comfortable and confident expressing what you find out with anyone you have sex with.

Ask an Expert

Is the hymen a real thing—and does it "break" during first-time penis-in-vagina intercourse?

When the vagina develops, it starts out as a canal that's closed. As that canal opens up and develops, the hymen is what's left—a natural anatomical structure that's essentially a remnant of human development. Then humankind made it weird by ascribing a cultural narrative to an anatomical structure and claiming an intact hymen is a sign of virginity. While the hymen *can* break during first intercourse, it also might not. The hymen can also tear with horseback riding or even walking—doing normal things. Most of us likely won't even know if our hymen is there or not or intact or not, and that's okay.

—Maria Uloko, MD, urologist, researcher, and comprehensive sexual medicine surgeon

What Is the "G-spot" or "G-zone"?

The G-zone is made up of five different parts that all work together, explains Dr. Uloko. These are:

- The clitoral crura, which are like legs of the clitoris that swell and enhance pleasure
- The clitoral bulbs, which also swell and add to sensations
- The prostate tissue around the urethra, which can produce pleasurable sensations and fluid release
- The urethra itself, which can also feel good when stimulated
- The front wall of the vagina, which is another area that contributes to pleasure

In simple terms, this entire area fills with blood when a person is aroused, which makes it much more sensitive to touch. When these parts are stimulated, they can create different types of orgasm, says Dr. Uloko.

"I believe the more we understand how this whole zone works, the more people can experience better and more satisfying orgasms," she adds.

Having trouble finding your G-zone? Emily Morse, host of the *Sex with Emily* podcast and author of *Smart Sex*, suggests exploring (on your own or with a partner) where it is after you've had a clitoral orgasm. This can make it easier to find the G-zone because the entire area engorges and swells with blood.

Hormones:
How They Turn Us On, Turn Us Off, and Otherwise Impact Our Sex Lives

While there's a lot more to sex than the rise and fall of certain hormones, these little chemical messengers are an important biological component of sex—and it can be helpful to know which ones are doing what at various points in a sexual experience. We'll take a deeper dive into all our hormones and how they work in chapter 8, but for now, here's a primer on the main ones in play when you have sex:

- **Estrogen.** During a sexual response, this hormone is associated with the control of blood flow to the genitals and helps enhance lubrication. Both women and men have estrogen—though women have comparatively higher levels of estrogen than men do—and it modulates sexual desire in all of us. And even though testosterone gets all the credit for our libido, higher levels of estrogen have a positive effect on sex drive.

- **Testosterone.** This is the hormone associated with desire: When you have a sexy thought or fantasy, or you start to feel aroused due to physical touch or some other sexual stimuli, your ovaries and adrenal glands start pumping out testosterone. (Yes, women make testosterone—in fact, before menopause, we have an average of ten times more testosterone coursing through our veins than estrogen!)

- **Dopamine.** This neurotransmitter is responsible for our seeking behavior—in other words, our desire for something (including sex). When you're doing anything that's pleasurable (like sex, hopefully), your brain releases a large amount of dopamine, which in turn prompts you to seek more of that feeling.

- **Oxytocin.** Sometimes referred to as the love hormone, oxytocin plays an important role during sexual arousal (it floods your body during sex and especially after an orgasm) and helps you feel bonded to the person you're with.

The Big Hormonal Shifts That Impact Women's Sex Lives

Knowing which hormones shift and when—plus how those changes can impact everything from your sexual desire and arousal to how sex feels—can help you normalize changes in your sex life when you find yourself in one of these transitions.

Let's go through each of these, one by one.

Puberty, as we learned in chapter 2, is the big swing "on" of the sex hormones that mark "sexual maturation"—the development of secondary sexual characteristics (like breasts and pubic hair in girls) and the onset of menstruation. During this transition, there's often an increase in sexual curiosity and desire, which are influenced by both an increased production of sex hormones and psychosocial factors.

Regular fluctuations in estrogen, progesterone, and testosterone occur with each **menstrual cycle**, and changes in sexual desire and arousal can happen based on the phase you're in. Menstruation happens during the first part of the follicular phase, and it's when estrogen and progesterone levels are low, which can mean a low libido. Menstrual discomfort (like cramps, bloating, and fatigue) can also kill your sex drive during this time. After your period, estrogen rises—a boost that can also increase your sexual desire and responsiveness. When you ovulate, estrogen and testosterone levels peak, which can boost your interest in sex. As you move into the luteal phase, progesterone rises as estrogen declines, which can lead to a gradual decline in libido.

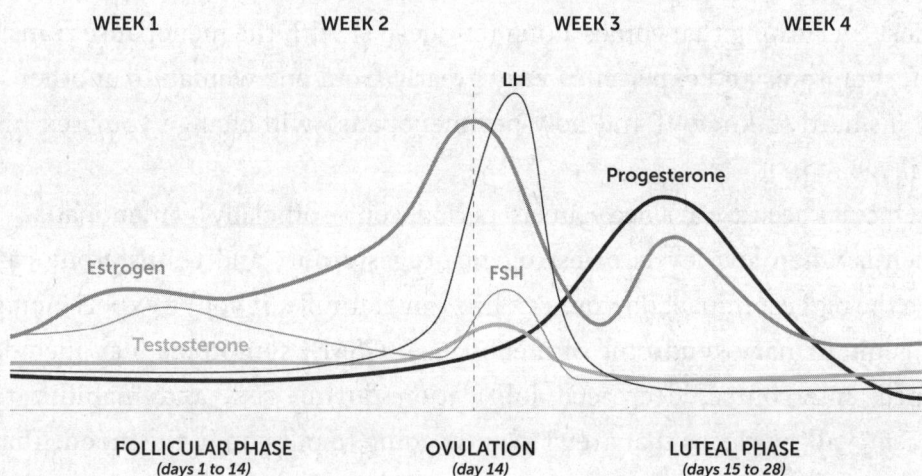

WEEK 1   WEEK 2   WEEK 3   WEEK 4

LH

Progesterone

Estrogen

FSH

Testosterone

FOLLICULAR PHASE
(days 1 to 14)

OVULATION
(day 14)

LUTEAL PHASE
(days 15 to 28)

The significant hormonal (and emotional) changes that come along with **pregnancy** can send your sex drive on quite the ride. During the first trimester, you get a rapid increase in human chorionic gonadotropin (hCG), progesterone, and estrogen—hormone changes that can cause symptoms like fatigue, nausea, and breast tenderness and prompt changes in sexual desire as a result. In the second trimester, sexual desire and arousal tend to increase for many women, which is often chalked up to increased energy and those first-trimester symptoms finally subsiding. As for the third trimester, further increases in estrogen can increase libido—though that can quickly be squashed thanks to discomfort from a large belly, body aches, and physical limitations that can prevent you from having sex as usual. It's also important to note that the pelvic floor muscles, which are quite active during sex, stretch and move during pregnancy, which can lead to changes in orgasm and physical comfort during sex and can impact your sex drive as a result.

After you give birth, you'll experience a sharp drop in estrogen and progesterone. Essentially, your **postpartum** hormones can look like those of a woman in menopause—and these changes can greatly impact both your desire and how sex feels due to the vulvovaginal symptoms that low estrogen can cause. Pair that with the stress of caring for a newborn, and it's easy to see how sex drive can tank.

Perimenopause, or the transition leading up to menopause, is characterized by big, unpredictable fluctuations in hormone levels that can lead to a wide range of symptoms (think hot flashes, unpredictable menstrual cycles, and vaginal dryness), which can impact how much we want or like sex. Like almost everything that comes along (or doesn't) with the menopause transition, symptoms and experience vary greatly from one woman to another—and it's hard to know if and how perimenopause will change your sex life until you're in it.

Once it's been a year since your last period, you've officially hit **menopause**—which is when low levels of estrogen, progesterone, and testosterone can have the biggest impact on your sex life. For example, if you're experiencing the genitourinary syndrome of menopause (GSM), symptoms may include painful intercourse, decreased lubrication during sex, and inability to orgasm—all scenarios that aren't exactly going to put you in the mood. That said, some women report having the best sex of their lives after menopause, when there's a newfound comfort in our bodies and no need to worry about pregnancy.

Sex Problems: What Can Go Wrong—and the Treatment Options That Can Save Your Sex Life

So many of us suffer through painful sex or an inability to have an orgasm thinking it's "normal," when it might actually be a dysfunction. Female sexual dysfunction is a common problem around the world, impacting an estimated 30 to 50 percent of women.[3] Yet research shows less than half of all women are screened by their healthcare clinicians for sexual dysfunction.[4]

"We've normalized sexual dysfunction in our society," says professor Sarah Cigna, MD. "Then we go to our doctors for advice—the ones who delivered our babies, doctors we trust—and those doctors haven't been trained to give women evidence-based advice."

If you're unhappy with your sex life, it can help to know what sexual dysfunction entails. This will give you the language to talk to your healthcare provider, who can help you find solutions.

To start, sexual dysfunction is usually classified in four different categories of disorders:

Desire: This can be summed up as a lack of interest in sex and low or no sex drive.

Arousal: If your sex drive is there but you're not able to become physically aroused (what's often referred to as getting "wet") or maintain arousal during sex, it may point to a sexual arousal disorder.

Orgasm: This is when you experience recurrent difficulty in having an orgasm despite sufficient sexual stimulation and arousal. It's important to note that not having an orgasm every time you have sex is completely normal. However, if you'd like to have orgasms but have persistent problems achieving them, you might talk to your healthcare provider about orgasmic disorder.

Pain: When you have pain associated with either sexual stimulation or vaginal contact—think stinging, burning, discomfort, or searing pain—you may be experiencing a sexual pain disorder. This becomes increasingly common as a woman hits perimenopause, when GSM can set in.

While sexual dysfunction tends to fall into one of these four categories, it's important to realize there is a lot of intersection among them. For example, if you're having pain during sex, your desire may wane and/or you may have trouble having an orgasm (because orgasms happen when your pelvic floor muscles can freely contract and relax—something that's unlikely if you're in pain).

Next up, we'll look at some of the medical and nonmedical treatments available. Remember, the most effective approach will vary from person to person; knowing your options is a great starting point for a conversation with your healthcare provider.

Treatment Options for Sexual Dysfunction

When it comes to talking to a clinician about what you can do to treat sexual dysfunction, it's helpful to remember that sex is biopsychosocial and that understanding what, specifically, you're struggling with can help you home in on the best treatment for your situation. For example, are you dealing with a biological issue such as pain? Are you experiencing depression or anxiety, which are psychological issues that could impact your sex life? Or are you realizing you were socialized as a child to associate sex with shame?

"Once you understand what the problem is, you can target the treatment accordingly," says Pelin Batur, MD, who specializes in sexual health and menopause. "However, it's also important to know that the vast majority of people with a clitoris need direct clitoral stimulation, typically for about twenty minutes, to have an orgasm. Most women won't have an orgasm with penis-in-vagina intercourse, and when I tell this to my patients, so many say, 'Oh! I'm good, I don't need treatment.'"

That said, it's important to know that there are options you can discuss with your healthcare provider. Here, Dr. Batur walks us through a few of those.

IF YOU'RE EXPERIENCING PAIN . . .

- **Pelvic floor physical therapy.** A pelvic floor physical therapist might perform manual therapy to address muscle tension that's causing pain during sex, or use other treatment techniques—from biofeedback that gives you real-time information on muscle activity and can help you learn to control your pelvic floor muscles to electrical stimulation that can help stimulate or relax muscles—to help you heal or manage your symptoms.

- **Menopause hormone therapy (MHT, formerly known as hormone replacement therapy).** This is prescribed to supplement declining hormone levels during and after the menopause transition and can help relieve vaginal dryness, improve vaginal lubrication, and boost libido. (For a lot more info on MHT and how it works, see pages 250–257.)

- **Localized hormone therapy, including topical estrogen and dehydroepiandrosterone (DHEA).** These topical hormones can improve sexual function by boosting vaginal elasticity and tone, increasing blood flow, and increasing lubrication. They can be used in premenopausal and postmenopausal women.

- **Ospemifene (aka Osphena).** FDA approved for use in postmenopausal women, this pill is used to help alleviate symptoms associated with genitourinary syndrome of menopause (GSM). It works like estrogen in the vagina and vulvar tissues to improve elasticity and lubrication in the area.

IF YOU'RE DEALING WITH LIBIDO ISSUES . . .

- **Talk therapy.** Whether sex therapy, couples counseling, or another form of therapy, working with a trained therapist or counselor can be a great way to explore the many issues often related to sexual dysfunction— from body image and self-esteem to relationship dynamics, past sexual abuse or trauma, and even the kind of everyday stressors that can impact your sex life. Therapy can help you learn more about your body and how to communicate your needs to your partner(s), and it can also help you address negative thoughts and beliefs that may be contributing to the issues you're facing.

- **Flibanserin (aka Addyi).** FDA approved for premenopausal women with hypoactive sexual desire disorder (HSDD), this is a pill that's taken daily and works by reducing serotonin (high levels of which are associated with reduced sexual desire) and increasing dopamine (which boosts feelings of pleasure, attraction, and anticipation and makes us seek out a "reward"—including sex).

- **Bremelanotide (aka Vyleesi).** Also FDA approved for premenopausal women with hypoactive sexual desire disorder (HSDD), this is an injectable medication you can give yourself forty-five minutes before sexual activity, which works by impacting several neurotransmitters that regulate mood, pleasure, and sexual desire, including dopamine, norepinephrine, and serotonin. (Note that both bremelanotide and flibanserin also work after menopause, though insurance typically doesn't cover the cost because these drugs aren't FDA approved in postmenopausal women.)

- **Androgen therapy (aka testosterone therapy and DHEA).** While testosterone is currently not approved by the Food and Drug Administration (FDA) for use in women, some clinicians prescribe it off label (a practice that's legal and common and means a clinician is prescribing a drug the FDA has approved to treat a condition that's different from yours) with instructions to use one-tenth the male dose.

Safe Sex: Preventing and Treating Sexually Transmitted Infections, Plus Healing After Sexual Abuse or Trauma

What You Need to Know About STIs

Understanding sexually transmitted infections (STIs)—what they are and how they spread, as well as their symptoms and treatments—is crucial, if admittedly not *sexy*. Because here's the truth: STIs are on the rise and show no signs of slowing down, according to the CDC.[5]

The more you know, the better able you'll be to protect yourself against these infections and get treatment if you contract one. Here, family physician Shannon Dowler, MD, explains what all of us need to know to take charge of our sexual health.

- **Talk to intimate partners about your sexual history (and get their history, too).** One of the best ways you can advocate for your sexual health is to have a conversation with anyone you're planning on being intimate with about your sexual health and theirs. Share any STI diagnoses you've received and ask them if they've ever been diagnosed with an STI as well. It's also important to get tested for STIs before having sex with a new partner and ask all new partners to get tested (and to show you the results).

    "Not everyone will be truthful, and not everyone will know what tests were done," says Dr. Dowler. "But *you* can be honest. Don't be afraid to ask your partner and doctors a lot of questions. It's the best way to advocate for yourself."

- **Know what is normal for your body (and not).** Many STIs can go undetected because symptoms are mild or look like something else. Dr. Dowler says she sees many women come into her office with what they assume is a benign symptom—say, an ingrown hair, a small cut from shaving, or vaginal discharge—when really it's an STI. What's more, a lot of STIs will appear to go away, but they actually don't—and then they cause long-term damage. The antidote: Look at your vulva in a mirror, touch yourself, know what's normal for you so you're more likely to recognize when something is different, and then go to a clinician to talk about it. "And pay attention to all exposed parts—mouths, throats, and anal areas should not be ignored," says Dr. Dowler.

- **Be truthful about your sexuality when you talk to healthcare providers**. Sex can prompt so much shame in even the most self-confident among us. Yet in the privacy of your healthcare provider's office, it's important to be forthcoming about your sexual history and practices. "This helps us know what STIs to test for and to test all the sites that are exposed," says Dr. Dowler. "You're not going to embarrass us, you're not going to make us feel uncomfortable. Lay it all out there— let us know what your risks and exposures are—so we can do a better job taking care of you."

- **Use condoms**. Consistent and correct use of barrier methods (like male condoms, female condoms, and dental dams) can significantly reduce your risk of exposure to an STI. Condoms provide a physical barrier between one partner's genitals or a sex toy and a vagina, anus, or mouth, preventing the exchange of bodily fluids like semen, vaginal secretions, and blood, all of which can contain STI pathogens, during sex.

- **Get the HPV vaccine**. There is a vaccine to prevent the most common STI in both women and men, and a cause of cervical cancer as well as head and neck cancers: HPV. The U.S. Centers for Disease Control and Prevention recommends eleven- to twelve-year-olds (both girls and boys) receive two doses of HPV vaccine six months to twelve months apart; teens and adults who start the series later (it's currently FDA approved for people up to age forty-five) need three doses. For those older than forty-five, the vaccine can be administered off label, though health insurance likely won't cover it.

  "Let's say you're fifty-five years old, you've been in a long-term marriage and just got divorced, and now you're back out there dating. It might be worth getting the vaccine," says Dr. Dowler. "If it was me, I'd get the vaccine. But it's an individual choice and important conversation to have with your healthcare provider." (For more information on HPV and the vaccine, see page 79.)

- **Get screened**. The CDC has clear guidelines on who should be tested and when. (Visit cdc.gov/sti/testing for those.) Dr. Dowler recommends that everyone get screened for STIs when establishing with a new healthcare provider. After that, screening can be done based on your risk factors. If you're in a lifelong monogamous relationship and you're 100 percent sure your partner isn't being intimate with anyone else, you probably don't need routine STI testing. If you have a partner change or you're intimate with multiple partners, you'll want to get tested more frequently. Talk to a healthcare provider about how often you should be tested based on your individual risk factors—and know that you should be tested for STIs at every site of exposure.

  "This is something a lot of providers miss, because they're not asking their patients if they're having anal or oral sex," says Dr. Dowler. If you are, it's important to discuss throat and rectal testing. Don't feel comfortable talking to your go-to clinician about your sex life and STI risk? Go to gettested.cdc.gov to find a clinic that provides free or low-cost and confidential testing near you.

- **Talk to your friends about STIs.** It's time to normalize the fact that STIs are something many of us deal with. And with rates continually rising, most of us in new relationships will deal with them, says Dr. Dowler. The shame and fear surrounding these common (and often treatable and curable!) infections prevent too many of us from getting tested and seeking medical care. The more we talk about STIs, the more we can collectively consider these infections like any other: something to be tested for and treated if contracted.

COMMON STIs, EXPLAINED

STI	CAUSED BY	HOW IT SPREADS
Human papillomavirus (HPV)	A group of viruses (approximately 150 types have been identified, and at least 40 affect the genitals) grouped into high- or low-risk	Many types of HPV are sexually transmitted through anogenital contact, mainly during vaginal and anal sex. HPV can also be transmitted during oral sex and via genital-to-genital contact without penetration.
Genital herpes	Two strains of the herpes simplex virus: HSV-1 (which often causes oral herpes and can result in cold sores or fever blisters on or around the mouth) and HSV-2 (which causes most cases of recurrent genital herpes)	Having vaginal, anal, or oral sex with someone who has the infection; it can spread even if a sex partner doesn't have a visible sore.
Syphilis	*T. pallidum* (bacteria)	Vaginal, anal, or oral sex without a condom with a partner who has syphilis. Sometimes sores occur in areas not covered by a condom, and contact with these sores can transmit syphilis. People can also pass syphilis to their baby during pregnancy.
Chlamydia	*C. trachomatis* (bacteria)	Vaginal, anal, or oral sex without a condom with a partner who has chlamydia; between mom and baby during childbirth if you have chlamydia while pregnant.

SYMPTOMS	TREATMENT	PREVENTION
Often asymptomatic. Anogenital warts may appear. Persistent infection is a risk factor for HPV-related cancers and precancers.	Many HPV infections resolve on their own without treatment; genital warts and/or precancerous lesions caused by HPV can be removed (though this doesn't treat the virus itself). Cancer treatment is necessary for HPV-associated cancers.	Vaccination up to age forty-five is FDA approved; barrier methods can reduce transmission.
Often asymptomatic. Symptoms may be mild and are often mistaken for other skin conditions (like an ingrown hair or pimple). Herpes sores usually appear as one or more blisters on or around the genitals, rectum, or mouth.	Antiviral medications can prevent or shorten herpes outbreaks and may make it less likely to pass the infection to your sex partner(s).	Consistent use of condoms and daily antiviral medications when a partner is known to be positive can be effective in preventing transmission.
There are four stages of syphilis (primary, secondary, latent, and tertiary), each with different signs and symptoms: *Primary stage*: You may notice a single sore or multiple sores that appear at the site where the bacteria entered the body, usually the penis, vagina, anus, rectum, lips, or mouth. *Secondary stage*: You may have skin rashes, hair loss, and/or white patches in your mouth, vagina, or anus. *Latent stage*: No visible signs or symptoms. *Tertiary stage*: This is when it can affect many different organ systems, including the heart, brain, and nervous system. Can cause brain, eye, and ear symptoms at any stage.	Syphilis is curable with the right antibiotics, usually injection(s) of long-acting benzathine penicillin G.	Barrier methods can reduce transmission. Doxycycline postexposure prophylaxis (doxy PEP) can help prevent infection.
Often asymptomatic. Symptoms in women can include abnormal vaginal discharge and burning during urination. Symptoms in men may include discharge from the penis, burning sensation when peeing, and pain and swelling in one or both testicles. It can spread to the liver and uterine tubes.	Chlamydia is curable with the right antibiotic, usually doxycycline.	Barrier methods can reduce transmission. Routine screening is recommended in all sexually active women twenty-four and younger and in women twenty-five and older who are at increased risk for infection. Doxycycline postexposure prophylaxis (doxy PEP) can help prevent infection.

STI	CAUSED BY	HOW IT SPREADS
Gonorrhea	*N. gonorrhoeae* (bacteria)	Vaginal, anal, or oral sex without a condom with someone who has gonorrhea; between mom and baby during childbirth if you have gonorrhea while pregnant.
Trichomoniasis (aka trich)	*T. vaginalis* (a parasite)	Having sex without a condom with a partner who is infected. In women, trich is most often found in the vulva, vagina, cervix, or urethra; in men, it's most often found inside the penis (urethra).
HIV/AIDS	Human immunodeficiency virus (HIV), which attacks the immune system	Vaginal or anal sex most commonly; sharing needles, syringes, or other drug-injection equipment. Only certain body fluids can transmit HIV, including blood, semen, preseminal fluid (aka "pre-cum"), rectal fluids, vaginal fluids, and breast milk.
Hepatitis B and C	Viruses that attack the liver	Hepatitis B is transmitted when you're exposed to blood, semen, or another body fluid from a person infected with the virus (most commonly through sex). Hepatitis C is spread when blood from an infected person enters your body (even in microscopic amounts). It can also spread through sex, though that's rare. Both hepatitis B and hepatitis C can be spread from an infected mother to her baby at birth.

Source: U.S. Centers for Disease Control and Prevention[6]
Medical review by Shannon Dowler, MD

SYMPTOMS	TREATMENT	PREVENTION
Often asymptomatic. Signs may include painful or burning sensation when peeing, increased vaginal discharge, and/or vaginal bleeding between periods. Men who have symptoms may experience a burning sensation when peeing, discharge from the penis that's white, yellow, or green, and/or painful or swollen testicles. It can spread to the skin, joints, eyes, and liver; it can also cause pelvic inflammatory disease (PID), which can lead to scar tissue that blocks the uterine tubes.	Gonorrhea is curable with the right antibiotic, usually an injection of ceftriaxone.	Barrier methods can reduce transmission; doxycycline postexposure prophylaxis (doxy PEP) can help prevent infection.
Often asymptomatic. Women may notice itching, burning, redness, or soreness of the genitals; discomfort when peeing; and a clear, white, yellowish, or greenish vaginal discharge with a fishy smell. Men may notice itching or irritation inside the penis; a burning sensation after peeing or ejaculating; and discharge from the penis.	Trich is known as the most common curable STI and can be treated with the right antibiotic, usually metronidazole.	Barrier methods can reduce transmission.
Can be asymptomatic. Most people have flu-like symptoms within two to four weeks of HIV infection. Without treatment, it can lead to acquired immunodeficiency syndrome (AIDS), in which case rapid weight loss, prolonged diarrhea, recurring infections, and even neurological symptoms may occur.	While there is no cure, taking antiretroviral therapy (ART) as soon as possible after diagnosis can control HIV and help prevent the progression to AIDS.	Barrier methods can reduce transmission. Pre-exposure prophylaxis (PrEP) is a daily medication that can prevent HIV infection. A long-acting injectable form of PrEP has also been approved by the FDA.
Often asymptomatic. Those infected can develop chronic infection that has no symptoms until disease progression. Without treatment, can lead to cancer, liver failure, and death.	For acute hepatitis B (occurs within the first six months after exposure) there's currently no available medication; medications for chronic hepatitis B can help prevent serious liver disease. Hepatitis C can be cured with antiviral medication.	Barrier methods can reduce transmission. There is a hepatitis B vaccine that can help prevent infection.

Sex After Abuse and Trauma:
Charting a Path Toward Sexual Healing

Over half of women and almost one in three men have experienced sexual violence, according to the CDC.[7]

What exactly constitutes sexual abuse? The answer is wide-ranging. It could be rape or incest; it could also be exposure to sexual acts or lewd comments at some point in your life. The definition isn't what's most important, says sex therapist Wendy Maltz, LCSW.

"If you are feeling upset about something inappropriate that happened to you around sex, it's important to acknowledge what happened," she says. "The recognition alone can be incredibly empowering and the key to beginning a recovery journey."

Here Maltz—who spent forty years as a sex therapist and wrote *The Sexual Healing Journey: A Guide for Survivors of Sexual Abuse*—shares the truths she wants every victim to know, and the steps involved in starting the healing process.

Making the connection between past abuse and current sexual issues is the first step in healing. It's a normal, understandable reaction to place sexual abuse experiences in the back recesses of our minds. It's a coping mechanism—something we do in the name of self-preservation. Yet it's important to understand that past sexual trauma and the issues it may still be causing in your life can surface at any time, even years after the abuse took place and in response to new conditions and experiences.

You might be reminded of what happened to you because of a specific event (like seeing someone who looks like your offender or even receiving sexual requests that remind you of ones you once inappropriately fielded) or a change (like having a child about the same age as you were when your abuse occurred). Memories can also surface if you're challenged to go to a deeper level of intimacy with a current, safe partner. All of this is normal, and acknowledging the abuse and identifying its impact on your life now are crucial.

"Without understanding that sexual issues you're experiencing today may be rooted in sexual abuse and trauma from your past, you can be in for years of unnecessary suffering," says Maltz.

The sex-related symptoms of previous sexual abuse are varied. If the connection between things that happened in the past and problems in your sex life today isn't exactly clear, it can help to know some of the common ways sexual assault and abuse can impact sexuality years later. Maltz says these are some of the most common sexual repercussions:

- Negative feelings (such as guilt, anger, or disgust) associated with touch
- Intrusive or disturbing sexual thoughts and/or images
- No interest in sex, avoiding sex, or approaching sex as an obligation
- Being emotionally distant or not present during sex
- Having pain during sex, difficulty having an orgasm, and/or difficulty becoming aroused or feeling sensation
- Engaging in compulsive or harmful sexual behaviors
- Difficulty establishing or maintaining intimate relationships

You are in charge of your healing and the way it unfolds. The work of healing from sexual trauma involves spending some time assessing what happened to you, how you feel about it, and how it's impacting you today. Additional steps include developing ways to handle negative reactions to touch, learning new approaches to touch and sex, and solving sexual problems.

Healing can be truly difficult, and it's important to approach this challenging work slowly and with the help of a therapist and intimate partner as needed. Be patient with yourself. Maintain compassion for what happened to you. Put a pause on areas you're not ready to look at and focus on the ones you do feel ready to address first.

"Ultimately, this work is about helping you see you are in charge of your own experiences now," says Maltz. "You are not alone. The abuse was not your fault. There is a path to recovery. Remember, with time and support it is possible to heal your sexuality."

Your Game Plan: How to Have Great Sex

After more than two decades as a sex educator, Emily Morse says she knows not to talk in absolutes—with one exception: "The vast majority of people don't take the time to really understand what they find truly pleasurable—and it keeps them from having great sex," she says. "We leave sex up to mystery! It's like each time we go to have it, we close our eyes and hope for the best." Here, Morse explains exactly where to start when it comes to changing that.

Take your personal sexual pleasure history. Think back in time and ask yourself: What were some of your biggest turn-ons, hottest moments, and most memorable sexual experiences? Write them down so you can see at a glance all the things that help you feel like your most vibrant sexual self—and then consider the ways you can work them into your current-day sex life.

Write a sexual bucket list. What interests you sexually? Where do you want to go with your sex life? Do you have fantasies or erotic desires that you haven't been able to express or have fulfilled? "Maybe you've always wanted to be tied up, or you've always wanted someone to talk dirty to you, and it's never happened," says Morse. "Getting honest about what you want your sex life to look like is the first step toward making it happen."

Start a mindful masturbation practice. The goal here is to breathe deeply and tune in to the sensations in your body as you touch yourself. "This isn't a 'hit it and quit it' session," says Morse. "For mindful masturbation, I recommend removing things like porn or anything else you typically use. It's not that there's anything wrong with that. It's just that in mindful masturbation, the goal is exploration—so I want you to get curious and intentionally explore what feels good." What part of your labia gets you going? Is your clitoris more sensitive on the left or right side? How long did it take you to really warm up? What were you thinking about as you touched yourself? Answering these questions can help you tee yourself up for pleasure again—whether solo or with a partner.

Attune to your body's sensations the next time you're having sex. Whether masturbating or with a partner, really clue in to what feels good. Ask yourself: *What do I need to be aroused? What does the environment need to look or feel like? What kind of connection do I need to feel if I'm with a partner?*

"Once you know what you need physically, mentally, and emotionally, you'll be better able to optimize these areas that contribute to having great sex," says Morse.

Identify your pleasure thieves. Is it stress? A history of sexual or emotional trauma? Shame? A big hormonal transition like perimenopause? What's keeping you from pleasure? It's not that you'll be able to completely eradicate these pleasure thieves, says Morse, but when you know they're there, you'll be better able to recognize them when they rear their ugly heads and make it hard for you to get aroused. Then you can consider if there's anything you might do to facilitate more desire and arousal.

· · · · ·

When you have the facts about your sexual health, it can help you feel more confident when you have sex—solo or partnered—and communicate with your partner(s) and healthcare practitioners about your sex life more effectively. Most important, you'll feel empowered knowing that having sex you genuinely enjoy is not only possible but the ultimate goal.

Chapter 4

Gynecology

What You Need to Know About the

Care and Keeping of Your Female Parts

> *Women and people dealing with gynecologic issues have suffered for thousands of years too long, and it's time to break the cycle. It's not hysteria, and it never was.*
>
> —Karen Tang, MD, MPH, *It's Not Hysteria: Everything You Need to Know About Your Reproductive Health (But Were Never Told)*

If you have a vulva, it's important to have regular gynecologic exams. These checkups are a chance to monitor your menstrual and reproductive health, get preventive screenings to help detect health issues early on, give you a chance to discuss birth control options and sexual health, and so much more.

Yet just as there are many reasons for a gynecologic exam, there are a similarly wide range of feelings that can bubble to the surface when you make that appointment. No matter why you find yourself in the exam room or what emotions are swirling as you change into that flimsy paper robe, here's the truth: The more you know about how the female reproductive system works and what to expect when you meet with your practitioner, the better.

In this chapter, we'll learn . . .

- **What to expect at your annual well-woman visit**, including some specific advice for those who don't identify as heterosexual, cisgender females.

- **The recommendations for cervical cancer screening**, so you have a clear understanding of the different screening options (Pap smear and HPV testing) and when and how frequently you need each.

- **Details about the menstrual cycle and vaginal discharge.** A staggering 47 percent of women don't know what ovulation is and 67 percent can't say when it happens, according to one study.[1] We're obviously missing out on some key information about the different phases of our cycles—not to mention how to know what's "normal" versus when something is wrong.

- **The many birth control options that exist, including how they work and their pros and cons.** On pages 87–100, you'll find crucial information about many methods so you can decide which options sound best for you and discuss them with your clinician.

- **Options for emergency contraception and abortion, how they work, and the best way to know your options based on where you live.** Because no matter how you feel about ending a pregnancy from a political or religious perspective, the fact is that it is a women's healthcare issue—and knowing the unbiased facts about the options available can help put a stop to the misinformation surrounding them.

Meet the Experts

Frances Grimstad, MD, associate professor of obstetrics, gynecology, and reproductive biology at Harvard Medical School and a member of the world's largest and oldest association of LGBTQ+ and allied healthcare professionals, GLMA

Margo Harrison, MD, ob-gyn, assistant adjoint professor at the University of Colorado School of Medicine, and CEO of Wave Bye, a femtech company aiming to revolutionize menstrual care

Genevieve Hofmann, DNP, WHNP-BC, women's health nurse practitioner at the University of Colorado with a special interest in contraception and family planning

Alison Edelman, MD, ob-gyn, with specialty training in complex family planning and professor of obstetrics and gynecology at Oregon Health & Science University School of Medicine

Sarah Cigna, MD, assistant professor of obstetrics and gynecology at The George Washington University and director of the first sexual medicine fellowship in the U.S. for ob-gyn physicians

Ushma Upadhyay, PhD, MPH, professor of reproductive health at the University of California, San Francisco

Stephanie Trentacoste McNally, MD, ob-gyn, certified menopause provider, and director of ob-gyn services at the Katz Institute for Women's Health

Your Annual Gynecology Visit: What to Expect and How to Get the Most Out of Your Appointment

The conversation: You'll probably have anywhere from twenty to thirty minutes with your provider, during which you'll be on the receiving end of questions about your menstrual cycle, sexual activity and partners, what you use for contraception, and even things like your drug and alcohol use. Given this time crunch and how much your clinician needs to cover in an annual exam, bring up what feels most pressing for you at the start—and know that you may need to schedule a follow-up appointment to go over specific concerns, symptoms, or exciting things like pregnancy planning if you don't have time to cover that ground during your annual visit.

The physical exam: There are a number of components of this portion of the exam, which your healthcare provider may or may not do depending on the purpose of your visit and the symptoms or concerns you've shared with them. These include a urine sample to test for pregnancy and various infections; a breast exam; an external abdominopelvic exam where your provider will palpate your abdominal area to feel for things like an enlarged uterus or other abdominal-area growths or abnormalities as well as look at your vulva; and an internal pelvic exam, where your provider will insert a speculum in the vagina so it (and your cervix) can be more easily seen.

The Pap smear: If you're due for a Pap, your provider may use a small swab to take a sample of cells from your cervix during the speculum exam. This test looks for precancerous cells on the cervix (or vaginal walls, in the case of the self-swab). While Pap smears used to be a regular part of every gynecologic annual exam, updated guidelines now state that cervical cancer screening can be done every three to five years. (More on this below.)

HPV testing: A narrow brush or spatula is used to collect a small sample of cervical cells, which is then tested to see if they're infected with the strains of HPV that are more likely to cause cancer. Here's the thing about HPV: It's super common. So common, in fact, that nearly all sexually active men and women get the virus at some point in their lives, according to the CDC.[2] Of the roughly two hundred types of HPV, about forty can be spread sexually—and twelve types are considered high-risk. Two of those high-risk HPV types (HPV 16 and HPV 18) are responsible for most of the HPV-related cancers. The good news is that most cases of HPV go away on their own; the immune system attacks the virus and clears it from your body. Sometimes, however, HPV persists—and because there's currently no way to predict who will clear the virus and who will continue to live with it over the long term, HPV testing is the best way to gauge cervical cancer risk.

Here's what the U.S. Preventive Services Task Force 2018 guidelines say about who needs HPV testing, a Pap smear, or both:[3]

- Women under age twenty-one probably do not need a Pap smear.

- Women ages twenty-one through twenty-nine should get a Pap smear every three years (even if they've been vaccinated against HPV).

- Women ages thirty through sixty-five can get an HPV test every five years or a Pap test every three years, or a combination (called the HPV/Pap co-test) every five years.

- Women ages sixty-five and older who've had regular screening in the past ten years and normal results don't need a Pap smear.

- People who have had a total hysterectomy (removal of the uterus and cervix) should stop screening (both Pap and HPV tests), unless they have a history of cervical cancer or serious precancer.

What to Know About the HPV Vaccine

While cervical cancer screening is crucial, it's also important to realize that there is a way to help *prevent* almost all cervical and other HPV-related cancers, which include head and neck cancers, as well as other cancers of the vulva, vagina, anus, and penis: the HPV vaccine. It is highly effective at protecting against nine HPV types, including two that cause 90 percent of genital warts (6 and 11) and two that cause about 70 percent of cervical cancer cases (16 and 18), as well as others that account for an additional 10 to 20 percent of cervical cancers (31, 33, 45, 52, and 58).

One major study out of Scotland found no cases of cervical cancer in women who were fully vaccinated against HPV between the ages of twelve and thirteen.[4] This timing is crucial, pointing to the importance of getting kids vaccinated before they become sexually active. And yes, boys can get vaccinated for HPV as well, as they can get infected with and spread the virus. In men, HPV causes head and neck cancers, as well as penile and anal cancer.

The goal is to complete the vaccine series before becoming sexually active, to help prevent contracting HPV. The CDC recommends getting kids vaccinated at age eleven or twelve, though kids as young as nine can get the vaccine. If you're between ages twenty-seven and forty-five, your clinician may discuss the HPV vaccine with you. While vaccination after exposure to HPV is thought to provide less benefit, having a conversation with your healthcare provider will help you decide if it might still be a good choice for you.

If You're Not a Heterosexual, Cisgender Woman . . .

It's important for all of us to find a provider who understands our health history and makes us feel comfortable while providing the care we need. Sadly, this can be tough to find—especially for those of us who aren't straight or cisgender.

"The field of gynecology was traditionally built around the premise that every person we care for identifies as a woman," says ob-gyn Frances Grimstad, MD. "Still, too many gynecologic clinicians assume all of their patients will get a period, have penile-vaginal sex, get pregnant, give birth, and go through menopause." For some LGBTQ+ people, that arc won't apply.

To ensure you get the care you deserve, it's important to find a clinician who doesn't make assumptions about your anatomy, identity, or behaviors. If you sense assumptions *are* being made, ask for clarification. Let's say your provider asks, "Are you sexually active?" You might reply, "What do you mean by that?"

"I think the most important thing to remember is that the field of gynecology is still evolving from a historically heterosexual framework," says Dr. Grimstad. "Until the majority of clinicians become better at not making assumptions about their patients, it's up to you to advocate for yourself about the care you may need, including screenings or vaccinations." To help you do that, here are some important factors to keep in mind.

IF YOU'RE LESBIAN . . .

- **You still need Pap smears**. Many healthcare providers incorrectly assume lesbian patients are at low risk of cervical cancer, based on the assumption that the patient hasn't previously had sex with men. In addition to that being an inaccurate assumption, cervical dysplasia has been reported in lesbians who haven't previously had intercourse with men—meaning routine cervical cancer screening is crucial.

- **You may be at increased risk for breast, cervical, and ovarian cancer compared with heterosexual women**, because you may be less likely to get screening exams if, due to fear of discrimination or past negative experiences with providers, you've skipped screening exams.[5] Create a cancer-screening plan with your provider, then stick to it.

- **You're at the same risk of STIs as heterosexual women.** Lesbians can transmit STIs to each other through skin-to-skin contact, vaginal fluids, mucous membrane contact, and menstrual blood. If you're sexually active, it's crucial you get screened for STIs, especially if you have more than one sexual partner.

- **You can experience intimate partner violence.** Some lesbian women may experience violence in their intimate relationships—yet clinicians don't always ask lesbian women about it as often as they ask those who identify as heterosexual.

IF YOU'RE TRANSGENDER . . .

- **You may have a tough time accessing healthcare.** Finding a clinician who knows how to treat trans people—and insurance that will pay for your treatments—may be very difficult. When looking for a provider, ask if they care for transgender people; you want your provider to have the knowledge and skills to provide care and be affirming of you.

- **You'll want to keep detailed medical records.** While this is important for everyone to do, it's especially important to share your health history with a provider you trust—including the medications you've taken, any surgeries you've had, and mental health issues you've faced.

- **You should be able to talk about gender-affirming hormone treatment.** There are a lot of considerations when it comes to taking hormones. For example, if you're a transgender woman, taking estrogen can put you at a higher risk for blood clots; if you're a transgender man, blood tests may be necessary to make sure your testosterone dose is safe.

- **You should talk to your provider about cancer screenings.** You'll want to make sure you're getting the recommended screenings of the sex organs or other body tissues you have.

- **You'll benefit from having an STI screening and prevention plan.** It's important to be able to have an honest conversation about the type of sex and number of sex partners you have so that you can come up with a screening plan that keeps you and your partner(s) healthy.

Your Period: What to Know About Your Cycle

Menstruation—aka your period—is something many of us experience for about five days at a time, yet there's a remarkable amount of confusion, stigma, and misinformation that exists about our periods. That's too bad, given the menstrual cycle is considered a vital sign, says Dr. Margo Harrison.

"Knowing the basics of how your menstrual cycle works gives you the context to make the sexual and reproductive health decisions that are right for you," says Dr. Harrison. "Yes, it's a complicated dance of hormonal interplay, but it doesn't have to be hard to understand." Here, Dr. Harrison breaks it down.

There are *two* phases of your menstrual cycle:

Phase 1: The Follicular Phase

When it typically happens: Days 1 to 14

What your hormones are doing: Estrogen and progesterone start out at their lowest levels. If you're not pregnant, a decrease in progesterone triggers blood vessels growing into your uterine lining to spasm and break open and also prompts the production of inflammatory molecules. This combination of blood and inflammation causes the top layer of the lining of your uterus to separate from the bottom layer and shed through your vagina—bleeding that you likely refer to as your period. From the end of your period through the rest of the follicular phase, estrogen rises, which signals the uterine lining to grow. You also get a bump in follicle-stimulating hormone (FSH), which triggers the growth of immature eggs in the fluid-filled sacs in your ovaries called follicles. This phase ends with ovulation, when a sudden surge in luteinizing hormone (LH) prompts the largest follicle to burst and release an egg into your uterine tube (aka Fallopian tube).

How you might feel: Low hormone levels coupled with bleeding can make you feel extra exhausted during the first week of this phase. What's more, you may be experiencing period pain or menstrual cramps, joint pain, and breast tenderness—and this physical discomfort can be associated with irritability, emotional distress, and decreased self-esteem. As estrogen rises, it'll likely make you feel happy, social, and energized. You may also notice you feel super sharp and articulate during the latter half of this phase (the brain loves estrogen) and experience a boost in libido.

Phase 2: The Luteal Phase

When it typically happens: Days 15 to 28

What your hormones are doing: During this second phase of your cycle, that ruptured follicle develops into a corpus luteum, which is a temporary structure that secretes hormones—primarily progesterone—preparing your uterine lining for pregnancy. If your egg is fertilized by sperm and attaches itself to your uterine wall, the corpus luteum continues to produce estrogen and progesterone. If fertilization doesn't happen, the corpus luteum deteriorates, estrogen and progesterone levels drop, and the cycle starts again.

How you might feel: If you don't get pregnant and you experience this dip in progesterone, estrogen, and testosterone, that can help explain why PMS symptoms like breast tenderness, cramps, acne, headaches, and mood swings set in.

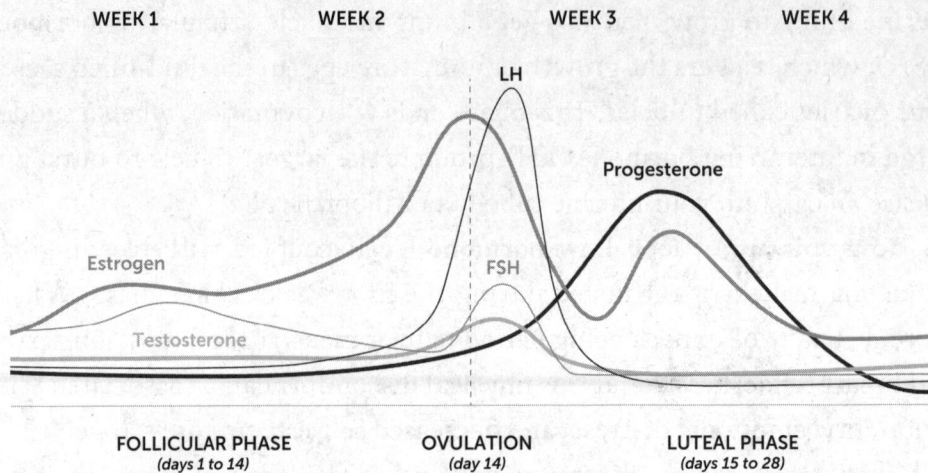

| WEEK 1 | WEEK 2 | WEEK 3 | WEEK 4 |

LH

Progesterone

Estrogen

FSH

Testosterone

FOLLICULAR PHASE
(days 1 to 14)

OVULATION
(day 14)

LUTEAL PHASE
(days 15 to 28)

It's important to note that these hormones fluctuate on different time frames for different women and can vary cycle to cycle, says Dr. Harrison. "This graph represents an average of what's happening to the hormones that regulate the menstrual cycle," she says. "It's fine—and can still be considered 'normal'—if your hormones fluctuate on a different cycle length."

What's a Regular Versus an Irregular Period?

Clinicians consider four aspects of your period when answering this question:

1. **How frequently you get your period.** The average cycle is twenty-eight days but is still considered "normal" if it's anywhere between twenty-four and thirty-eight days.

2. **How regularly you're getting your period.** There should be no more than seven to nine days' difference between your shortest and longest cycle. (You can calculate your cycle length from the first day of your period to the first day of your next period.)

3. **How many days you bleed.** Up to eight days of bleeding in a single menstrual period is considered regular.

4. **How much you bleed.** While your blood "volume" is subjective, it's typically considered regular if it's not interfering with your physical, social, emotional, and/or material quality of life.

The most important thing you can do is get to know your cycle and track what the experience is like for you, says Dr. Harrison. Make a note of the length of your cycle, how many pads and/or tampons you use during a day (to help gauge how much you're bleeding), and any pain you experience before, during, or after your period. This information will arm you with the facts your health-care provider will need when assessing your cycle.

Ask an Expert

Is period blood toxic?

No—menstrual blood is regular blood. It's not filled with toxins or hormones that need to be excreted, as some social media influencers would have you believe. Just as all of your organs have a blood supply, so does your uterus. Period blood may look different from the blood you see if you get a cut, because technically, it's menstrual fluid: In addition to blood, it also contains some endometrial tissue, inflammatory fluid, and mucus from the lining of your uterus—and on its way out of your body, it picks up cervical mucus and vaginal discharge as well.

—Margo Harrison, MD, ob-gyn, assistant adjoint professor at the University of Colorado School of Medicine, and CEO of Wave Bye, a femtech company aiming to revolutionize menstrual care

Wetness and Discharge:
What's Going On and What It Means

Your vagina is lined with membranes that produce mucus, so there is always some level of wetness inside—and that wetness changes based on where you are in your cycle, how sexually aroused (or not) you feel, and whether your body is dealing with an infection. This is why knowing the difference between what's usual for you (and what's not) can alert you to something possibly being off and whether it's time to schedule an appointment with your practitioner.

What we call wetness or discharge is actually one of three main types of fluid:

1. Lubrication

This discharge is related to sexual arousal, which aids in pleasure during sexual activity. There are two types of glands that produce lubrication: the *greater vestibular glands* (aka Bartholin's glands), which are located on either side of the vaginal opening, and the *lesser vestibular glands* (aka Skene's glands) located on either side of the urethra.

2. Cervical Fluid

Sometimes called cervical mucus, this type of discharge changes in texture, volume, and color throughout your cycle. As you near ovulation, a rise in estrogen increases the quantity and quality of cervical mucus, making it stretchy. That's because the mucus helps sperm pass through the cervix and into the uterus and uterine tubes, where fertilization commonly happens.

Cervical mucus can have a strong odor, but it shouldn't be overwhelming or bad smelling. Also, while everyone with a cervix will produce mucus in different amounts, varieties, and odors, there are some generalities in how it appears at different times of your cycle.

TIME OF THE MONTH	YOUR CERVICAL MUCUS
During your period	You likely won't notice any mucus due to your bleeding.
Right after your period	Discharge is almost entirely absent, which means you'll be drier than usual these days.
The days before ovulation	Mucus production increases, and it's usually yellow, white, or "cloudy" and feels sticky.
Right before and during ovulation	This is when you'll usually have the most mucus, and it becomes clear and feels slippery and may even look like raw egg whites.
After ovulation	You'll likely notice less mucus, and it'll get sticky and cloudy again. You may also have more dry days, when you don't notice any cervical mucus.

Source: Planned Parenthood[6]

3. Infection

Your discharge can help signal if there's an infection. Here are some common infections and the type of discharge associated with each.

TYPE OF INFECTION	WHAT MUCUS OR DISCHARGE MAY LOOK LIKE
Bacterial vaginosis (BV)	Creamy white or grayish mucus with a strong, fishy smell
Yeast infection	Thick white mucus that resembles the texture of cottage cheese
Chlamydia	White, yellow, or gray discharge that may be smelly
Trichomoniasis	Clear, white, yellowish, or greenish discharge with a fishy smell

Contraception Basics: Your Options, How They Work, and Tips on Choosing the Right One for You

When it comes to birth control, your choices can seem endless. There are hormonal and nonhormonal options. There are pills, patches, vaginal rings, injections, and intrauterine devices. Then there's the fact that many of these forms of birth control aren't strictly used for pregnancy prevention. Do you have heavy periods? Severe PMS? Acne? There's a birth control method that can help to treat each one of those symptoms (and many more)—and if the first one you try doesn't help or makes you feel worse, there's a good chance another option exists that might work better.

Yet despite the many excellent methods of contraception available to us right now, more than 40 percent of pregnancies that occur in the U.S. are unplanned.[7] This is scary stuff—and points to a major need for more education around what the options are (including ones for men), how they work, and how to use them effectively.

The best place to start is by knowing your options and having a conversation with your healthcare provider about your specific needs, medical history, and lifestyle so together you can figure out the best contraceptive fit for you. You'll want to talk about your relationship status, if you want to have kids (and roughly when, if you do), your health history (including whether you have a history of high blood pressure or smoking), as well as questions like whether you have a track record of forgetting to take a daily birth control pill or not using a condom in the heat of the moment.

When you see just how many choices you have, it can be easy to feel overwhelmed. But you're more likely to land on a method that feels right for you when you have an informed conversation with your healthcare provider. You'll find the intel you need on many of the currently available options here, as well as expert guidance from Genevieve Hofmann, DNP, WHNP-BC.

Contraceptive options tend to fall into one of these categories:

1. Hormonal methods

2. Intrauterine devices (IUDs)

3. Barrier methods

4. Fertility awareness

5. Permanent methods

6. Emergency contraception

Let's go through some of the basics in each of these categories to help you have an informed conversation with your practitioner about which option may be best for you.

Hormonal Methods

These contain synthetic forms of the hormones progesterone (progestin) and/or estrogen (ethinyl estradiol is the most common estrogen in oral contraceptives), which work in multiple ways to prevent pregnancy and control the menstrual cycle.

- *Progestin* stops or suppresses ovulation (depending on the type you're taking), thins the lining of the uterus, and thickens the cervical mucus so it's harder for sperm to travel into the uterus and uterine tubes (where sperm typically meet egg for fertilization).

- *Ethinyl estradiol* also helps to stop ovulation by suppressing the production of luteinizing hormone, which also results in a thinner lining of the uterus and leads to a lighter menstrual cycle.

There are a number of hormonal contraception methods, and each one comes with different pros, cons, and rates of effectiveness.

» ORAL CONTRACEPTIVE PILLS (AKA THE PILL)

How they work: By preventing ovulation and thickening the mucus in the cervix, which makes it harder for sperm to get into the uterus and reach an egg. Oral contraceptives may also thin the lining of your uterus so there's less chance of a fertilized egg implanting and being able to grow (and you'll likely have a lighter period, too).

Oral contraceptive pills are either combined estrogen-progestin or progestin-only. You are instructed to take one pill every day for twenty-eight days. With most combined oral contraceptives, the pills you take on days twenty-two through twenty-eight don't contain any hormones (which will prompt you to have "withdrawal bleeding" that will feel like your period). Most progestin-only pills (such as Opill, the over-the-counter birth control pill option) do not include hormone-free pills, and you don't take a break between packs. If you're taking an extended-use pill, you take the active hormones for three months, then the hormone-free pills for a week.

The upsides and downsides: With many different combinations of hormones (and varying strengths of hormones), there's a good chance you can find a method that gives you the effect you're hoping for with few noticeable side effects. If you have high blood pressure, if you smoke, if you have a history of blood clots, or if you get migraine headaches with aura (seeing flashing lights or zigzags), you may not be a good candidate. It's also important to keep in mind that this method of birth control relies on you taking the pill around the same time every day, and it becomes less effective almost immediately after a couple of "Oops, I forgot to take my pill" moments.

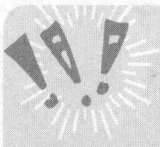

WHAT DO I DO IF I MISS A DAY OR TWO (OR MORE) OF MY "ACTIVE" BIRTH CONTROL PILL?

Take your missed pill as soon as you remember, even if it means taking two pills in one day. If you miss two pills in a row, take two pills the day you remember and two pills the next day, then resume taking one pill per day as usual. Keep in mind that missed days make pregnancy more likely, so it's important to use additional forms of contraception (like condoms) until you start a new cycle of pills.

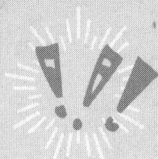

» THE PATCH

How it works: Similarly to combined oral contraceptive pills, as it contains both estrogen and progestin. You'll place a small patch on your upper arm, lower abdomen, or butt once a week for three weeks (which is when it releases hormones through your skin) and not wear the patch the following week (which prompts bleeding to start).

The upsides and downsides: You only have to remember to put on a new patch once a week versus remembering to take a pill every day. However, skin irritation where the patch is placed is a possibility. In addition to contraindications similar to those that come with use of the pill (high blood pressure, blood clotting, smoking), it's also important to note that the patch may be less effective in those who weigh more than 198 pounds.

» VAGINAL RING

How it works: When you place this small, soft, plastic ring inside your vagina, the ring releases a continuous dose of the hormones estrogen and progestin into the bloodstream. You'll leave the ring in your vagina for twenty-one days, then remove it for a seven-day ring-free week (which prompts bleeding to start).

The upsides and downsides: It's an easy-to-use option you have to think about only twice a month, when it's time to insert and remove the ring. You also have a choice between disposable options and reusable rings. However, you may not be a candidate if you have certain contraindications, including high blood pressure, unmanaged diabetes, a history of blood clots, or if you smoke. And like all estrogen-containing methods, if you get migraines with aura, the ring may worsen symptoms.

» THE BIRTH CONTROL SHOT

How it works: Often referred to by the brand name Depo-Provera or called the Depo shot, this is a progestin-only birth control method that suppresses ovulation and makes cervical mucus thicker. It's administered as a shot into the muscle of your upper arm or butt once every three months by a clinician. There is also a self-administered version that's delivered subcutaneously (under the skin).

The upsides and downsides: If remembering to take a daily pill or replace a patch or ring on a regular schedule has proved difficult for you, this is an option. But given the three-month time frame of the shot, this method isn't as reversible as other forms of birth control—meaning it may not be right for you if you want to get pregnant within three to ten months.

Ask an Expert

Is it okay to skip periods if I'm on hormonal birth control?
You may have heard that taking a "break" from the hormones in your pill pack—taking the week of placebo pills, which prompts you to

have a period—is good for you. However, the truth is that the period you have on the pill isn't actually a natural period. It's called withdrawal bleeding because it's caused by not taking the hormones. In fact, the only reason having a week of bleeding while taking the pill is even an option is that the scientists who created the pill thought women would find it more natural to have a period each month.

There's no medical reason that you need a cycle if you're taking oral contraceptives. Regular, monthly bleeding while on hormonal birth control doesn't provide any benefits. Actually, for women with medical disorders like menstrual migraines, endometriosis, or polycystic ovarian disease, it's better to *not* have that period week, because it could reactivate symptoms or cause other problems. Skipping periods when you're on hormonal birth control doesn't affect fertility in the future and doesn't increase the risk of side effects, like blood clotting. The one downside to skipping a period is that some individuals can experience breakthrough spotting or bleeding, which isn't dangerous but can be annoying.

The bottom line: If you're on hormonal birth control, your cycle is happening because of the medication you're taking—and it's not medically necessary or even beneficial for your health. So go ahead and enjoy not having a period if that's your preference.

—Alison Edelman, MD, ob-gyn with specialty training in complex family planning and professor of obstetrics and gynecology at Oregon Health & Science University School of Medicine

Intrauterine Devices (IUDs)

These are small, T-shaped devices that your healthcare provider will insert into your uterus to prevent pregnancy. There are hormonal and nonhormonal IUD options. The nonhormonal IUD can remain in place for up to ten years, while the hormonal IUD can remain in place for up to eight years, depending on the brand. But either option can also be removed by your provider at any time.

» HORMONAL IUD

How it works: By releasing progestin, which prevents pregnancy by thinning the lining of the uterus, suppressing ovulation, and thickening the mucus in the cervix to inhibit sperm movement and viability.

The upsides and downsides: This is a set-it-and-forget-it method that you won't have to think about for five to eight years, and the amount of systemic hormone absorption is much lower than with other hormonal methods. Keep in mind irregular bleeding can happen at first (this often improves after three to six months) and side effects can include breast tenderness, mood changes, headaches, acne, and cramping or pelvic pain. In rare cases, insertion of an IUD causes perforation of the uterus—a risk that may be higher when the IUD is inserted during the postpartum period. Also, you'll need to have an appointment for both insertion and removal of an IUD, both of which can be painful. That said, pain management is and should be available, and it's something to discuss with your clinician. (For more info on pain-management options during an IUD insertion, flip to page 94.)

» NONHORMONAL COPPER IUD

How it works: This T-shaped plastic device is wrapped in copper, which changes the way sperm move and prevents them from swimming to an egg.

The upsides and downsides: The copper IUD can be left in your uterus for up to ten years, making it a great option if you want a highly effective, nonhormonal birth control option that you don't have to think about. It can make your periods heavier and cause cramping, especially in the first three to six months after it's inserted. And just like the hormonal IUD, insertion and removal of the copper IUD can be painful, and you'll need an appointment for both.

Ask an Expert

I've heard IUD insertion can be excruciatingly painful. Do I have options for pain management during the procedure?

You have many options for pain management during an IUD insertion. But it can be challenging to find a provider who will offer them to you. I've personally had four IUDs and would never have one inserted without pain medication. In fact, I tried the no-pain-medication approach after I had a baby, because everyone tells you having an IUD inserted after a baby is less painful. Within seconds, I was like, *Nope!*

So many patients don't even know pain-management options exist, because they aren't widely available, which makes it especially important to know your options. They include:

- A high dose of over-the-counter pain reliever like ibuprofen (Advil, Motrin) or naproxen (Aleve) before the procedure. Your healthcare provider will tell you how much to take.

- Prescription pain medication, which a practitioner may prescribe if they feel stronger pain meds would be beneficial to take preprocedure.

- Antianxiety medication, which can help calm your nerves, ease stress, and relax your whole body—including your pelvic floor muscles, which are more likely to clench if you're stressed.

- Local anesthesia, such as a paracervical block that's injected on either side of the cervix and numbs some of the cervical nerves. This can ease the pain associated with the dilation that often needs to happen during the insertion of the IUD.

- Systemic anesthesia, or IV sedation, during which a patient is not awake and the IUD insertion happens in an operating room. It's important to note, however, that many insurance companies deem systemic anesthesia "unnecessary" and will not cover it.

- Nitrous oxide (commonly referred to as laughing gas), just like the stuff on offer at many dentists' offices—though many ob-gyn offices do not offer this as a pain-management option.

Here's the truth: Pain during IUD insertion varies greatly among patients. I have some patients who get an IUD with nothing and barely feel it. (Though full disclosure: I call them unicorns.) For most patients, this is an incredibly painful procedure and offering a spectrum of pain-management options should be the standard of care. Until that happens, talk to your clinician about these options, and if you're dismissed for bringing them up, find a new provider.

—Sarah Cigna, MD, assistant professor of obstetrics and gynecology at The George Washington University and director of the first sexual medicine fellowship in the U.S. for ob-gyn physicians

Barrier Methods

These are excellent methods of contraception that work just like they sound: They create a barrier so that sperm are less likely to enter the uterus.

» CONDOM

How it works: When placed on a penis before penetrative sex, the condom traps sperm and prevents them from entering the uterus. Internal condoms (often referred to as female condoms) are inserted into the vagina up to eight hours before penetrative sex and also trap sperm, preventing them from entering the uterus.

The upsides and downsides: Not only do both male and female condoms protect against pregnancy, but most also protect against some sexually transmitted infections (STIs). This is why condoms are recommended if you have a new sex partner, even if you're using another method of birth control. One of the biggest downsides is that in the heat of the moment, using a condom can seem like an extra step that kills the vibe. Condoms can also break and come off during sex. And if you're using lube, make sure it's water- or silicone-based; oil-based lubes can make condoms break.

» CONTRACEPTIVE DIAPHRAGM AND CERVICAL CAP

How they work: These are small, reusable devices made of soft silicone and designed to be inserted into the vagina before penetrative sex, and they work by blocking the cervix so sperm can't reach an egg. Both devices should always be used with spermicide, a chemical that immobilizes or kills sperm so they can't swim into your uterus. The main difference between the two is that a cervical cap is smaller and can be left in place longer.

The upsides and downsides: These are barrier methods of birth control that *you* get to control, that come with few side effects, and that take immediate effect. And they don't interrupt sexual spontaneity like condoms can, as you can insert a diaphragm up to two hours before sex and a cervical cap up to six hours before sex. However, unlike condoms, diaphragms and cervical caps do not protect against STIs and may contribute to an increased risk of urinary tract infections. You'll also have to use water- or silicone-based lube, as oil-based products can damage the material, making it more likely to break or tear.

» SPERMICIDE

How it works: This comes in various forms (including gels, creams, foams, suppositories, sponges, and films) and works by immobilizing or killing sperm on contact, preventing them from reaching and fertilizing an egg. A new nonhormonal prescription birth control method (called Phexxi) used in a similar way to spermicide lowers the pH in your vagina when sperm is there, making it hard for sperm to move and lowering the chance that fertilization will happen as a result.

The upsides and downsides: These are hormone-free options that you can control. Spermicide and Phexxi must be placed in the vagina about ten to fifteen minutes before sexual intercourse, and they don't protect against STIs. When used alone, spermicide is less effective than other contraceptive methods, though its effectiveness improves when combined with another barrier method.

Fertility Awareness Methods

These fall under the "natural family planning" category and typically involve tracking your menstrual cycle to determine when you are most fertile. Then you'll either use a barrier method of contraception or avoid sex during that time. It's worth noting that while many use the "pull-out" method (a form of birth control where the partner with a penis withdraws it from the vagina before ejaculation to prevent sperm from entering the uterus), it has a failure rate of about 20 percent. More reliable options include the following.

» CALENDAR-BASED, BASAL BODY TEMPERATURE, AND CERVICAL MUCUS METHODS

How they work: These methods involve tracking your menstrual cycle, basal (resting) body temperature, and/or cervical mucus changes over several months, typically using a period-tracking app, to determine the average length of your cycle—and therefore the most likely days of ovulation. In an average twenty-eight-day cycle, ovulation happens around day 14, though tracking your period in an app will give you a better sense of your ovulation time frame. Basal body temperature can increase slightly after ovulation (giving you a sense of your fertile window), and cervical mucus becomes thin, stretchy, and clear around the time of ovulation. Tracking these changes helps you know when you're most fertile, during which time you can either use a barrier method or avoid sex if you don't want to get pregnant.

The upsides and downsides: These methods cost nothing, don't have side effects, and don't require a visit to a healthcare provider (though that's recommended if you want to learn how to properly track your cycle and interpret the signs of fertility). They're also a good option if you hope to become pregnant soon—or if it wouldn't feel like the end of the world if you did conceive. It's important to keep in mind these methods require a significant amount of consistency and diligence to be effective, and you'll need your sexual partner(s) to cooperate. It's also important to note that the effectiveness of these methods is among the lowest of all contraception options.

Permanent Methods

There are two main types of permanent birth control, also known as sterilization. They both involve surgical procedures that permanently block or remove the uterine tubes (in women) or the vas deferens, the tubes that carry sperm from the testicles to the urethra (in men).

» TUBAL LIGATION OR SALPINGECTOMY (AKA FEMALE STERILIZATION)

How it works: The uterine tubes are blocked or cut (tubal ligation—sometimes referred to as getting your tubes tied), preventing eggs from traveling from the ovaries to the uterus, in a surgical, usually laparoscopic and outpatient procedure. Increasingly, healthcare providers are urging women to consider the removal of the uterine tubes (bilateral salpingectomy) rather than tubal ligation, to reduce the risk of ovarian cancer. That's because the most common type of ovarian cancer may originate in the uterine tubes, according to research. This procedure does not put you into menopause or alter your menstrual cycle.

The upsides and downsides: If you're sure you don't want to become pregnant, this is a permanent, highly effective option that'll make it so you never have to worry about contraception again. If you opt to have both tubes removed, you can also rest assured that you've helped reduce your risk of ovarian cancer.[8] Of course, there are risks associated with any surgical procedure, and tubal ligation and bilateral salpingectomy are no exception.

» VASECTOMY (AKA MALE STERILIZATION)

How it works: This outpatient surgery involves closing off the vas deferens—two tubes located near each testicle that carry sperm out of the body. During the procedure, usually performed by a urologist, the ends of the vas deferens are closed off by being tied, clipped, or seared with heat (cauterized).

The upsides and downsides: This procedure is almost 100 percent effective at preventing pregnancy—though not right away. A vasectomy is not effective until two to three months (or about twenty ejaculations) after the surgery, which is about how long it takes for sperm cells to clear the vas deferens. To be sure the procedure worked, a semen sample will be tested to make sure it's free of sperm. While rare, risks and complications of a vasectomy include infection, bleeding, and chronic pain in the scrotum.

Emergency Contraception

This category often doesn't get the airtime it deserves, but it's become increasingly important to understand your options and how they work, thanks to continually changing laws, which vary from state to state.

- **Levonorgestrel (aka the morning-after pill, Plan B One-Step, Next Choice, Take Action, among others).** These are over-the-counter pills that work by giving the body a dose of levonorgestrel, a synthetic hormone that prevents a woman's egg from fully developing. A big myth here is that they work only the morning after you had unprotected sex. In fact, some can be taken up to five days after unprotected sex. (Though the sooner you take any of these options, the better.) However, levonorgestrel won't work if you've already ovulated.

- **Ulipristal acetate (aka Ella).** This is a prescription-only pill that can be taken up to five days after unprotected sex and works by preventing or delaying ovulation (ulipristal acetate modulates progesterone to do this).

- **Copper IUD.** This is the most effective form of emergency contraception, as it prevents fertilization or implantation of a fertilized egg in the uterus. It can be inserted by a healthcare provider up to five days after unprotected sex. You can also get a hormonal IUD (specifically a progestin-releasing IUD that contains levonorgestrel, such as Mirena or Liletta) within five days after having unprotected sex.

Reproductive Rights: Understanding Your Options and Finding the Care You Deserve

No matter how you feel about abortion from an ethical perspective, the fact is that it's a common medical procedure: One analysis of data found that nearly one in four women in the U.S. will have an abortion by age forty-five.[9] Sadly, too many of us also have an inaccurate understanding of abortion. According to one poll, 70 percent of respondents thought most abortions occur eight weeks or later into a pregnancy, and few knew that fewer than 5 percent of abortions happen more than twenty weeks into a pregnancy.[10]

So let's put aside the religiously and politically fueled debates on the topic long enough to look at the facts about this healthcare service. Ushma Upadhyay, PhD, MPH, a professor of reproductive health, shares what all of us need to know.

Your Options for Ending a Pregnancy

There are two ways of terminating a pregnancy: the abortion pill (aka medication abortion) and the procedural abortion (aka in-clinic abortion or surgical abortion).

- **The abortion pill** is actually a two-drug combination that can be taken up to eleven or twelve weeks after the first day of your last period. The first pill you'll take is a drug called mifepristone, which blocks progesterone—a key hormone when it comes to sustaining a pregnancy. The second pill is a drug called misoprostol, which is taken up to forty-eight hours after taking mifepristone and causes cramping and bleeding that prompts the uterus to empty.

- **The procedural abortion** is a medical procedure that involves emptying the uterus using either a gentle suction (also called vacuum aspiration) or suction and a spoon-shaped medical tool that scrapes out the lining of the uterus (called a D&E, dilation and evacuation, or a D&C, dilation and curettage). Suction abortion is the most common type of in-clinic abortion and is usually used until about fourteen to sixteen weeks after your last period. You'll likely need a D&C if it has been sixteen weeks or longer since your last period.

Timing is everything when it comes to this decision. In 2021, about 93 percent of abortions happened during the first trimester, according to the CDC.[11] This means the vast majority of women will have both options available to them, if allowed by the abortion laws in the state in which they live. After the twelve-week mark, options will likely be more limited.

One reason for this is that many states have gestational bans—laws that prohibit abortion after a specific point in pregnancy. Another reason is that providers may be uncomfortable performing abortions later than a certain week of gestation, which may be related to concerns they have about their training. (Because fewer patients get abortions at later gestational stages, the majority of clinicians performing procedural abortions won't have extensive experience doing them on later-stage pregnancies—and so they'll refer patients to clinics that do more of them, where the outcomes will be better.) Finally, many hospitals have a complex approval process for abortions after twelve weeks, even in states where abortion is legal.

Where you live may affect your choices as well. In 1973, the landmark Supreme Court case ruling in *Roe v. Wade* established a constitutional right to abortion in the U.S. This ruling made it so that a state law banning or severely restricting abortion was unconstitutional. In 2022, the Supreme Court overturned *Roe v. Wade* in the *Dobbs v. Jackson Women's Health Organization* decision. The ruling returned to individual states the power to either protect or restrict abortion.

After the ruling overturning *Roe v. Wade*, many states banned or severely restricted abortion. Some states now have laws restricting abortion after certain gestational limits; others have state-mandated ultrasound requirements or extended waiting periods. Still other states have banned using telehealth services for abortion. This is why you have to get clear on the state laws that affect you.

While laws are continually changing, two nonprofit websites offer up-to-date information on the abortion laws in every state: ineedana.com and abortionfinder.org. You can plug in your city or zip code, your age, and the number of weeks since your last period (if you know it), and these sites will let you know everything from your state's laws to what your options are.

Telehealth abortion may be possible, also depending on your location. Before the global COVID-19 pandemic, FDA regulations required that patients see a certified clinician in person at a clinic or hospital to get the pills needed for a medication abortion. Then in 2021, the FDA changed some of those regulations, which made it legal for the abortion pill to be sent in the mail and administered via a telehealth appointment. (Because a procedural abortion requires an actual physical procedure, it can't be done via telehealth.)

A telehealth abortion involves a few basic steps: You'll find out if you're eligible and, if so, review your medical history with the provider. Then you'll either receive your pills via mail or pick them up. Finally, you'll take the pills as prescribed—and the provider who prescribed them should be available to you throughout the process if you have any questions or concerns.

It's important to note that the FDA has deemed the abortion pill safe and effective, even when prescribed to patients in a virtual appointment, and Dr. Upadhyay's research looking at abortion pills prescribed via telehealth has also found them safe.[12] In fact, Dr. Upadhyay's research shows that patients who choose an asynchronous telehealth abortion (where all communication happens via secure messaging) feel more cared for than those who opt for a synchronous option (which is more standard telehealthcare that includes a video consultation at the start of the process).

To find out if it's an option for you, visit ineedana.com or abortionfinder .org for state-by-state guides. And keep in mind that just as it's legal to travel to get an abortion, it's also legal to travel to get a telehealth abortion.

What to Keep in Mind If You're Considering an Abortion

Given the evolving nature of the legal issues you may run into depending on where you live, it's important to **do some online research to understand your options before you call a clinic.**

When you do talk to a provider, feel free to **ask questions as you would with any healthcare practitioner,** including things like what to expect, any side effects that may happen after the treatment, and anything else that's on your mind.

If you make an appointment at an abortion clinic, make sure it's actually an abortion clinic and not a "crisis pregnancy center," which often pose as abortion clinics yet don't actually provide abortions or provide unbiased counseling. These centers outnumber abortion clinics in the U.S. The best way to tell if you've reached one is to ask this question: Do you provide abortions at your site? If the answer is no, you know they're not an abortion clinic.

Finally, try to **remember that the old tropes about who gets abortions in America—"promiscuous women," "irresponsible teens"—are inaccurate.** The typical patient is a mother in her twenties who likely has a college background, is in her first six weeks of pregnancy, and is having an abortion for the first time.

"The same people who become pregnant and give birth are the same people who have abortions at different points in their lives," says Dr. Upadhyay. "No matter how you feel about the issue, this is true. And when abortion is treated as a political issue instead of healthcare, it affects people's lives."

Your Game Plan:
How to Make the Most of a GYN Exam

No matter the reason for the appointment—whether it's your annual exam or you have a specific question or concern you want to discuss—there are a number of things you can do to optimize your visit, says Dr. Stephanie Trentacoste McNally. Here's where to start.

Find a provider who specializes in your stage of life. Most women see one ob-gyn from their teenage years through menopause. These visits may include conversations about birth control, preconception, labor and delivery plans, and care well past a woman's reproductive window. Yet as your health-care needs change, there may be an opportunity for you to find a clinician who specializes in what you're going through. If you're an adolescent, you might consider seeing a pediatric and adolescent gynecologist specialist (PAGS). Are you experiencing the symptoms of hormonal changes that start to happen during perimenopause? A Menopause Society Certified Practitioner (MSCP) may provide more comprehensive and specialized care during later decades. And that's okay, says Dr. McNally.

"What's most important is to be honest about your healthcare needs at the various stages of your life and then seek out a specialist in those issues," she says.

Hatch a plan for your important screenings. While guidelines exist for gynecologic and breast cancer screenings, your healthcare provider may suggest more frequent screenings, including mammograms or breast MRIs, based on your medical or family health history. Have a conversation about this and make sure you're on the same page.

Know your personal and family health history. A comprehensive health history is one of the most important aspects of a well-woman visit, and you can help your provider tremendously if you're able to answer the range of questions that create this important part of your chart. If you have access to it, come to your visit knowing your family history, which will provide insight into your personal risk factors for disease. Show up to your appointment ready to talk about any symptoms you're experiencing, medication you're taking, or allergies to medications you may have. (For a helpful guide to creating a personal and family health history, see page 600.)

Make sure you feel comfortable talking about the more intimate aspects of your life—without feeling judged. Maybe one day we'll live in a world where all of us feel A-OK talking openly about our genitals and sexual health the same way we talk about other aspects of our bodies. But until that time, it's crucial to find a healthcare practitioner you feel you can talk to about anything, even if it's the kind of stuff you'd rather not share with anyone.

· · · · ·

When we come to our gynecology appointments more informed about our bodies, we can more accurately talk about how we're *really* doing and get the kind of care we need and deserve to feel our best at every stage of life.

Chapter 5

A Guide to Gynecologic Conditions

Understanding the Health Issues That Can

Affect the Female Reproductive System

> *There's nothing wrong, or bad, or embarrassing about a yeast infection or a UTI. It's just a body being a body. We talk about so many other aspects of bodies being bodies. But because of a stack of taboos related to sexual organs and the materials that come out of them, there's often a limited amount of resources—particularly the sort of casual ones that actually make you feel better—about the various conditions related to them.*
>
> —Anne Helen Peterson, "Welcome to Colonoscopy Land" in her *Culture Study* Substack

For an area of the body able to sustain new life and provide so much pleasure, our genitals and reproductive organs can also be the source of a lot of pain. What's worse, figuring out what's causing that pain—which can range from annoying discomfort to debilitating agony—often leads many women down a yearslong path of confusion, uncertainty, and not feeling heard.

Take endometriosis, for example, a disease where the tissue that forms the inner lining of the uterus is found in places it shouldn't be—like the uterine tubes, ovaries, bladder, intestines, and even lungs. The condition can cause a range of symptoms, from intense menstrual cramps and heavy periods to chronic pain in the pelvic region and digestive distress. Yet despite these serious symptoms—and the fact that having endometriosis increases a patient's chance of developing ovarian cancer—it can take women up to eleven years to get an official diagnosis.[1] That's right: A condition that impacts 10 to 15 percent of all women of reproductive age can take more than a decade to diagnose.[2]

The news isn't much better for a host of other common gynecologic conditions. Polycystic ovary syndrome (PCOS), which affects an estimated one in ten women of childbearing age, can take more than two years and appointments with more than three healthcare professionals to be diagnosed.[3]

The gynecologic conditions we'll be covering in this chapter often take a toll on both our physical and our mental health. They can wreak havoc in our personal and professional lives, as pain and sometimes embarrassment can keep us from spending time with friends and talking with others (including our doctors) about the extent of what we're dealing with.

So if you're experiencing pain, read on to find expert information to help you understand what might be happening and better advocate for yourself when something feels wrong.

In this chapter, we'll learn . . .

- **What a "normal" period looks like (it's a pretty big range!) so you're better able to assess irregularities and spot menstrual disorders**—and, even better, have the language you'll need to talk to your healthcare provider about your symptoms.

- **The most common noncancerous gynecologic conditions, their symptoms, and how each is diagnosed and treated**. The more you know about what can possibly go wrong with your reproductive system, the better positioned you'll be to pursue answers if you start having symptoms.

- **Why UTIs happen**, why women get them up to thirty times more than men, and the best prevention and treatment strategies.

- **What you need to know about getting a hysterectomy**, the second-most-common surgery for women in the U.S. (just behind Cesarean sections).

- **How to talk to your clinician about your symptoms**, and recommended steps to take if you're diagnosed with one of these gynecologic conditions.

Meet the Experts

Ashley Winter, MD, board-certified urologist trained in sexual medicine, with extensive experience in sexual medicine for all genders

Indira Mysorekar, PhD, professor of medicine at Baylor College of Medicine

Sadaf Lodhi, DO, ob-gyn, menopause-certified practitioner, intimacy coach, and host of *The Muslim Sex Podcast*

Lauren F. Streicher, MD, professor of obstetrics and gynecology at Northwestern University Feinberg School of Medicine and author of *The Essential Guide to Hysterectomy*

Stephanie Trentacoste McNally, MD, ob-gyn, certified menopause provider, and director of ob-gyn services at the Katz Institute for Women's Health

Period Problems: When Your Cycle *Isn't* Normal

Irregular periods. Debilitating PMS. Heavy bleeding. Cramps. Far too often, we power through these symptoms because we think what we're experiencing is normal—"just one of the downsides of being born with a uterus"—or because many healthcare providers don't ask the kind of detailed questions that would lead to further investigation.

Part of what makes menstrual disorders tough to spot and diagnose is that, as we've learned, there's no such thing as "normal" bleeding. If you've ever wondered if your period is "normal"—for example, whether your bleeding would officially be deemed "heavy" or if your PMS symptoms are extreme—bring it up with your healthcare provider. To help you come to that discussion prepared, read on.

Premenstrual Syndrome (PMS)

What it is: Physical or mood changes during the days leading up to your period that happen month after month and may affect your ability to live life as you'd like. Common emotional symptoms include depression, irritability, anxiety, social withdrawal, sleep issues, and changes in libido. Common physical symptoms include breast tenderness, food cravings, aches and pains, skin woes (like acne), gastrointestinal symptoms, abdominal pain, and fatigue.

Why it happens: Researchers believe it's due to estrogen and progesterone levels falling dramatically (if you're not pregnant) in the days after ovulation.

Premenstrual Dysphoric Disorder (PMDD)

What it is: A severe type of PMS that affects a small percentage of women but can be serious. It increases the risk of a suicide attempt sevenfold and the risk of suicide ideation almost fourfold compared with women without the disorder.[4] Common symptoms include markedly depressed mood, feelings of hopelessness, and/or anxiety, tension, or feeling "on edge"; marked anger or irritability that persists; increased interpersonal conflicts; decreased interest in usual activities; changes in ability to concentrate, appetite, and/or sleep; physical changes such as breast tenderness, headaches, joint or muscle pain, and bloating.

Why it happens: While the exact causes aren't fully understood, research indicates that hormonal changes throughout the menstrual cycle could be a factor, as well as the brain chemical serotonin. You may also be more prone to PMDD if you've experienced trauma, smoke cigarettes, or have obesity.

Dysmenorrhea

What it is: Pain associated with your period. For some women, this pain can be severe and come along with other symptoms, including nausea, vomiting, headache, dizziness, and diarrhea. Dysmenorrhea may be referred to as primary or secondary.

Why it happens: Primary dysmenorrhea is caused by hormonelike substances called prostaglandins that are made in the lining of the uterus and cause the muscles and blood vessels in the uterus to contract. Secondary dysmenorrhea is often caused by a medical condition, such as endometriosis, uterine fibroids, pelvic inflammatory disease, or possibly even an IUD.

Amenorrhea

What it is: The absence of menstruation. It may be referred to as primary, which occurs when a girl doesn't begin to menstruate by age fifteen, or secondary, which occurs when periods that were previously regular stop for three months or more.

Why it happens: Outside of normal causes of skipped or irregular periods—such as some forms of hormonal birth control, pregnancy, breastfeeding, and perimenopause—amenorrhea is associated with a few factors. Primary amenorrhea can be due to a genetic condition; problems with the development of the uterus, vagina, or hymen; problems with the hypothalamus or pituitary gland; or a delay in puberty. Reasons for secondary amenorrhea may include rapid weight loss; eating disorders; polycystic ovary syndrome (PCOS); problems with the hypothalamus, pituitary gland, and/or thyroid gland; premature ovarian failure; stress; and chronic medical conditions such as inflammatory bowel disease (IBD) and kidney failure.

Menorrhagia

What it is: Heavy or excessive menstrual bleeding. You may be diagnosed with menorrhagia if you have periods lasting longer than a week; have to change your pad or tampon every hour for several hours back to back; have to change pads in the middle of the night; can't do your go-to activities when you have your period; and/or pass blood clots the size of a quarter or larger several times a day.

Why it happens: Causes include hormonal imbalances; ovulation problems (when ovulation doesn't occur, progesterone levels drop, which can cause heavy bleeding); noncancerous growths in your uterus, such as fibroids; endometriosis (where the cells that line the uterus grow outside of the uterus); pregnancy complications (such as miscarriage or ectopic pregnancy); some sexually transmitted infections (including trichomoniasis, chlamydia, and gonorrhea); and certain medications, including menopause hormone therapy and contraceptives.

Hypomenorrhea

What it is: Abnormally light periods with little bleeding, usually characterized by menstruation that lasts two days or less.

Why it happens: One reason for a lighter period is going on hormonal contraception, but anything that prompts a change in your hormone levels—like significant weight loss or gain, stress, an overactive thyroid, or entering perimenopause—can also prompt your monthly bleeding to become shorter and lighter.

Oligomenorrhea

What it is: Irregular and inconsistent menstrual periods that occur more than thirty-five days apart or four to nine menstrual cycles in a year. This is common in early adolescence (when girls first start getting their period, it's often irregular) and is something about 13 percent of those who menstruate may experience at some point in our lives.[5]

Why it happens: Health conditions that cause hormone imbalances in the body—such as PCOS, hyperthyroidism, and type 1 diabetes—are often to blame for oligomenorrhea. It can also be a side effect of certain medications, such as antipsychotics and antiseizure medications, and oral contraceptive pills.

A Guide to the Dreaded UTI:
Why They Happen, How to Treat Them, and the Myths About How to Prevent Them Every Woman Needs to Know

If you've ever had a urinary tract infection (UTI), you likely shudder at the memory of the telltale signs: the burning feeling when urinating; an urge to pee that doesn't go away; the unsatisfyingly tiny amount of (possibly cloudy, bloody, or strange-smelling) pee you're able to pass despite feeling like you could "go" all the time. These infections are something nearly half of all women will experience at least once in their lifetime, and nearly half of those infections will recur.[6] What's more, even if you spent your reproductive years largely avoiding UTIs, there's a chance you'll get them during the menopause transition and after, when certain factors make you more prone to infection.

Here, urologist Ashley Winter, MD, answers some of the most common questions about these infections.

Why Do UTIs Happen?

A UTI is when some sort of pathogen, most commonly a bacterium related to your gastrointestinal tract, enters your urethra, travels up into your bladder, and invades the lining of the bladder. This generates an immune system response, which you may experience as blood or pus in your urine and possibly even a fever (a sign your body is fighting the UTI).

Why Do Men—Who Also Have Urethras—Never Seem to Get UTIs?

First, it's important to note that men do get UTIs, just much less frequently than women. In fact, we get them up to thirty times more than men![7] Mostly, this is due to anatomical differences. In women, the openings to the urethra, vagina, and rectum are very close together, which makes it easy for an organism to move from the anus or vagina to the urinary opening. Plus, the female urethra is much shorter than a male's, which means organisms don't have as far to travel to get to the bladder and cause problems.

Another, less-talked-about factor in female susceptibility to UTIs is the delicate balance of our vaginal microbiome. You can think of the lactobacilli that thrive in the vagina and give it its acidic pH as bodyguards that also hang out around your urethra to prevent bad bacteria from getting in, explains Dr. Winter. But because that balance of flora in the vagina can be disrupted by so many things, it can lower your defenses against infection. For example, the pH of menstrual blood is high, which can be disruptive to your vaginal flora. (It's why you could be more susceptible to a UTI if you have penetrative vaginal sex while menstruating.) The type of hormonal contraception you use can also disrupt your vaginal flora.

The hormonal changes women go through during the menopause transition can also increase the likelihood of getting a UTI. As estrogen production falls, vaginal tissue can get thinner and drier and your vaginal canal can narrow and shorten, a combination that makes UTIs more likely. That drop in estrogen also causes changes in the vaginal microbiome. Estrogen prompts your vaginal epithelial cells to make glycogen, which is what those healthy lactobacillus bugs (your urinary tract's "bodyguards") need to thrive. This makes it more likely for bad bacteria to enter and stay in your bladder, making recurrent UTIs more common.

What Are the Best Ways to Prevent UTIs?

When it comes to staving off these painful infections, the advice often focuses on hygiene—like wiping front to back and peeing immediately after sex. But tips like these are antiquated and can do more harm than good, says Dr. Winter.

"There is no consistent data that wiping causes UTIs," she says. "What woman is smearing feces into her vulva when she wipes back to front? That just doesn't happen. And focusing on old advice like this distracts us from looking at the underlying cause of many UTIs—like low estrogen—and from talking about effective interventions like using topical hormones when appropriate."

As for urinating after vaginal penetrative sex, there's some data that shows it can be helpful, but it's probably not the kind of crucial UTI-prevention tactic that most of us have been taught it is, adds Dr. Winter.

Instead, double down on these basics that are proven to help:

- **Empty your bladder when you have the urge.** When urine hangs out in the bladder rather than being pushed out, it's more likely that bacteria will grow. If you're getting recurrent UTIs, keep a bladder diary. You can download an app that lets you track things like what fluids you drank and when over the course of your day and when you urinated—all information that can help your healthcare provider get to the bottom of why you're experiencing recurring UTIs.

- **Stay well hydrated.** Drinking enough fluids throughout the day means you're more likely to urinate regularly, which helps flush out the urinary tract.

- **Consider vaginal estrogen.** If you're over age forty and you've started to get recurrent UTIs, talk to your clinician about vaginal estrogen—a safe, effective, and often underutilized treatment that helps raise the level of healthy bacteria that normally live in your vagina and make you less susceptible to UTIs. "Using low-dose vaginal estrogen is the standard of care for recurrent UTIs in women over forty, and if your provider isn't talking to you about this treatment option, they're not following the American Urologic Association's guidelines," says Dr. Winter.[8]

If these interventions fail, there are other strategies to discuss with your clinician, says Dr. Winter, including methenamine (a drug that's not an antibiotic but that can help prevent UTIs caused by E. coli), drinking cranberry juice or taking a supplement (cranberries contain a substance called proanthocyanidins that helps prevent bacteria from sticking to the walls of the bladder), antibiotics, and even a UTI vaccine.

What's the Best Way to Treat a UTI?

If you suspect you're dealing with a UTI, it's important to call your healthcare practitioner, who will likely order a urinalysis or urine culture (you'll pee in a cup so technicians can look for bacteria or other signs of infection in your urine). If it's a UTI, there's a good chance you'll be prescribed an antibiotic, as most UTIs need antibiotics to go away.

Ask an Expert

Why are recurrent UTIs more common as we enter menopause?

Among the many changes that can happen during the menopause transition is recurrent UTIs. In addition to the drop in estrogen causing a change in the vaginal environment, it can also decrease the muscle strength of your bladder.

That's right: Your bladder is a muscle that expands when it fills with urine and contracts to excrete that urine. And just as the precipitous drop in estrogen after menopause can weaken other muscles, it can also weaken your bladder, urethra, and pelvic floor muscles. The result? Not all of the urine in your bladder will be emptied—which makes it more ripe for infection. Just as little pools of water in a garden are likely to start growing things, it's the same in our bladder when urine hangs around that shouldn't be there.

The cells that line your bladder also become less robust. A strong bladder lining plays a number of roles when it comes to preventing UTIs. It acts as a physical barrier that prevents bacteria and other harmful stuff in the urine from migrating into the bloodstream; these barrier cells also have natural antimicrobial properties and secrete substances that can kill bacteria and prevent them from growing; and they can even recognize bacteria and recruit immune cells to help fight infection. When the bladder lining is weakened, these protective functions don't work as well as they were designed to, making it easier for bacteria to attach to the bladder wall and spark a UTI.

As we age, immune cells also tend to congregate in the bladder. As they accumulate, they form structures known as tertiary lymphoid tissue, which you can think of like little pools of immune cells. Sounds like this should be a good thing, right? However, as we get older, our immune cells get older as well—and they don't work as accurately or efficiently as they used to. In fact, these pools of immune cells in the menopausal bladder tend to overreact, which leads to inflammation. And if you have these tertiary lymphoid tissue structures in your bladder, you're more likely to have recurrent UTIs with a shorter time between the infections. Not only that, but they can lead to a lot of discomfort—many women describe it as a feeling of "heaviness" in their abdomen.

My advice for all women who've reached menopause is to talk to your healthcare provider about any discomfort, pain, or other changes in urination you're experiencing rather than assuming they're just another part of the aging process. Yes, these changes can happen with age, but that doesn't mean that they're inevitable or that you have to suffer.

—Indira Mysorekar, PhD, professor of medicine at Baylor College of Medicine

Gynecologic Conditions to Know About: What to Keep on Your Radar

Maybe you made an appointment with your gynecologist due to a symptom like painful urination or crazy-heavy periods. Or perhaps you scheduled your annual appointment expecting to hear the usual, cheery "Everything looks great!" and instead are told you need further testing because your doc suspects uterine fibroids. The fact is that at some point in most women's lives, we'll face a concern that leaves us with a slew of questions—and very little time to ask them.

Here is a brief overview of some of the most common gynecologic conditions women face during their reproductive years. These descriptions aren't exhaustive, and they're not meant to diagnose your medical issues. This information is meant to give you a starting point for a conversation with your healthcare provider if you're experiencing symptoms.

Polycystic Ovary Syndrome (PCOS)

This is a common hormonal problem among reproductive-aged women, affecting one in ten women of childbearing age. It's usually identified when someone is having trouble conceiving. While there's no clear understanding of what causes PCOS, experts believe several different factors may contribute to it, including insulin resistance, higher-than-normal levels of androgens (sex hormones that are usually present in small amounts in women), and genetics. It's important to note that despite what the name suggests, you don't have to have cysts on your ovaries to have PCOS.

» SYMPTOMS

A diagnosis of PCOS is made when you have two out of three of the following symptoms:

- irregular or absent ovulation
- signs of elevated androgens, including excess facial and body hair (hirsutism), severe acne, male-pattern baldness, and/or lab tests that show elevated androgens
- polycystic-appearing ovaries (which your clinician will be able to diagnose only via an ultrasound); alternatively, if anti-Mullerian hormone (AMH) is elevated, it can be indicative of polycystic ovaries

Other signs of PCOS may include:

- infertility
- weight gain or difficulty losing weight
- dark or thick patches of skin on the back of the neck, in the armpits, and under the breasts
- skin tags (small flaps of skin, usually in the armpits or neck area)

If you're experiencing any of these symptoms, talk to your healthcare provider. Not only can PCOS be physically painful and interrupt your family-building plans, but it can also put you at higher risk for some serious health problems. More than half of people with PCOS develop type 2 diabetes by the time they reach age forty, and the condition also puts you at risk for high blood pressure, heart problems, and gynecologic cancers.[9]

» TREATMENT

Managing PCOS is mostly focused on lifestyle changes, like healthy eating, regular exercise, getting enough sleep, and stress management. Other treatments should be used based on a patient's goals (for example, do you need and/or want to lose weight, and are you hoping to have kids, and if so, when?) or health risks (do you have insulin resistance, anemia, elevated cholesterol, or fatty liver disease?). Medications such as birth control pills and/or diabetes medication can help treat the underlying cause of PCOS, as well as symptoms.

Ovarian Cysts

You can still develop cysts on your ovaries if you don't have PCOS. In fact, an estimated 10 percent of women will have them.[10] One reason ovarian cysts are so common is that in your reproductive years, your ovaries already grow small cysts (called follicles) each month. When that follicle keeps growing, it's known as a functional cyst. But there are many more types of ovarian cysts, and they can be either benign or malignant.

Smaller ovarian cysts can be "functional," meaning they can come and go and may not cause symptoms, says ob-gyn Sadaf Lodhi, DO. Larger ovarian cysts (typically five centimeters in diameter or bigger) can cause pelvic pain, a feeling of fullness or bloating in your abdomen, pain during intercourse, and/or painful periods. Sometimes a cyst can burst open (rupture), causing severe pain and sometimes bleeding in the pelvis. A large cyst may also twist on itself, which can be painful and is a medical emergency, as this can cut off the blood supply to that ovary.

» TREATMENTS

If your healthcare provider suspects you have an ovarian cyst, they'll likely prescribe a pelvic ultrasound to make the diagnosis. If your cysts require treatment, options may include medications containing hormones to stop ovulation and prevent future cysts from forming or surgery to remove the cyst(s).

Uterine Fibroids

Also known as leiomyomas or myomas, these are almost always benign (noncancerous) growths that develop in or on the wall of the uterus. Up to 80 percent of women will have a fibroid by age fifty.[11] Black and Asian women can have a two- to threefold higher prevalence of fibroids than white or Hispanic women.[12] While experts don't know exactly why they form, they do know that age, genetics, ethnic origin, and hormonal fluctuation can be contributing factors. For instance, fibroids are more common during a woman's thirties and forties and up to menopause, at which point they are much less likely to form and usually shrink if present. (Estrogen "feeds" fibroids and makes it easier for them to grow, and the drop in estrogen after menopause is thought to make them shrink.)

There are three main types of fibroids:

- *Subserosal*, which form under the outermost (serosal) layer of the uterus and can bulge outside the uterus

- *Submucosal*, which originate in the layer closest to the cavity of the uterus and can bulge into the uterine cavity

- *Intramural*, which grow within the muscular wall of the uterus (if they grow outside the wall of the uterus, they become subserosal; if they grow toward the uterine cavity, they become submucosal)

If submucosal or subserosal fibroids hang from a "stalk" inside or outside the uterus, they're called pedunculated.

» SYMPTOMS

Because fibroids vary in size and location, they can cause a range of symptoms— or none at all. Some of the most common signs are:

- heavy bleeding and clots during your menstrual cycle
- painful periods
- bleeding between periods
- pain during sex
- low-back pain
- a feeling of fullness or bloating in the abdomen
- constipation
- difficulty urinating or frequent urination due to pressure in the abdomen
- constipation, rectal pain, or difficult bowel movements
- abdominal cramps
- pregnancy complications
- infertility

» TREATMENT

If you or your healthcare provider suspects fibroids, there are multiple tests that can confirm the diagnosis, including a pelvic ultrasound (which uses sound waves to create an image of the uterus and other pelvic organs), hysteroscopy (in which a thin device is inserted through the vagina and cervix to see the inside of the uterus), or MRI.

If your fibroids cause symptoms, treatment options to discuss with your healthcare provider include:

- Medications, such as hormonal contraception (which can help control heavy bleeding and pain but don't treat the fibroids themselves), gonadotropin-releasing hormone (GnRH) agonists (which stop the menstrual cycle and can shrink fibroids), and tranexamic acid (a medication used to treat heavy bleeding).

- Procedures aimed at shrinking or removing fibroids, such as a myomectomy (surgical removal of fibroids while leaving the uterus in place), uterine artery embolization (where tiny particles are injected into the blood vessels that lead to the uterus to cut off the blood flow to the fibroid, causing it to shrink), and radiofrequency ablation (which uses energy and heat to shrink fibroids).

- Hysterectomy, which is the removal of the uterus and typically used as a treatment for fibroids when other treatments haven't worked or aren't possible or when the fibroids are very big (for more information on this common surgery, see page 131).

Endometriosis

This condition, which occurs in about one in ten women of reproductive age,[13] happens when the tissue forming the inner lining of the uterus, called the endometrium, is found outside of the uterus. Endometrial tissue is most often found in the following places: the membrane that lines the abdominal cavity and surrounds the abdominal organs (called the peritoneum); ovaries; uterine tubes; and outer surfaces of the bladder, uterus, intestines, rectum, and ureters (the tubes that lead from each kidney to the bladder).

» SYMPTOMS

There are many symptoms of endometriosis, the most common being pelvic pain (though it's important to note that there can also be no symptoms). Other symptoms include:

- Severe menstrual cramps

- Chronic low-back pain, abdominal pain, and pain when peeing or pooping

- Pain during sex

- Irregular bleeding (including heavy bleeding during periods or spotting between periods)

- Digestive issues like diarrhea, constipation, bloating, and nausea

» TREATMENTS

While there's currently no cure for endometriosis, there are a number of science-backed treatments that work depending on the severity of symptoms, your desire for fertility, and other factors. Some of the most common treatments include:

- *Pain medication*: Over-the-counter nonsteroidal anti-inflammatory drugs (NSAIDs) and prescription pain medication won't treat the cause of your pain, but they can help you manage the discomfort associated with endometriosis.

- *Birth control methods*: Contraceptives such as pills, IUDs, vaginal rings, implants, injections, and patches can help manage endometriosis symptoms by reducing menstrual bleeding, pelvic pain, and inflammation.

- *Gonadotropin-releasing hormone (GnRH) agonists*: These medications suppress ovarian function and induce a temporary menopause-like state, leading to a decrease in estrogen levels in the body that may help shrink endometriosis lesions and alleviate symptoms.

- *Laparoscopic surgery*: This is used to both definitively diagnose endometriosis and remove endometrial tissue, adhesions, and scar tissue.

- *Hysterectomy*: In severe cases of endometriosis and when preserving fertility isn't a concern, surgical removal of the uterus and sometimes the ovaries may be the best treatment option.

Adenomyosis

This condition occurs when the tissue lining the uterus (the endometrium) grows into the muscular inner wall of the uterus (the myometrium). This tissue responds to hormones and thickens and bleeds with the monthly hormone cycle, and it causes the uterine wall to become thicker.

While the cause of adenomyosis isn't known, some theories suggest it may be related to hormonal imbalances, previous uterine surgeries, or inflammation. Unlike endometriosis, which can be more common in women who've never had children, adenomyosis primarily affects women in their thirties to fifties and can be more common in those who've had multiple pregnancies or who've had a procedure on their uterus, such as a C-section or surgery to remove a fibroid.

» SYMPTOMS

Common signs of adenomyosis may include all or some of the following:

- heavy menstrual bleeding (menorrhagia)
- severe menstrual cramps (dysmenorrhea)
- pelvic pain or pressure
- enlarged uterus
- pain during sex (dyspareunia)

» TREATMENTS

Clinicians use many of the same tactics for adenomyosis as they do for endometriosis, including pain medications like NSAIDs and hormonal contraceptives. If your pain is severe and none of these tactics work, you might consider a hysterectomy.

Yeast Infection (aka Candidiasis)

The fungus candida (typically *Candida albicans*) is always present in small amounts in the vagina. However, under certain circumstances—such as a weakened immune system, hormonal changes, or the use of antibiotics—the balance of bugs and fungus in the vagina can be disrupted. The result? Candida can multiply, causing this common infection. (Other things can throw off the delicate balance of bugs and fungus in your vagina as well, including the use of scented products, douching, and wearing synthetic or nonbreathable underwear.)

» SYMPTOMS

Common signs of a yeast infection may include all or some of the following:

- itching and irritation of the vagina and vulva
- redness and swelling of the vulva
- burning sensation of the vulva that may get worse during urination or sex
- thick, white, cottage cheese–like, usually odorless vaginal discharge

It's tempting to assume you have a yeast infection if you have one or more of these symptoms, but the truth is that not all vaginal infections or symptoms are caused by an overgrowth of candida. Other conditions, such as bacterial vaginosis (more on this next) or even some STIs can cause similar symptoms, which is why it's never a good idea to self-diagnose a yeast infection—even if you've had multiple infections in the past.

» TREATMENTS

Treatment usually involves antifungal medications (creams, suppositories, or oral tablets), many of which you'll find over the counter. But if you suspect you have a yeast infection, don't just go straight for an OTC remedy.

Get in touch with your provider for an official diagnosis and to discuss the best treatment plan for you.

Bacterial Vaginosis (BV)

This is a common condition caused by an imbalance in the natural bacterial flora of the vagina. In healthy vaginas, beneficial bacteria (such as lactobacilli) keep harmful bacteria in check, creating a delicate balance of good and bad bacteria. In BV, there's an overgrowth of harmful bacteria, leading to an imbalance that can cause infection.

While more research is needed to understand the exact causes of BV, experts do know that certain factors can put you at an increased risk for developing the condition, including multiple sexual partners, having a new sex partner, douching, and using scented hygiene products that can disrupt the balance of bacteria in your vagina.

» SYMPTOMS

The most common symptom of BV is a grayish-white vaginal discharge with a distinctive, "fishy" odor that's particularly noticeable after sex. You may also experience vaginal itching or irritation, as well as a burning sensation when you pee. However, it's important to note that many people with BV have no symptoms at all, which underscores the importance of routine gynecologic exams.

» TREATMENTS

Treatment for BV typically involves taking either oral or topical antibiotics. While BV isn't considered an STI, it's more common in women who are sexually active—and having BV puts you at a higher risk of getting an STI. If left untreated, BV can also lead to pelvic inflammatory disease and an increased risk of preterm birth in pregnant women.

Pelvic Inflammatory Disease (PID)

PID is an infection that can happen when sexually transmitted bacteria—most commonly chlamydia and gonorrhea—spread from your vagina to your upper reproductive organs (including the uterus, uterine tubes, or ovaries) and cause infection and inflammation. When left untreated, PID can lead to pockets of infected fluid (abscesses) in the reproductive tract, which can cause permanent damage.

» SYMPTOMS

Common signs you may be experiencing PID include:

- lower abdominal or pelvic pain or tenderness (the most common symptom)
- abnormal discharge that may have an unusual color (usually yellow or green) or odor
- pain during sex
- irregular periods or having spotting or cramping throughout the month
- fever, fatigue, nausea, and/or vomiting
- burning sensation when you pee

You're at higher risk of developing PID if you've had it in the past, have an STI (especially gonorrhea or chlamydia), or have multiple sexual partners (or have a partner who has multiple partners). It's important to get PID looked at ASAP, as it can have serious consequences if left untreated, including scarring and damage to the organs in your pelvis, infertility, and an increased risk of ectopic pregnancy.

» TREATMENTS

The good news is that treatment is usually straightforward. After your healthcare provider diagnoses PID (usually using a combination of your medical history, a physical exam, and lab tests), you'll take antibiotics to eliminate the infection.

Vulvar Lichen Sclerosus (LS)

This is a chronic, inflammatory skin condition that primarily affects the vulva. LS can also extend to the tissues around your anus, which can lead to skin changes similar to those seen in the vulvar area (thinning and whitening of the skin, as well as itching and pain). It's also associated with an increased risk of vulvar cancer when it goes untreated.

While the exact cause of LS is unclear, evidence suggests it's an autoimmune disorder with a genetic component. It's important to note that many experts believe LS is underreported, because while it happens in women of all ages, it's more common in postmenopausal women (who may be less likely to go for regular gynecology appointments). Good reason to regularly look at your genitals using a hand mirror, so you're more likely to notice any changes in the appearance of your vulva and talk to your doctor if you do.

» SYMPTOMS

Some of the most common signs include:

- intense itching, soreness, burning, and/or pain in the vulvar region
- skin changes, where the vulvar skin becomes thin and white
- fragile skin that bruises or cracks easily
- pain and difficulty with urinating and/or having sex

» TREATMENTS

A gynecologist or dermatologist can diagnose LS by looking at your vulva. Sometimes a skin biopsy will be needed to rule out other conditions and confirm an LS diagnosis.

While there is no cure for LS, treatments can help control the symptoms and inflammation in the skin. The most common treatment is topical corticosteroids.

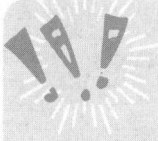

WHAT IS VAGINITIS?

You might hear the term vaginitis *in the context of a number of gynecologic conditions. That's because this term broadly refers to inflammation of the vagina. Some of the most common types of vaginitis include bacterial vaginosis (BV), yeast infections, and sexually transmitted infections (STIs). The type of treatment for vaginitis depends on the cause.*

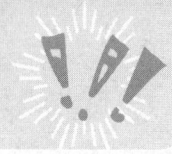

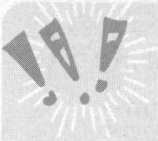

WHAT IS VULVODYNIA?

Vulvodynia *is a blanket term used when there is persistent pain or discomfort in the vulva, typically described as stinging, burning, irritated, sore, or raw. Pain may be localized to a specific area of the vulva, or it can be more generalized and affect the entire vulvar region. For many women, the pain is often provoked by pressure, touch, sex, inserting tampons, and even sitting for long periods. In some cases, the pain can occur without any apparent trigger. There can be multiple contributing factors, including inflammation of the vulva, injury or irritation of the nerves that transmit sensations to and from the vulva, pelvic floor muscle dysfunction, or even some genetic factors. Vulvodynia is often a "diagnosis of exclusion"—in other words, it's diagnosed only after other conditions are ruled out—which means it can take a while to get diagnosed. Treatment options depend on what's causing your pain and the severity of your symptoms.*

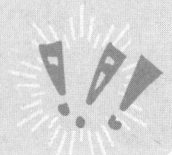

Gynecologic Cancers

One of the most important reasons to get regular gynecology checkups is that they include screenings for gynecologic cancers and a discussion with your clinician about your risk factors, which can help your provider catch cancer in its earliest stages, when it's most treatable. In addition to cervical cancer (which we discussed in chapter 4), here's what to keep on your radar:

- **Endometrial cancer**, which originates in the lining of the uterus (endometrium), occurs when endometrial cells start to grow too rapidly. There is no routine screening for uterine cancer, though a pelvic exam and transvaginal ultrasound (as well as other procedures) can help assess any abnormalities if there's cause for concern.

- **Ovarian cancer** is referred to as a silent killer because symptoms often aren't noticeable until the cancer has reached an advanced stage. However, upward of 90 percent of people with ovarian cancer have at least one symptom, such as abdominal pain, bloating, and changes in bowel movements[14]—all common digestive woes that too often go unreported by women and may be overlooked or misdiagnosed by their doctors. While early detection remains challenging, certain risk factors are associated with ovarian cancer, including a family history of ovarian, uterine, colon, or breast cancer; a personal history of breast cancer; mutations in BRCA1 and BRCA2 genes; never having had children; infertility; and endometriosis.

- **Vulvar and vaginal cancer**, which originates on the vulva (the external genitalia) and in the vagina (an internal organ) respectively. Signs and symptoms of vulvar cancer may include itching, burning, or bleeding on the vulva that doesn't go away; changes in the color of the skin of the vulva; sores, lumps, or ulcers on the vulva that don't go away; and/or pain in your pelvic area. Persistent HPV infection and a history of cervical precancer or cancer are risk factors for vulvar cancer. Vaginal cancer symptoms may include vaginal discharge or bleeding; pain in your pelvis, especially when you pee or have sex; having blood in your urine or stool; a feeling of constipation; and/or needing to go to the bathroom more often than usual.

Hysterectomy, Explained:
What You Need to Know About This Common Surgery in Women

If you're diagnosed with uterine fibroids, endometriosis, uterine prolapse, abnormal uterine bleeding, or a gynecologic cancer, you may be faced with the decision to have a hysterectomy, a surgical procedure to remove the uterus and/or the uterine tubes and cervix. Yet even though hysterectomy is second only to Cesarean section in how common it is for women in the U.S., few of us know about the choices we have when it comes to the procedure.[15]

"Hysterectomy doesn't have to be the same for everyone—you can think of it as à la carte," says Lauren F. Streicher, MD. "The more you know about your options, the better able you'll be to ask the right questions and come to a shared decision with your surgeon that feels right for you." Consider this your crash course to prepare you for that appointment.

Types of Hysterectomy

These terms define what is removed during a hysterectomy, which can include any number of different combinations:

- **Total hysterectomy** is the removal of the uterus and cervix, which can be done with or without removing the uterine tubes or ovaries.

- **Subtotal hysterectomy (aka supracervical hysterectomy or partial hysterectomy)** is the removal of the upper part of the uterus while leaving the cervix.

- **Oophorectomy** is the removal of one or both of the ovaries.

- **Salpingectomy** is the removal of one or both of the uterine tubes.

- **Radical hysterectomy** is the removal of the uterus, cervix, ovaries, uterine tubes, and possibly upper portions of the vagina and lymph nodes.

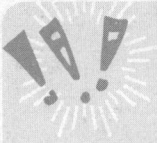

. . . there's a good chance your surgeon will suggest removing your uterine tubes during hysterectomy. And if this isn't discussed, ask. "There is no benefit to leaving your tubes," says Dr. Streicher. In fact, the potential cancer prevention that comes along with bilateral salpingectomy (the removal of both uterine tubes) has prompted many physicians to recommend it when women have other abdominal surgical procedures, such as gallbladder surgery or hernia operations.

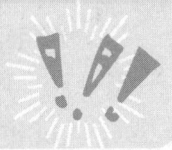

Surgical Options

Hysterectomies aren't differentiated just by what's removed but also by *how* the various organs are removed. If you're scheduled to have a hysterectomy, your surgeon will talk through these options with you. Going into that appointment with the basic knowledge of each can help you ask the right questions and better understand the procedure.

- **Abdominal hysterectomy** is when the uterus (and/or the uterine tubes, ovaries, and cervix) is removed through an opening in the lower belly (the abdomen).

- **Vaginal hysterectomy** is when the uterus and cervix (and/or the uterine tubes and ovaries) are removed through the vagina. Note that a vaginal hysterectomy always includes the removal of the cervix, which is attached to the upper end of the vagina and therefore must be removed in order to remove the uterus above it.

- **Abdominal laparoscopic hysterectomy** is when a surgeon makes small incisions in the abdomen to remove the uterus (and/or the uterine tubes, ovaries, and cervix). The uterus is then removed in sections through a laparoscope tube; if a total hysterectomy is planned, the uterus and cervix can be removed through the vagina (called a laparoscopically assisted vaginal hysterectomy, or LAVH).

- **Robotic-assisted laparoscopic hysterectomy** is a laparoscopic hysterectomy with one difference: The surgeon uses a computer to control the surgical instruments used to remove your uterus (and/or the uterine tubes, ovaries, and cervix).

Ask an Expert

Will I go into early menopause after a hysterectomy?

If your hysterectomy involves the removal of your ovaries (bilateral oophorectomy) before you've reached menopause, you'll enter what's called surgical menopause and may experience symptoms caused by a lack of estrogen and progesterone. If your ovaries are left in place during your hysterectomy, they will continue to produce hormones. That said, you may go into menopause a year or two earlier than you otherwise would've. That's because the surgery to remove your uterus impacts blood flow to your ovaries, which may in turn impact hormone production. However, that's just one hypothesis, which is hard to tease apart from this fact: A common time for a woman to have a hysterectomy is in her forties, which also happens to be when women naturally enter perimenopause.

—Lauren F. Streicher, MD, professor of obstetrics and gynecology at Northwestern University Feinberg School of Medicine and author of *The Essential Guide to Hysterectomy*

Your Game Plan: What to Do If You Suspect You Have—or You've Been Diagnosed with— a Gynecologic Condition

As we've seen so far, many gynecologic disorders are notoriously difficult to diagnose and can be challenging to treat. What's worse, the pain and other life-altering symptoms these conditions often cause is far too often dismissed—by ourselves and even our care providers. Here, Dr. Stephanie Trentacoste McNally shares her best advice on the steps to take if you're worried you have a gynecologic disorder, or if you've received a diagnosis and want to hatch a plan for how to approach your next steps.

Educate yourself on the condition you have (or think you have) and bring that data with you to your appointment. Going to a doctor's appointment with information is power, says Dr. McNally. Go ahead and do some internet searching based on what symptoms you have and take notes on what the results turn up. This isn't self-diagnosis; it's crucial research that can help point your clinician in the right direction.

"Once you've done your research and you're at your appointment, go ahead and say something like 'I have data to suggest that maybe I have endometriosis or PCOS, and I'd like to go over this with you,'" says Dr. McNally. The more information you have about all the possible reasons for your symptoms, the more empowered you'll feel when it comes to advocating for yourself at your appointments.

Find a clinician who listens—and makes decisions *with* you. If you feel you've been dismissed by your doctor or feel that the severity of your symptoms has been downplayed, you need a new provider, says Dr. McNally.

"In an ideal world, you'll have a doctor who practices relationship-centered communication and shared decision-making," she says. "That means your provider asks you to list all of your concerns up front and really listens, doesn't cut you off when you're talking, follows up with the kind of questions that prompt you to accurately describe what's happening to you, and asks for your thoughts on suggested treatment plans."

Once you have a diagnosis, find someone who specializes in that specific condition. These gynecologic conditions aren't just tricky to diagnose; they can also be complicated to treat. Take endometriosis, for example. You have to look at hormonal regulation, pain management, mental health, and possible pelvic floor dysfunction, and you may need to involve a fertility specialist. Not only do you want to find a practitioner who knows the condition you're dealing with inside and out, but you also want one who works with other practitioners who can help you manage all of the possible implications of your condition.

"Try to find a community of physicians who work collaboratively, which makes it more likely that all the pieces of the puzzle can be put together seamlessly," says Dr. McNally. "You want a team who really champions what you need."

• • • • •

Until more funds and focus are devoted to studying women's bodies, it's up to us to be aware of what can go wrong, speak up when symptoms arise, and stay committed to getting the care we need and deserve.

Chapter 6

Fertility and Pregnancy

*How Fertility Works,
Preparing for Conception, and Teeing Yourself Up for
the Healthiest Pregnancy Possible*

> *Knowledge and authority about pregnancy and birth—which make
> up our individual and collective histories and guarantee our future—
> shouldn't be held exclusively by people with certificates, degrees, or
> high-profile publishing platforms. It should be something that all
> women talk about openly and have access to, without cost.*
>
> —Angela Garbes, *Like a Mother: A Feminist Journey Through the
> Science and Culture of Pregnancy*

Most of us who were born with ovaries spend the majority of our adult reproductive years trying not to get pregnant. By the time we reach our twenties, we've been given some form of "the talk"—the one about how sex works and babies are made. Yet while that talk usually contains some helpful advice on how to use condoms (if you're lucky!), it often stops well short of fully explaining how human fertility actually works. This lack of education about fertility not only puts us at greater risk of accidentally getting pregnant but also can lead to a lot of unnecessary confusion (and delay) for those of us who want to get pregnant.

The information in the following pages will not only help you understand how your body's reproductive system works but also provide the science-backed steps you can take to prepare for pregnancy if and when you want to have a baby. It'll also give you the knowledge you need to ask the right questions and make the best decisions for you and your growing baby.

In this chapter, we'll learn . . .

- **How women's fertility works**, from the hormones your body releases to prompt ovulation to the timing of conception if it happens (as well as what happens if you don't conceive).

- **What infertility actually is and why age really does matter when it comes to your fertility.** We'll also debunk a number of myths that still exist around the process of getting pregnant.

- **Options for preserving your fertility, as well as the assisted reproductive technologies available if you're having trouble conceiving.** From egg and embryo freezing to fertility medications, IUI, and IVF, we'll break down what's available and when to consider using each.

- **The science-backed steps you can take *before* you conceive**—a period of time known as preconception—to increase your odds of a healthy pregnancy, delivery, and baby.

- **How to navigate pregnancy**, including a guide to prenatal visits, the most common pregnancy complications, and how to manage health-care appointments when you're pregnant and considered overweight.

Meet the Experts

Randi Heather Goldman, MD, reproductive health and infertility specialist at Northwell Health Fertility and the program director for its reproductive endocrinology and infertility fellowship program

Noa Sterling, MD, ob-gyn and founder of Sterling Parents, an online subscription that supports women as they navigate pregnancy, birth, and postpartum

Melinda Henne, MD, double board-certified ob-gyn and reproductive endocrinology and infertility specialist

Tara Harding, DNP, family nurse practitioner and fertility coach

Afrouz Demeri, ND, former director of functional medicine at the University of California, Irvine's School of Medicine and creator of the Trimester Zero online course

Stephanie Waggel, MD, MS, PMH-C, medical director of Improve Life PLLC, a clinic specializing in perinatal psychopharmacology, which is the treatment of mental health challenges during and after pregnancy

Nicola Salmon, fat-positive fertility coach and author of *Fat and Fertile: How to Get Pregnant in a Bigger Body*

Getting Pregnant: How Fertility Works, Options for Preserving Yours, and What to Know About Fertility Treatments

If you're trying to conceive, it can be one of the most hopeful, exhilarating times of your life. It can also be extremely stressful, frustrating, and disappointing. Understanding some biological details (beyond the sperm-meet-egg basics) can help you go into your journey toward building a family—or not—better informed, says reproductive health and infertility specialist Randi Heather Goldman, MD.

"When you know how fertility works and what to expect, it empowers you to make decisions that are right for you," says Dr. Goldman. Here, she walks us through the basics.

How Fertility Works in Women: Understanding the Basics

- You are born with all the eggs you'll have in your lifetime. However, they're not fully developed and degenerate rapidly—and you'll go on to ovulate only a fraction of the eggs you start out with. As fetuses, we've got about six to seven million eggs; when we're born, that egg count is around one to two million; by the time we hit puberty, we have about three hundred thousand to four hundred thousand eggs. Over the course of our reproductive lifespan, we ovulate about four hundred eggs. And by the time we reach menopause, we have fewer than one thousand eggs.

- During the first half of your monthly menstrual cycle (starting with day 1 of your period and lasting until you ovulate), your pituitary gland releases follicle-stimulating hormone (FSH). FSH "recruits" anywhere from five to twenty of your ovarian follicles—each of which contains an immature egg—to get pulled to the surface of your ovary, where they develop further.

- Multiple follicles start to mature, but only one (though occasionally more, such as in the case of fraternal twins) becomes the "dominant" follicle, which has more FSH receptors and becomes more sensitive to the hormone, ultimately allowing it to grow faster than the others.

- As the dominant follicle grows, it starts producing increasing amounts of estrogen, which signals the pituitary gland to slow down its FSH production. This decrease in FSH prompts the smaller, nondominant follicles to stop growing. Eventually, they disintegrate.

- The size of the "cohort" of follicles that get pulled to the surface of your ovary each month depends on how many eggs you have overall. The younger you are, the more eggs you have at any given point—and the more follicles get pulled to the surface. As you get older and your egg supply dwindles, fewer follicles are pulled to the surface of your ovaries. You can think of it like your body rationing its egg supply.

- As that dominant follicle gets bigger and produces more estrogen, that rising estrogen level triggers the release of luteinizing hormone (LH) from the pituitary gland. This LH "surge" causes the ovary to release the egg into the uterine tube. In the average twenty-eight-day cycle, this happens around day 14.

Fun Fact

Ovulation doesn't always alternate from one ovary to the other each month. It can be completely random! Which means you could ovulate from one side multiple times in a row.

- After ovulation, the empty follicle transforms into the corpus luteum, which secretes progesterone and some estrogen—a hormone combination that supports the uterine lining, preparing the uterus for a potential pregnancy.

- If the egg is not fertilized, the corpus luteum degenerates, leading to a stop in the production of progesterone. Estrogen decreases as well. This prompts the top layers of the uterine lining to shed—aka your period has arrived—and the cycle starts all over again.

- After your egg is released from your ovary, it hangs out in your uterine tube (aka Fallopian tube), where it can survive for roughly twelve to twenty-four hours (after which time it's reabsorbed by your body). That means sperm, which can survive in a woman's reproductive tract for up to five days, should be present in the uterine tube for the best chance of fertilization happening.

- Sperm travel into the reproductive tract via semen, and once it hits your cervical canal, the sperm get trapped in cervical mucus and swim upward through the uterus and into the uterine tube, while the (now spermless) semen flows out of you. Translation: If you're hoping to get pregnant, don't be alarmed if a load of semen leaves your body after intercourse. There's a good chance the sperm are swimming toward your uterine tubes, which is where they need to be.

- While millions of sperm may make the journey toward your uterine tubes, only a few hundred reach the vicinity of your egg. Enzymes from the sperm head digest the outer layer of the egg, allowing one sperm to penetrate. Once that sperm enters the egg, the egg's surface changes to prevent any other sperm from entering.

- Your egg is officially fertilized, which usually takes place in the widest section of the uterine tube, called the ampulla.

- Immediately after the sperm penetrates the egg, the nuclei of the two start to fuse and combine their genetic material, each usually contributing twenty-three chromosomes. The result is a zygote with a complete set of forty-six chromosomes—a genetic combination that determines things like sex, eye color, and other traits.

- The zygote then begins to divide and multiply through a process called mitosis, and it moves down the uterine tube toward the uterus.

- Several days after sperm meets egg, the rapidly dividing group of cells (now called a blastocyst) reaches the uterus, where it must implant into the lining of the uterus. If this implantation happens (and only about half of fertilized eggs will implant),[1] the blastocyst develops into an embryo and later into a fetus. Once implantation happens, your body starts producing a hormone called human chorionic gonadotropin (aka hCG or the pregnancy hormone), which tells your ovaries to hold off on producing another egg.

Why Age Matters When It Comes to Your Fertility

As much as we like to consider age as "just a number"—and we are radically reframing what it means to be an older woman in our society in so many ways—the fact is that age is a significant factor in your fertility. Here's why:

- Egg quantity declines over time, gradually at first and then more rapidly in our mid-to-late thirties.

- Egg quality also declines with age. Older eggs have a higher chance of becoming an embryo with chromosomal abnormalities.

- Ovulation can become less regular, and this irregularity can make timing conception more challenging.

- Your risk of health issues that can negatively impact fertility (such as uterine fibroids) increases with age.

- Your risk of pregnancy complications, including gestational diabetes, high blood pressure, preeclampsia, and ectopic pregnancy (when a fertilized egg implants and begins to grow outside the uterus, most often in one of the uterine tubes), increases with age.

The American College of Obstetricians and Gynecologists says significant fertility decline starts at age thirty-two,[2] and you're considered "advanced maternal age" (aka AMA) if you're thirty-five or older. (This term may not feel great, though it's an improvement on "geriatric pregnancy," which is the phrase clinicians used to use!) While AMA pregnancies are associated with a higher risk of complications, it's important to remember that many women older than thirty-five have healthy pregnancies and babies. If this is you, know that you'll likely receive a higher level of monitoring throughout your pregnancy, such as more frequent prenatal visits and ultrasounds as well as additional screening for genetic abnormalities, blood pressure, and gestational diabetes.

Yet along with the increased risks and monitoring you might be in for, it's also important to remember the benefits of being an older parent, says ob-gyn Noa Sterling, MD.

"The reasons we delay childbearing—to get an education, focus on our careers, marry later because we want to find the right partner—can be hugely beneficial for your kids' health and wellness," says Dr. Sterling. "Yes, there are risks to conceiving when you're older, but there's a lot we can do to mitigate those risks—and upsides to being an older parent that we don't talk about nearly enough."

What Is Infertility?

Infertility is defined as not being able to get pregnant after twelve months of trying if a woman is younger than thirty-five or after six months of trying to conceive if a woman is older than thirty-five.[3] It's also more common than you might think: Nearly 20 percent of married women with no prior births are unable to get pregnant after a year of trying, and about one in four women in this group struggles to get pregnant or carry a pregnancy to term.[4]

While infertility often gets blamed on women, only about one-third of infertility cases are caused by fertility problems in women. Another third of cases are caused by male reproductive issues, and another third are due to a mix of both female and male issues or, unfortunately, go unexplained.[5] In women, the most common cause of infertility is problems with ovulation. In men, sperm disorders, structural issues (like a block in the genital tract where sperm flows), erectile dysfunction, or premature ejaculation may be to blame.

Ask an Expert

My infertility is prompting a lot of stress, which I know isn't great for my chances of getting pregnant. How can I deal with this Catch-22 scenario?

We live in a very stressful world. There's job stress, money stress, social stress—the list goes on. And infertility ranks up there with divorce, death of a family member, job loss, and a cancer diagnosis as one of the most stressful things you can go through. Most of us are used to being able to assert some form of control over most things in our lives, and infertility can feel like a situation where we're decidedly not in control.

First, remind yourself that stress is a normal reaction to what you're going through. If you're struggling with infertility and trying to get pregnant, you're likely going through a process that involves lots of instructions about precise timing and dosing of fertility medications, while also recognizing that none of this is guaranteed to be successful. Of course you're going to have scary, uncomfortable emotions while you're going through that! I tell all my patients to ignore all the people who tell you to "just go on vacation and relax," because that's usually just not possible—and stressing about how stressed you are isn't going to help.

Next, think about just one step you can take to try to control your response to your stress. Therapy can be helpful, and there are actually fertility-certified psychotherapists who are trained specifically to help people manage the range of emotions that often surfaces during fertility struggles. Also, think about how you can minimize any other big stresses in your life so you don't feel completely overwhelmed.

Finally, try to think about the stress you're feeling right now as a reminder of how badly you want to have a baby. Your fear and worry are showing you what you want most and can remind you that you're doing everything in your power to succeed in getting it.

—Melinda Henne, MD, double board-certified ob-gyn and reproductive endocrinology and infertility specialist

Miscarriage, Explained

Miscarriage, or the loss of a pregnancy that's in the uterus, is common. It happens in about 10 percent of people who know they're pregnant. Most miscarriages (about 80 percent) happen in the first trimester, which is also when a miscarriage may be referred to as spontaneous abortion or early pregnancy loss. Here, fertility coach Tara Harding, DNP, walks us through what we need to know.

» WHAT CAUSES A MISCARRIAGE?

The reasons are varied and often not fully understood, but here are some of the primary reasons why miscarriages happen:

- **Chromosomal abnormalities.** This is the most common cause of miscarriage during the first trimester and can result from errors during cell division that lead to too many or too few chromosomes or structural problems with the chromosomes. These issues can prevent the embryo from developing normally.

- **Anatomical issues.** Abnormalities in the uterus or cervix (such as uterine fibroids or polyps and weak cervical tissue) can interfere with the implantation or growth of the embryo or lead to the premature opening of the cervix.

- **Untreated medical conditions.** Chronic diseases such as uncontrolled diabetes, thyroid disease, and lupus can impact your ability to maintain a pregnancy. A serious infection or injury can also cause miscarriage.

It's important to note that most miscarriages are isolated events, and many women go on to have successful pregnancies afterward. In fact, research shows that even with a diagnosis of recurrent pregnancy loss (aka RPL) and as many as four or five prior pregnancy losses, a patient is more likely to carry her next pregnancy to term than to go through another miscarriage.

» WHAT DO I DO IF I SUSPECT I'M HAVING OR HAD A MISCARRIAGE?

If you're pregnant and start to notice any bleeding, call your healthcare provider. While some light bleeding or spotting can occur in early pregnancy and isn't always a sign of miscarriage, any bleeding should be evaluated by a clinician immediately. If you've had a miscarriage, your next steps will depend on your stage of pregnancy and symptoms, as well as other health factors.

There are three main approaches to managing a miscarriage, any of which your healthcare provider might recommend based on your particular situation:

1. Wait for your body to naturally expel your pregnancy tissue. This is often feasible only if you don't show any signs of an infection. It's also important to know that it usually takes up to two weeks and can take longer in some cases.

2. Take medication (such as misoprostol) that causes the uterus to contract and expel pregnancy tissue. This is often recommended for those who'd like to avoid surgery but want a more predictable process than waiting to expel pregnancy tissue naturally.

3. Have a surgical treatment, such as a vacuum aspiration, that removes the contents of the uterus with a suction device inserted through the cervix. A dilation and curettage (D&C) may be recommended if there's heavy bleeding or if not all of the pregnancy tissue has been expelled.

Regardless of the approach, follow-up care is important to make sure the miscarriage has been completed without complications. Emotional support is also key.

"If you're having a difficult time processing this loss, that's understandable," says Dr. Harding. "Miscarriage may be common, but it's a physically and emotionally difficult experience and one that's important to discuss with your healthcare provider and lean on others for support." (For more on common pregnancy complications, jump to page 164.)

Fertility Preservation: What to Know About Your Options

Egg and embryo freezing was considered "experimental" until 2013. Now the procedures are mainstream, and many healthy people who want to put off having kids until they're older are freezing their eggs and embryos. Here's an overview of what's involved with each procedure.

» EGG FREEZING (AKA OOCYTE CRYOPRESERVATION)

This procedure involves retrieving eggs and freezing them, a process that takes around two weeks.

HOW IT WORKS

- A fertility specialist will test your FSH and AMH levels, as well as perform a vaginal ultrasound to gauge how many eggs they think they might be able to get after you've taken fertility hormones.

- Some specialists require women to use birth control pills prior to an egg-freezing cycle so they can manipulate the timing of the menstrual cycle and help suppress the growth of ovarian cysts, which can interfere with the egg-retrieval process.

- When your doctor decides you're ready, you'll start giving yourself daily hormone injections (two to three hormone medications per day for ten to twelve days, often injected into skin you pinch around your belly or thigh). The goal of these medications is to get *all* of the eggs recruited to the surface of your ovary to mature—not just the one that would normally mature. When you start taking these fertility drugs, you'll also start going into the office for frequent blood work and vaginal ultrasounds, which help to give your doctor a sense of how your egg follicles are maturing.

- When your follicles are ready, your doctor will tell you to give yourself a "trigger shot," which prepares the eggs in those follicles to fully mature.

- Exactly thirty-six hours later, you'll go in for the egg retrieval: While you're under anesthesia, a doctor will do another vaginal ultrasound, this time with a needle attached to the probe that passes through the vaginal wall and into the ovaries to collect the egg from each mature follicle—a procedure called a transvaginal ultrasound aspiration.

- An embryologist will put your follicles in a liquid that keeps them alive while their quality is assessed. Then your eggs will be placed in an incubator that replicates the living conditions inside your body to fully develop.

- Your eggs will be immersed in a tank of liquid nitrogen, a "flash-freezing" method to prevent them from developing ice crystals, which can damage the egg and ultimately impact its quality. Once the eggs are frozen, they'll stay in a tank of liquid nitrogen until you're ready to use them.

Success rate: The survival rate of thawed frozen eggs ranges from 80 percent to 90 percent. One large study found that 70 percent of women who froze eggs when they were younger than age thirty-eight and thawed at least twenty eggs at a later date had a baby.[6]

Average cost: $10,000 to $15,000 per cycle, plus the cost of egg storage. Some employers offer coverage for this procedure, so it's worth checking to see what your health plan might cover.

» EMBRYO FREEZING (AKA EMBRYO CRYOPRESERVATION)

This procedure involves retrieving eggs, fertilizing them with sperm, and freezing the resulting embryos so they can be implanted at a later date.

HOW IT WORKS

- You'll go through all of the steps involved in egg freezing until the "flash freeze" part.

- After your eggs are retrieved, they're fertilized with sperm in a lab—either by combining them with sperm in a culture dish (in vitro fertilization, or IVF) or by injecting a single sperm directly into each egg (intracytoplasmic sperm injection, or ICSI). IVF is typically used when there are no significant male-factor fertility issues (such as low sperm count, poor sperm motility, or abnormal sperm shape or *morphology*); ICSI is more common when there are male-factor fertility issues, or if previous IVF attempts have resulted in failed fertilization.

- After fertilization, the embryos are cultured in an incubator for a few days to allow them to further develop. Embryos are monitored closely during this time to assess developmental progress and quality.

- Embryos are graded based on size, symmetry, and number of cells. This helps embryologists select the highest-quality embryos for freezing.

- Selected embryos are then flash frozen with liquid nitrogen and thawed when ready to use.

Success rate: Pregnancy after embryo transfer can approach up to 70 percent, depending on multiple factors.[7]

Average cost: $10,000 to $15,000 per cycle.

Fertility Treatments: Understanding Some of the Most Common Interventions

» FERTILITY DRUGS (AKA OVULATION-INDUCTION DRUGS)

These medications are used to stimulate ovulation. This chart describes some of the most common.

NAME OF DRUG	HOW IT WORKS
Clomiphene citrate (Clomid or Serophene)	Induces ovulation by blocking estrogen receptors, essentially tricking your body into thinking estrogen levels are low, which stimulates the production of more follicle-stimulating hormone (FSH)
Human menopausal gonadotropin (Pergonal, Humegon, Repronex)	Stimulates egg development in women who don't ovulate spontaneously or who ovulate irregularly, thanks to its being comprised of FSH and luteinizing hormone (LH)
Follicle-stimulating hormone (Follistim, Gonal-F, Bravelle)	Stimulates the recruitment and development of multiple eggs
Human chorionic gonadotropin (Profasi, Pregnyl, Ovidrel)	Helps with the final maturation of eggs and triggers the ovaries to release mature eggs; stimulates the secretion of progesterone, which prepares the lining of the uterus for implantation of a fertilized egg
Leuprolide (Lupron)	Suppresses the brain's secretion of LH and FSH to prevent the recruitment of a dominant follicle, enabling the ovaries to respond with the recruitment of multiple follicles; prevents premature ovulation

» INTRAUTERINE INSEMINATION (IUI, ARTIFICIAL INSEMINATION, OR "THE TURKEY BASTER METHOD")

During this procedure, healthy sperm are placed into a woman's uterus around the time she's ovulating to increase the odds of pregnancy.

HOW IT WORKS

- You may receive fertility medication to stimulate ovulation.

- On the day of the IUI procedure (which will be timed within your expected ovulation window), the sperm donor provides a semen sample. That semen then goes through "sperm washing," where the highly motile and healthy sperm are separated out from the seminal fluid. This concentrated sperm sample is what's used for insemination. Note that sometimes frozen sperm is used, and research shows no significant difference in IUI outcomes between frozen and fresh sperm.[8]

- Your provider will insert a speculum into the vagina, followed by a thin, flexible catheter attached to a syringe containing the concentrated sperm sample. The sperm is released directly into the uterus. The goal: increasing the number of sperm that reach the uterine tubes to increase the chance of fertilization.

- Following the IUI, you may be prescribed progesterone supplements or other medications to support the luteal phase of the cycle (which prepares the uterine lining for implantation of a fertilized egg).

- Approximately two weeks after the IUI, you can take a pregnancy test.

Success rate: Generally ranges from 10 to 20 percent per cycle, depending on various factors (such as age, reason for infertility, and whether fertility drugs were used).[9]

Average cost: About $300 to $1,000.

» IVF (IN VITRO FERTILIZATION)

IVF is a treatment that uses both medications and surgical procedures to help sperm fertilize an egg and help implant that fertilized egg (aka embryo) in your uterus. It involves multiple steps, known as an IVF cycle.

HOW IT WORKS

- IVF is a process that may begin with birth control pills or injections that are used to control the timing of your menstrual cycle.

- You'll take fertility medications that stimulate the development of multiple follicles in the ovaries. You'll also take drugs that prevent premature ovulation, to ensure the eggs have sufficiently developed before retrieval. Your response to these medications is monitored through blood tests and ultrasounds.

- When your eggs have sufficiently matured (something your clinician will be able to tell based on your blood work and ultrasound), you'll give yourself a "trigger shot" to trigger the ovaries to release the eggs. About thirty-six hours later, your eggs will be retrieved.

- The retrieved eggs are then mixed with sperm in a culture dish. When a sperm successfully penetrates an egg, the egg is considered fertilized. The resulting embryos are monitored in a lab for about five days and assessed for growth and quality. The best-quality embryos are usually frozen. (In some cases, clinicians will do a "fresh embryo transfer," inserting a never-been-frozen embryo into your uterus five days after fertilization. However, most clinicians prefer freezing embryos.)

- You'll likely take hormones to prepare your uterus to accept an embryo prior to your embryo transfer. Typically, this involves fourteen to twenty-one days of oral medication followed by six days of injections, as well as appointments with your fertility specialist for blood tests and ultrasounds.

- When your uterus is ready, one or more of the best-quality embryos will be selected for transfer into the uterus via a thin catheter. (This procedure typically takes less than ten minutes and doesn't require anesthesia.)

- Around twelve days after your IVF procedure, you can take a pregnancy test.

Success rate: Varies greatly based on multiple factors, with age at the time of egg retrieval being the major predictor. You can use the CDC's "IVF Success Estimator" (cdc.gov/art/ivf-success-estimator) to get a sense of your chance of having a live birth using IVF.[10]

Average cost: Up to $15,000 or more per cycle.[11]

Most Common Questions LGBTQ+ Couples Have About Getting Pregnant, Answered

For same-sex couples and transgender men and women, seeing a fertility specialist is often an important step when it comes to understanding your options for growing your family. Here are some of the most common questions about the process, answered by fertility specialist Melinda Henne, MD:

- **Whose sperm will we use?** For same-sex female couples, this may involve using a sperm bank or a known sperm donor. For same-sex male couples, it typically involves deciding which partner's sperm to use. Depending on your decision, you'll also want to talk through some important scenarios: Do you want your child to have biological siblings, and if so, how many? (Your answer can help you decide how many vials of sperm you order from the same donor, for example, or whether a same-sex male couple alternates sperm with each pregnancy attempt.) If you're using a known sperm donor, what are the rights, responsibilities, obligations, or lack thereof that the sperm donor will have?

- **Whose ovaries will we use for eggs, and whose uterus will we use to carry the baby?** Same-sex female couples often have multiple options when deciding how to answer this question. You may want to do artificial insemination with a sperm donor, with or without ovulation medications. In this case, the egg will be from the same person who will carry the pregnancy. You can do IVF where the person who carries the pregnancy will also supply the egg. You can also use an egg from one partner, fertilize it with donor sperm, and then transfer the embryo to the other partner's uterus to carry the pregnancy. (This is called reciprocal IVF.) Fertility workups on both partners can help inform the decisions you make. For example, testing on egg quantity / ovarian reserve may dictate whose eggs you use. Or, if a transvaginal ultrasound on one partner shows anatomical issues (such as uterine fibroids) that could make carrying a baby challenging, the decision on who will carry your baby may be made for you.

    For same-sex male couples and single men, you'll need an egg donor and someone to carry the baby (gestational carrier). This is an important decision with multiple legal issues involved, so it's important to consult an attorney to walk you through important documentation you'll want to have in place.

- **Am I comfortable with the various steps involved if I want to preserve my fertility?** If you're a transgender man and have already started hormone therapy, you may be asked to stop taking that treatment to preserve your eggs. You'll also need procedures such as a vaginal ultrasound, which you may not be comfortable having. For transgender women, fertility preservation is a bit easier, as it involves sperm collection and storage. That said, it's still important to think through your family planning goals— even if the idea of having children feels far away—and ideally, meet with a gender-affirming fertility specialist to talk through the fertility-preservation process. Then get honest with yourself about what feels feasible (or not) for you.

Preconception Basics:
The Research-Backed Ways to Prepare Your Body for a Baby

If you think about having kids, you likely ask a ton of questions. What will the baby look like? How should we decorate the nursery? What books will best prepare me for everything that could possibly come up during pregnancy and those first few months of new parenthood?

But there's an even more crucial question most of us don't even know we need to ask: What do I need to know and do *before* I get pregnant?

Here's an important fact about conception that gets missed far too often: You and your partner have a window of opportunity in the three months before you conceive—a period known as preconception—to not only increase your odds of a successful pregnancy but also impact your future child's health for the better.

"Your nutrition and lifestyle choices *before* you conceive have an impact on the developmental programming—aka epigenetics—of your baby, which is how genes turn 'on' or 'off' to influence a child's susceptibility to chronic disease later in life," says Afrouz Demeri, ND. That's not to say a surprise pregnancy means your child's health is doomed. There's plenty you can do once you find out you're pregnant to get your health in order and optimize your baby's health. But if you're starting to think about growing your family, following this advice can be helpful:

- **Schedule a preconception evaluation.** Making sure you're in good health increases your odds of a healthy pregnancy and baby. Do you get headaches every day? Are you struggling with anxiety? Are you dealing with an overall feeling of *meh* most days rather than feeling vibrantly healthy? So many of us walk around with symptoms of various health conditions, and while we may get used to them, it's important to address these issues before you get pregnant.

  "Think of your body like a house that's going to be home to your growing baby," says Dr. Demeri. "And just like you'll look at the roof, the basement, and every room of a house before moving in to make sure everything is in the best shape possible, that's what you want to do with your health."

- **Have your male partner's health (and sperm) assessed**. The recommendation to have a preconception visit is almost always focused exclusively on the woman. But it's just as important for a male partner or sperm donor to be assessed.

   "Men are half the equation when it comes to conceiving—a fact most of us don't really think about," says Dr. Demeri. "So many of my female patients blame themselves for their miscarriages or infertility and don't realize that their male partner's health issues or sperm count and/or quality could very well be contributing to their fertility issues."

   Sperm counts have plummeted nearly 60 percent since 1973, according to one large, multicountry study.[12] There has also been a decline in sperm quality, which is assessed by looking at sperm shape (aka morphology). There are several theories to explain this; exposure to environmental toxins, poor diet, and obesity are thought to be some of the potential causes.

   "This is a big problem that most of us don't even consider until we have trouble conceiving," says Dr. Demeri. "Being proactive about the health of your sperm before you try to get pregnant is great, because there a lot of things you can do to boost sperm quality and quantity."

- **Double down on your healthy habits**. For both men and women, the healthy lifestyle advice you've heard a million times before really can go a long way toward improving your chances of conceiving *and* sustaining a healthy pregnancy. Dr. Demeri suggests starting with the basics: Stop smoking (both nicotine and marijuana), exercise regularly, keep stress in check, and make sure you're getting good sleep. Do what you can to avoid environmental toxicants—things like pesticides and herbicides in nonorganic food, plastics in food packaging, and volatile organic compounds found in things like cleaners, candles, and some personal care products.

   For both women and men, good nutrition can go a long way when it comes to boosting the quality of both eggs and sperm. Folate is important for everything from ovulation to fetal growth, and vitamins C and E have been shown to boost egg quality and lead to better IVF outcomes. Making sure your male partner or sperm donor is getting enough antioxidants is also key, because sperm are particularly prone to oxidative damage. Key antioxidants for male fertility include CoQ10, NAC, L-carnitine, alpha-lipoic acid, zinc, selenium, and vitamins C, E, and D.

- **Start taking a prenatal vitamin.** Every woman of childbearing age should consider taking a prenatal supplement, even if you're not considering getting pregnant in the near future, says Dr. Demeri. There are also prenatal vitamins men can take in the months before conception, which can help boost their stores of those key antioxidants before trying to conceive. This is important because nearly half of all pregnancies in the U.S. are unplanned.[13] For many couples, this means they find out they're pregnant a few weeks *after* they've conceived, which is after a period of early embryo development that requires key nutrients in high amounts, says Dr. Demeri. Another reason to build up these nutrient stores before you get pregnant is that many women experience food aversions and nausea during their first trimester, and your diet will likely take a turn for the worse as your body adjusts to growing a tiny human. Taking a prenatal vitamin means you'll still get enough of these important nutrients, even when all you can stomach is simple carbs.

There's a big bonus that comes along with taking these steps for your health before you try to conceive or soon after you get pregnant, says Dr. Demeri: It tees your family up for better health for the rest of your lives.

Ask an Expert

Do I need to go off my depression or anxiety medications when I want to start trying to get pregnant (or find out I'm pregnant)?

While every person is different and you need to have a conversation about your specific situation with your healthcare provider, in general the answer is no: You probably don't have to stop taking the prescription medication(s) you take for your mental health when trying to conceive or when you find out you're expecting. One big exception is valproate (Depakote), which is used to treat certain psychiatric conditions (such as bipolar disorder) and seizure disorders, as well as for the prevention of migraine headaches. This medication is associated with an increased risk of neural tube defects, decreased IQ scores, and neurodevelopmental disorders—and because of this, it should not be prescribed to women of reproductive age.

I can't tell you how many women tell me that they'd rather suffer from mental illness than risk their baby being exposed to their mental health medication. But here's the truth: Your uncontrolled mental illness during pregnancy can have very real impacts on both you *and* your fetus. Going off a medicine that's been helping you feel steady and happy can prompt your stress hormones to skyrocket, and your baby's exposure to that flood of cortisol can affect her brain development and even lead to an increased susceptibility to cognitive and behavioral problems later in life. It also has the potential to lead to preeclampsia, hemorrhage, premature delivery, and stillbirth—scenarios that can have serious health complications.

I see a lot of patients who assume that decreasing the dose of their antidepressant will be better for the baby, but this is misguided as well. The right dose is crucial when it comes to how well these medications work. If you decrease the dose, your baby will still be exposed to the medication—*and* the effects of your uncontrolled mental illness.

If you really want to go off a medication you're taking for your mental health, talk to your clinician. They can help you navigate the potential risks and benefits of taking psychiatric drugs during pregnancy, help you taper off what you're taking, and come up with a realistic plan for treating your mental health during pregnancy and beyond. If you are interested in continuing your medication, please see a clinician who has training in perinatal psychopharmacology. You can find prescribers with this training at postpartum.net/get-help/provider-directory/.

—Stephanie Waggel, MD, MS, PMH-C, medical director of Improve Life PLLC, a clinic specializing in perinatal psychopharmacology, which is the treatment of mental health challenges during and after pregnancy

You're Pregnant: A Road Map for Prenatal Visits and Pregnancy Complications to Keep on Your Radar

A Guide to Prenatal Visits: The Appointments and Tests You Need at Every Stage

Good prenatal care is an important step you can take to optimize the health of both you and your baby, and a key component to this is regular medical checkups and consultations with healthcare providers throughout your pregnancy. While your clinician will schedule these appointments for you when they need to happen, it helps to have an overview of the timing and goals of each visit.

WEEKS OF PREGNANCY	FREQUENCY OF PRENATAL VISITS
Weeks 4 to 10	Your initial checkup. (Though if you find out you're pregnant later than that, it's okay; call and make an appointment as soon as you learn that you're expecting.)
Weeks 4 to 28	One checkup a month
Weeks 28 to 36	One checkup every two weeks
Weeks 36 to 41	One checkup every week

Source: March of Dimes[14]

Note: Your individual health picture—including your age, preexisting health conditions, and any medical problems that develop during pregnancy—can impact your recommended prenatal visit schedule.

The Initial Appointment: What to Expect and How to Prepare

During this appointment, your clinician will do a wide range of tests and exams to confirm your pregnancy, calculate your due date, assess your health via a medical history and physical exam, and order lab tests to check for things like your blood type, Rh factor (a protein on the surface of some red blood cells that can cause issues if it's incompatible with the Rh factor of your baby), red blood cell and platelet counts, and infections. You'll also have a chance to discuss genetic screening and prenatal testing options, as well as nutrition, lifestyle, and exercise guidelines.

To prepare for this visit, be ready to talk about:

- The first day of your last menstrual period, which will help your clinician calculate the baby's due date
- Health conditions you have, such as diabetes, high blood pressure, and depression
- Your family health history
- Your pregnancy history, including if you've had a miscarriage, stillbirth, or premature baby

It's also great to bring to the appointment a record of your vaccinations, if you have it, as well as a list of all medications you take (including prescription and over-the-counter medicines, as well as supplements and herbs).

After this first visit, your appointments may follow a pattern each time you're at your clinician's office. Your healthcare team will likely check:

- How you're feeling
- The growth of your baby and uterus
- Your blood pressure
- Your baby's heartbeat (after about ten to twelve weeks of pregnancy)

Prenatal Tests to Expect—and When

Here are some of the screening and diagnostic tests your provider will offer you throughout your pregnancy.

TIMING	RECOMMENDED TESTS, SCREENINGS, AND VACCINATIONS
First trimester	• Carrier screening for genetic conditions (a blood or saliva test) • Blood tests to check your baby's DNA (cell-free fetal DNA testing), which is examined for certain genetic conditions, such as Down syndrome • The "first-trimester screening" that includes a blood test and an ultrasound to check for chromosomal disorders or a heart defect in the baby • Early ultrasound (aka first-trimester ultrasound) to "date" your pregnancy so you know how far along you are • Chorionic villus sampling (CVS), usually done at ten to thirteen weeks, that checks placenta tissue to see if your baby has a genetic condition
Second trimester	• Anatomy ultrasound, usually done between eighteen and twenty-two weeks, to check your baby's growth and development, and can usually tell you the baby's sex • Maternal blood screening, usually done at fifteen and twenty-two weeks and checks your blood to see if your baby is at risk for birth defects • Glucose screening test, usually done at twenty-four to twenty-eight weeks, to check for gestational diabetes • Amniocentesis, usually done at fifteen to twenty weeks, to see if your baby has a birth defect or genetic condition
Third trimester	• Test for group B strep (GBS), usually done at thirty-five to thirty-seven weeks, which looks at your cervical fluid for a bacterium that can colonize the vagina and rectum and infect the baby during childbirth

Source: March of Dimes[15]

Ask an Expert

Can I refuse a prenatal test my clinician recommends?

It is absolutely your right to deny prenatal testing your doctor recommends. That said, there's not a lot of unnecessary testing that happens during pregnancy. And while I know that prenatal screenings can cause a lot of anxiety and worry, try not to let fear drive your decisions.

Prenatal genetic testing is a group of screenings that's most likely to get some pushback from patients, especially if you know you wouldn't terminate your pregnancy no matter the results. However, I like to plant this seed in my patients' minds: Discovering something like a genetic abnormality for the first time when you're newly postpartum can be incredibly hard to navigate. Getting those results while you're pregnant isn't necessarily easier, but it does give you some time to wrap your head and heart around the reality before you also have the added pressure of taking care of a newborn.

Many patients also question the gestational diabetes screening. I get that the test isn't fun; I have three kids and I hated drinking that sugary liquid, too. But we know that undetected diabetes during pregnancy can lead to serious complications—many of which happen after giving birth. I've cared for patients who denied the glucose test and then felt immense guilt that the health complications their baby faced were due to a choice they made.

If you're tempted to deny a test your doctor is recommending, I'd urge you to consider what's at the heart of your reasoning. If it's fear of the results, talk through those fears with your provider.

—Noa Sterling, MD, ob-gyn and founder of Sterling Parents, an online subscription that supports women as they navigate pregnancy, birth, and postpartum

Healthy Pregnancies for *Every* Body: How to Find a Size-Friendly Specialist

When you live in a larger body, finding fertility and pregnancy care that's nonstigmatizing can be challenging. Many fertility clinics won't even see people over a certain body mass index (BMI), citing weight as a barrier to success.

Yet while a BMI over 30 is associated with some health risks related to pregnancy, it's just one factor—and shouldn't be the sole focus of your fertility and prenatal visits. (For a deep dive into the ways BMI is flawed, better measurements, and how to navigate the weight stigma baked into our healthcare system, which still uses BMI as a measure of health, see page 560.) In fact, many women in larger bodies don't struggle with infertility and go on to have healthy pregnancies.

If you live in a larger body and find out you're pregnant, early and regular prenatal care is an important step that'll ensure your clinician is able to watch for signs of the conditions you may be at increased risk for and treat them before they become serious. And if you do struggle with infertility, finding a size-inclusive provider who can help you get to the bottom of why you're having trouble getting pregnant can make all the difference when it comes to realizing your dream of having kids.

Nicola Salmon, a fat-positive fertility coach, offers tips on how to advocate for yourself with your healthcare providers and find clinicians who take a weight-neutral approach to their care.

- **Acknowledge that we live in a culture where weight stigma is prevalent**. When you live in a larger body and have trouble getting pregnant—or you've been told not to even try to conceive until you lose weight—it can be tempting to blame yourself for your struggles. This isn't the mindset you want to have when it comes to advocating for yourself, says Salmon. "Naming the systems at play and the medical bias against fat folks in our healthcare system is a great first step, because it can help you unload the heavy weight of blame and shame you may be carrying with you."

- **Get vulnerable with your providers and share your experience of weight stigma**. When you're meeting with a clinician, tell them that you've had a lot of negative experiences with healthcare providers who've made assumptions based on your size. Acknowledge the trauma it caused and say something like "I'd love to know if you're open to helping me in more of a weight-neutral way." Then clue in to their response, which should give you a good sense of the type of care they provide.

- **Set boundaries with your clinician that feel right for you**. For example, you can express your wish to not be weighed unless medically necessary, or that you'd prefer not to talk about weight loss or dieting. When you make these requests, ask that they be recorded in your chart so other clinicians you might see can access this information and you don't have to express these wishes on future visits.

Some of the Most Common Pregnancy Complications, Explained

In an ideal scenario, you find out you're pregnant and have nine months of smooth sailing—a pregnancy that unfolds by the book. In reality, many pregnancies involve or end in a complication, which can happen for a variety of reasons or even sometimes go unexplained. This can be especially difficult to navigate, given our expectations (not to mention the messages we're bombarded with from society at large) about what pregnancy *should* look like.

Knowing some of the most common conditions and diseases that can surface during pregnancy will help you keep symptoms on your radar and talk to your clinician as needed, as well as navigate the emotional toll so many of these complications can take.

EARLY PREGNANCY COMPLICATIONS

- **Miscarriage**, also known as pregnancy loss, which happens in about 10 to 20 percent of all pregnancies (usually due to genetic or chromosomal abnormalities) and most often within the first trimester.[16]

- **Ectopic pregnancy**, which happens when a fertilized egg implants and starts growing outside the uterus, usually in one of the uterine tubes.

- **Hyperemesis gravidarum (HG)**, which is extreme and persistent nausea and vomiting during pregnancy that typically occurs during the first trimester and can lead to dehydration and weight loss, and may require medical intervention to manage symptoms and prevent complications.

- **Gestational diabetes**, a type of diabetes that develops during pregnancy that can happen when the placenta's hormones block the mom's insulin, leading to insulin resistance.

- **Preeclampsia**, a blood pressure condition that develops during pregnancy (typically during the last trimester) and can lead to serious health complications for both mom and baby. It's one of the leading causes of maternal mortality in the U.S. and a top cause of maternal death among Black women. The U.S. Preventive Services Task Force recommends that women who are at high risk for this condition start taking baby aspirin between twelve and twenty-eight weeks of gestation (optimally before sixteen weeks), which can reduce the risk of preeclampsia. Aspirin is thought to improve blood flow to the placenta and decrease the risk of blood clots forming there, ultimately reducing the risk of this dangerous condition.

- **Infections during pregnancy**, particularly urinary tract infections (UTIs), group B streptococcus (GBS), cytomegalovirus (CMV), and sexually transmitted infections (STIs), which can increase the risk of complications for both mom and baby.

- **Iron-deficiency anemia**, which happens when you don't have enough red blood cells to carry adequate amounts of oxygen throughout your body and causes symptoms like fatigue, weakness, breathing difficulties, and fainting as a result. If left untreated, it can increase the risk of complications, including fetal growth problems, preterm birth, and low birth weight.

- **Placenta previa**, a condition where the placenta partially or completely blocks the cervix, which can lead to severe bleeding before, during, or after childbirth.

- **Placental abruption**, which occurs when the placenta separates from the uterine wall before childbirth, leading to bleeding, pain, and potential fetal distress.

- **Fetal growth restriction**, a condition that happens when a fetus is much smaller than expected for its gestational age.

- **Preterm birth**, which is defined as babies born before thirty-seven weeks of pregnancy.

Your Game Plan:
How to Tee Yourself Up for a Healthy, Happy Pregnancy

When you're trying to get pregnant or find out you're expecting, it can feel like you're drinking from a fire hose of information. There's endless data to geek out on to inform all kinds of decisions, big and small. However, before you order all the books and subscribe to the newsletters, start with these big-picture to-dos, says Dr. Sterling.

Find a healthcare provider you vibe with. You want the clinician you see throughout your pregnancy to be someone you have a good, collaborative relationship with. You want someone who asks good questions and really listens to your answers. You want someone who understands your health history, gets to know who you are, and can guide you when it comes to what's best for you and your growing baby.

"This is a practitioner who's going to carry you through one of the most difficult and transformative periods of your life," says Dr. Sterling. Which means you'll want to home in on a provider you really like.

To do this, choose a clinician who delivers babies (say, an ob-gyn or a midwife) for your annual exams a few years before you know you want to get pregnant, and consider these appointments like trials. Do you feel comfortable with the practitioner? Do you trust her and feel heard when you bring up your concerns? Do you like the clinic's office staff? The answers to these questions (and others that help you get at what feels most important to you) will help you land on a clinician who feels like a true ally.

Take an honest look at your stress. Stress matters when it comes to how your body functions, including your fertility and how good (or not) you feel once you get pregnant.

"All of the things that make you feel like you're at your max right now—

whether it's an overwhelming job, a toxic relationship with your mom, or another big stressor in your life—will almost certainly feel *more* stressful when you get pregnant and then when you have a baby," says Dr. Sterling. "Doing what you can to be kinder to yourself, to learn how to draw boundaries that ensure your well-being is prioritized, and to start to listen to your voice and what's most important to you will serve you well now *and* later, because these things become really important in pregnancy and parenthood."

Flip your perspective on the anxiety you'll undoubtedly experience. Feeling worried or anxious about having a baby may be normal, but that doesn't make it any less distressing. Anxiety can create very real, very uncomfortable physical sensations, and it can be a tricky emotion to tame when what you're worried about feels so precious to you. Unfortunately, the reality is anxiety tends to ramp up even more after giving birth, as the fear center of your brain gets larger in order to protect your newborn from potential harm. Dr. Sterling sees this as an opportunity to hone your get-calm skills *before* your baby arrives.

Think about it this way: Those who have very little anxiety during pregnancy and experience it after they give birth have no tried-and-true techniques to help them ease their anxiety—not exactly what you want when a new baby has turned life upside down. Anxiety during pregnancy is an opportunity to figure out a plan that helps you manage your emotions before you give birth, so that once your baby is here, you know how to ride the waves of worry that will undoubtedly come as you find your way as a parent.

Let yourself feel all the feels. Pregnancy can feel exciting and leave you in complete awe of how your body can transform. It can also feel overwhelming, painful, exhausting, and even miserable.

"When you're expecting, everyone always asks, 'Are you excited?' but I try to remind my patients that it's okay to *not* feel excited all the time and that the societal pressure to feel excited can lead to a lot of unnecessary guilt," says Dr. Sterling. "No matter where you find yourself on the emotional spectrum, remember that you're working incredibly hard, twenty-four hours a day, seven days a week right now—and that is an accomplishment to be celebrated."

For something many of us think of as one of the most natural things the body is capable of doing, it can be quite a challenge to conceive—and then to know what information to trust (and what to ignore) when you do get pregnant. The antidote: arming yourself with the facts you need to take charge of your reproductive life and to tee yourself up to have a healthy, happy pregnancy.

Chapter 7

Childbirth and Postpartum Health

Preparing for Labor and Delivery, Plus How to

Navigate Your Transition into Motherhood

> *In giving birth to our babies, we may find that we give birth to new possibilities within ourselves.*
>
> —Myla and Jon Kabat-Zinn, *Everyday Blessings*

Few moments in life carry as much significance—and uncertainty—as labor and delivery. In addition to the excitement you may feel when you think about meeting your baby for the first time, there's a good chance you're experiencing a range of other emotions as you prepare for the day. You likely have a ticker tape of questions running through your mind, too.

The postpartum period also has its unknowns. It's a time when reality often feels vastly different from our expectations as we navigate the physical and emotional challenges of caring for a newborn. And sadly, the one postpartum checkup many new moms receive six weeks after giving birth—the one where many of us are sent home with the go-ahead to start exercising and having sex again and a handful of reassurances that everything else we're experiencing is "normal"—can't possibly cover all there is to address.

The truth is that when a baby is born, so is a mother. There are so many shifts that come along with this transition—changes in our identity, relationships, emotions, hormones, bodies, and brains that are considered so significant, this phase of a woman's life actually has a name: *matrescence*. (And yes, it sounds like and can feel just as big as another major transition you went through: adolescence.)

Given the enormity of this transition, feeling prepared is key. So let's get into the nitty-gritty of what you need to know.

In this chapter, we'll learn . . .

- **How to feel prepared for labor and delivery.** We'll go over the stages of labor and what to expect during each, as well as a detailed explanation of Cesarean sections.

- **How to create a birth plan.** From whom you want with you in the birthing room and an explanation of your labor pain-management options to the important role doulas can play, we'll run through the different points you'll want to consider before the big day (including the importance of not getting too attached to your plan due to the utter unpredictability of labor and delivery).

- **Why the Black maternal mortality rate in this country is so high**, and the specific steps every Black woman can take to turn fear into action before giving birth.

- **The physical changes that happen after childbirth**, including what happens to your hormones, the things nobody tells you about your postpartum body, and common complications after delivery.

- **What perinatal mood and anxiety disorders (PMADs) are**, which includes the more talked-about postpartum depression (PPD), as well as conditions like anxiety, scary thoughts, and other common mental health conditions that can surface in pregnancy and the first year after childbirth.

- **How to navigate the transition to motherhood**—a truly transformational time in your life.

Meet the Experts

Nicole Rankins, MD, MPH, ob-gyn and host of the *All About Pregnancy & Birth* podcast

Maren Oser, MSN, CRNP, CNM, certified nurse midwife and women's health nurse practitioner in the Special Delivery Unit at Children's Hospital of Philadelphia

Jamila K. Taylor, PhD, president and CEO of the Institute for Women's Policy Research, who developed some of the most promising policy solutions to address the U.S. Black maternal health crisis

Carrie Pagliano, PT, DPT, doctor of physical therapy who specializes in women's pelvic floor health, spokesperson for the American Physical Therapy Association, and CEO of Carrie Pagliano Physical Therapy

Karen Kleiman, MSW, LCSW, maternal mental health expert, founder of the Postpartum Stress Center, and author of *Good Moms Have Scary Thoughts*

Linda Dahl, MD, otolaryngologist, breastfeeding specialist, and author of *Better Breastfeeding* and *Clinician's Guide to Breastfeeding*

Nicole Pensak, PhD, clinical psychologist certified in postpartum mental health and author of *Rattled: How to Calm New Mom Anxiety with the Power of the Postpartum Brain*

Labor and Delivery: What You Need to Know to Feel Prepared for the Big Day

The Stages of Labor: How Your Body Changes to Give Birth

As you embark on the incredible journey of childbirth, understanding the stages of labor can help you feel more prepared and empowered. Here's what to expect:

- **Early labor.** This stage is characterized by mild contractions that become more frequent and intense over time. These contractions cause the cervix to open (aka dilation) as well as soften, shorten, and thin out (aka effacement). These changes allow your baby to move into your birth canal. How long early labor lasts is unpredictable and has a frustratingly wide range (from hours to days) but it tends to be shorter if you've had a baby before. If you're not considered a high-risk pregnancy, you may be able to spend most of your early labor at home and go to the hospital only when contractions start to get more frequent and intense. That said, it's crucial to talk to your healthcare provider about when to leave for the hospital or birthing center.

- **Active labor.** This is when your contractions will become stronger, last longer, and arrive closer together (typically about three minutes apart), all of which can really ramp up your pain. Your cervix will continue to dilate. During the last part of active labor (aka transition), contractions come very close together and can last sixty to ninety seconds. This is also when you may experience pressure in your lower back and rectum, and you'll be asked to push when you're fully dilated. Active labor often lasts four to eight hours (or more).

- **Your baby's birth.** You'll deliver your baby during what's known as the second stage of labor, which is when your clinician will instruct you on when and how to push. While you may be asked to push when you feel the urge to, there may be other times when you're told to push when you don't feel like it (you may hear the phrase *bear down*, which essentially means to push like you do when you're pooping), hold back from pushing, or push more gently (which can give your vaginal tissue time to stretch and prevent tearing). Once your baby's head is delivered, the rest of their body should follow pretty quickly.

- **Delivering the placenta.** This typically happens within thirty minutes of giving birth. You'll continue to have mild, less painful contractions that are close together, which prompt the placenta (the entirely new organ your body created to sustain your pregnancy and help your baby grow) to detach from the uterine wall and move into the birth canal. You might be given medication before or after the placenta is delivered, to either encourage contractions that will help you deliver it or minimize bleeding once it's out of you. Even after you've delivered the placenta, you'll likely still feel your uterus contracting. These contractions are helping it return to its normal size and decrease bleeding. This is also when any tears that happened during birth (or episiotomy, which is a surgical cut made at the opening of the vagina during birth) will be repaired.

Understanding Cesarean Sections: What's Involved and the New Thinking on When They're Needed

A Cesarean section (aka C-section)—delivery of a baby through surgical incisions made in the belly and uterus—may be performed when it's safer for the mother, the baby, or both. Considering about one in three babies are delivered by C-section in the U.S., it's helpful to know what's involved so you can prepare yourself for this possibility.[1]

» WHAT'S HAPPENS IN A C-SECTION?

Before a C-section, you'll get an IV in your hand or arm to give you fluids and medicine, and receive regional anesthesia (most commonly an epidural or spinal block to numb the lower half of your body while you stay awake). A catheter will be inserted into your bladder to drain urine during the procedure. When you're numb, your clinician makes the first cut (usually just above your pubic bone), followed by another cut in the uterus. Next, your provider opens the amniotic sac and takes out the baby, and you may feel some pulling or pressure when this happens. The umbilical cord is cut, the placenta is removed, and the incisions are closed with stitches or staples. Most women stay in the hospital for a few days after a C-section, to monitor for complications and make sure recovery is happening as it should.

» WHEN ARE C-SECTIONS NECESSARY?

There's a growing awareness of the importance of avoiding unnecessary C-sections, due to their increased risk of infection and bleeding, and longer recovery times after birth compared with vaginal delivery. However, there are situations when a C-section may be necessary, including:

- The baby isn't in a head-down position (aka the baby is breech)

- Contractions do not open the cervix enough for vaginal delivery

- Labor monitoring shows fetal distress (which can happen if the umbilical cord is pinched or compressed) or fetal monitoring detects an abnormal heart rate

- You have certain health conditions that make vaginal birth risky, such as an active genital herpes infection or certain heart conditions

- There are issues with the placenta, including placenta previa—a condition where the placenta partially or completely covers the cervix, increasing the risk of complications such as hemorrhage

- The baby is very large

- You're having more than one baby, like twins or triplets, which can increase the chances of preterm birth or make it less likely that your babies are in an optimal position for vaginal delivery

» WHAT IS RECOVERY REALLY LIKE?

While Cesarean section is the most common surgery performed in the U.S., it's still a major surgery that involves cutting or parting multiple layers of tissue. In many cases, your surgeon will move organs surrounding the uterus (such as the bladder and intestines) aside to more clearly see your uterus. This information isn't meant to scare you but rather to help explain why recovering from a C-section can feel really challenging and take anywhere from four to six weeks.

After a C-section, you may not be able to stand up straight without pain, or you might need help sitting up in bed. Even everyday activities, like getting dressed or changing your baby's diaper, can feel challenging. If this is the case, talk to your clinician about your pain. Physical and occupational therapists can help you figure out how to adjust your movements in ways that will make it easier to navigate daily life as you recover.

If you've had a previous C-section, you may consider a vaginal birth after Cesarean (VBAC) for future deliveries. However, the decision to try for a VBAC depends on various factors, and it's important to talk these through with your healthcare provider.

Labor Pain Management: Knowing Your Options Can Help You Choose What's Right for You

For many pregnant women, anticipating the pain that accompanies childbirth can be anxiety-provoking. But it's important to remind yourself that labor pain is different from other types of pain, it comes and goes in mostly predictable intervals, and you know it's going to end, says ob-gyn Nicole Rankins, MD.

"Having the right mindset about the pain can help you work with your body contraction by contraction, which can make it easier to manage than if you're fighting and fearing the pain," she says.

Above all, remember there's no "right" way to manage your labor pain. The path you choose is personal—and decisions can feel easier to make when you know your options.

» MEDICATION-FREE PAIN MANAGEMENT

Even if you're planning on requesting medication to ease your pain, Dr. Rankins says it's important for all women to be familiar with at least a few medication-free pain-management techniques, because there will likely be some period of time during labor—either before you're able to receive medication, while you're waiting for it to kick in, or if labor progresses quickly or delays happen—when you'll have to manage pain. Here are some of the most common strategies:

- **Focused breathing techniques**. Deep breathing, patterned breathing, and relaxation techniques that incorporate breathwork can help you ride the waves of discomfort and pain that come with labor.

- **Movement and positioning.** Changing how your body is positioned during labor not only can help you find what feels more comfortable but also can help your labor progress. Walking, swaying, rocking, and bouncing or leaning on an exercise ball can be helpful.

- **Massage.** Gentle massage, counterpressure, and other types of supportive touch from your "support person" (a partner, friend, or doula who's with you in the delivery room) can be a pain reliever.

- **Hydrotherapy.** Immersing yourself in warm water, such as a shower or birthing pool, can provide soothing relief.

- **Self-hypnosis.** Often referred to as hypnobirthing, this is a technique that involves using relaxation, visualization, and positive affirmations to manage pain and reduce anxiety.

- **Transcutaneous electrical nerve stimulation (TENS).** TENS units deliver mild electrical impulses to nerve endings, which can help block pain signals. This is a noninvasive pain relief option that can be used throughout labor and has no known effects on the baby.

» MOST COMMON MEDICATIONS USED DURING LABOR AND DELIVERY

- **Intravenous (IV) opioids.** Opioids, such as fentanyl or morphine, may be administered via IV or intramuscularly (with an injection) to reduce labor pain, helping birthing moms relax by taking the edge off the pain of contractions. These are typically used in early labor or as a supplement to other pain relief methods. It's important to note that all opioids cross the placenta and get to the baby—and the baby will clear the medication from their system the same way we do, it just takes a little longer.

- **Nitrous oxide (aka laughing gas).** When inhaled, nitrous oxide (which, when used for labor pain, is most often a mixture of 50 percent nitrous oxide and 50 percent oxygen) provides short-term pain relief and is often used in early labor or during specific procedures that can be painful, such as a cervical check or an epidural shot. It's cleared from your system quickly and has no known risks for the baby.

- **Epidural analgesia.** This involves placing a catheter into the outermost part of the spinal canal (aka the epidural space), through which a combination of a local anesthetic and opioid medication can be inserted to numb the lower body and provide pain relief during labor.

"This generally provides the best pain relief; however, it's not a guarantee," says Dr. Rankins. "For a small percentage of people, it doesn't work or provides pain relief on just one side."

- **Local anesthetic injection.** With this option, medication is inserted directly into the nerves that carry feeling to a particular area, such as the vagina or vulva. It's most commonly used during the later stages of labor—particularly during an episiotomy or repair of a tear after delivery.

How to Create a Birth Plan: Key Components to Include

A birth plan is a written document that outlines your preferences and priorities for your childbirth experience. It's important—there to serve as a guide for your healthcare team.

"Many women give birth in a healthcare system that too often takes away power from women over what happens in their own bodies, and a birth plan can help you advocate for yourself within that system," says Dr. Rankins.

That said, it's also important to understand that you may have to ditch your plan if your baby's delivery takes an unexpected turn. "The only predictable thing about giving birth is that it's unpredictable," says Dr. Rankins. While it's great to have preferences about how you'd like your labor and delivery to unfold, try not to stay too attached to your wishes and remember that being flexible is important.

So what should be included in your birth plan? Here's what to think about and talk through with your clinician:

- **Your support crew.** Whom do you want with you in the delivery room? Your partner? Another loved one? A doula?

- **Delivery room details.** What kind of atmosphere do you want? What's your preferred lighting, music, or even photos you might want to bring with you?

- **Cultural preferences.** Are there social, religious, or cultural practices you'd like to make sure are honored?

- **Pain management.** Do you want to have access to hydrotherapy? Would you like to make sure you can move around freely and change birthing positions as needed? Do you have a preference as to what type of pain relief you'd like your healthcare team to use?

- **Requests for newborn care.** Would you like skin-to-skin contact ASAP? Do you plan to breastfeed?

While this isn't an exhaustive list, it's a starting point when it comes to talking through your options with your healthcare team. Also, Dr. Rankins says it's important to have these conversations early on in your pregnancy and over multiple prenatal visits. This will help you make sure the facility where you plan to give birth can accommodate your wishes and that your provider is on board with—and will help facilitate, when possible—the various aspects you'd like your birth experience to entail.

Ask an Expert

What is a birth doula, what do they do, and should I consider hiring one?

Laboring to bring a baby into the world can be a truly transformative experience—and one that can be unpredictable, overwhelming, and physically and emotionally demanding. In an ideal world, the clinician taking care of you during labor and delivery would be in the room with you for long stretches of time, supporting you through every contraction. But the fact is that we're often taking care of multiple patients at once and can't always stay with you as long as we'd like to. This is where a birth doula comes in.

A birth doula is a professional who is specifically trained to offer support during labor. It's important to note that doulas are not medical professionals, which means they can't perform medical exams or give medical advice. However, a doula can be there alongside healthcare providers to support a birthing person—as well as their support team, such as a partner, family member, or friend. Here are some of the ways doulas do that:

- **They know what's important to you and advocate for you.** Usually, a doula will meet with the birthing person a few times prior to labor so they have a clear sense of what's most important to you. They can also help you think through your birth plan, asking you questions you may not have considered that can help inform your preferences. During labor, your doula will then speak up about those preferences and help you communicate your needs and desires to the clinicians delivering your baby.

- **They provide emotional support.** You can think of a doula as a compassionate ally, offering encouragement and reassurance and also helping you navigate any fears, anxieties, or uncertainties that may surface.

- **They provide physical support, too.** This can include massage or positioning suggestions during labor, as well as help with breathing and relaxation techniques. Doulas often help create a calm and supportive birth environment as well, taking charge of things like dimming the lights, playing your favorite music, or using aromatherapy.

- **They can give your support person a much-needed break.** One of the key roles of a birth doula is to stay with you through active labor. This can also be super helpful for the person you've asked to support you, who will likely need breaks to get some rest or something to eat.

- **They can help support you in those first, important moments with your baby.** After childbirth, a doula may offer help when it comes to breastfeeding, bonding with your infant, and even processing your birth experience. They can also be a great resource for postpartum care. In fact, some doulas work with their clients up to a couple of months after delivery, helping to support your recovery process and adjust to life with a newborn.

Having a birth doula in the delivery room has been shown to have many benefits. Research shows that people who use a doula are less likely to use pain medications or have a Cesarean delivery.[2] Birthing people who have continuous labor support are also more likely to be happy with their birth experience. In fact, doulas can improve outcomes for both the birthing person and the baby so much that they are increasingly seen as playing a critical role in addressing the biases that contribute to our Black maternal health crisis.[3]

To find a doula, you might ask the clinician who'll deliver your baby for a referral or talk to moms in your area for their recommendations. DONA International, which is the first and largest doula training and certification organization, also has a database of certified doulas (dona.org). Then take time to interview one or more birth doulas, asking them things like their philosophy or approach to their work, what's included in their services, and their fee (doulas can cost anywhere from a few hundred to a few thousand dollars, and insurance usually doesn't fully cover this service). It's also crucial to make sure your hospital or birth center allows a birth doula to be in the room with you.

—Maren Oser, MSN, CRNP, CNM, certified nurse midwife and women's health nurse practitioner in the Special Delivery Unit at Children's Hospital of Philadelphia

Overcoming Racial Disparities:
A Black Woman's Guide to Giving Birth

The Black Maternal Mortality Crisis: Why Is Pregnancy and Childbirth Deadlier for Black Families?

The research is shocking and upsetting: The U.S. maternal mortality rate has increased for all racial and ethnic groups, and Black women are three times as likely to die from pregnancy-related causes as their white counterparts.[4] Why?

Jamila K. Taylor, PhD, president and CEO of the Institute for Women's Policy Research, which has developed some of the most promising policy solutions to address the U.S. Black maternal health crisis, says that to answer that question, we must consider our country's long history of medical racism and gaslighting of people of color, particularly Black people—factors that still exist within our medical system today.

Take one survey of white medical students that showed nearly half held unscientific beliefs that Black patients' skin is thicker and therefore Black patients don't experience pain with the same intensity as their white counterparts.[5] Another study found Black pregnant patients were more likely to receive a urine drug test during labor and delivery than white patients, regardless of their history of substance use.[6] Nearly one in four women of color reports mistreatment by healthcare providers, and women of color are around twice as likely as white women to report that a clinician ignored them, refused a request for help, or failed to respond to requests for help in a reasonable amount of time.[7]

"It's clear that our Black maternal health crisis is a result of this country's long history of racial inequality and structural racism," says Dr. Taylor. "This crisis is happening due to racism, not race."

Steps You Can Take as a Black Woman Giving Birth

Here, Dr. Taylor shares her top tips for taking ownership of your health and advocating for yourself in a healthcare system that's stacked against you if you're Black.

- **Prioritize your physical and emotional health.** When you find out you're pregnant (or ideally, before you even start trying), schedule a checkup with a primary care practitioner or ob-gyn to get an overall assessment of your health. If you have a chronic condition, it's important to talk through the potential implications of that condition during the perinatal period—and come up with a plan to manage the condition throughout your pregnancy. For example, controlling high blood pressure in the prenatal and postpartum periods lowers your risk of complications like preeclampsia, which is also a significant risk factor for heart disease later on. It's also important to make sure you're caring for your mental and emotional health and to seek help managing stress, depression, or anxiety. If your risk for physical and/or mental health–related complications is high, talk to your clinician about continued care and monitoring after you give birth.

- **Find a healthcare provider who feels like a partner in your care.** While it can take a lot of legwork and trial and error to find a maternal healthcare clinician you really like, it's worth the effort.

  "There's a chilling effect that often happens when you don't have a good experience with a clinician, and that can lead to not going to a provider for prenatal care," says Dr. Taylor. Try to find a clinician who takes into account any cultural considerations that feel important to you, who listens to your concerns and takes them seriously, and who responds to you in a timely way. You want your provider to make you feel like you're in a shared-power relationship.

  "We're socialized to think that whatever a doctor says is gospel, but it's important to know that you have power in the doctor-patient relationship as well," says Dr. Taylor. "When talking through your health, what you want to feel is a calling in as opposed to the provider calling you out."

- **See a family medicine practitioner if you live in a maternity-care desert.** If there's no obstetrician near where you live, it's still important to get prenatal and postpartum care—and that care can come from a primary care physician if necessary. Midwives and doulas are also great sources of support, and you can also look into accessing maternity care via telehealth.

- **Consider hiring a doula.** The research is clear that if a woman has a doula, it leads to better pregnancy and birth outcomes.[8] If you can't afford to hire a doula or there isn't one in your area, bring a friend or a loved one to your prenatal care appointments, and plan on having them in the delivery room with you.

- **Bring someone with you to your prenatal appointments.** Whether a partner, mom, sister, auntie, or bestie, someone in the room with you during your healthcare appointments and when you give birth can provide support as you advocate for yourself—or even step in and speak up for you, if needed. For example, your loved one might reinforce what you're telling your clinician about something not feeling right to you and can offer additional context when it comes to what's normal for you (think things like mood or pain tolerance) and what's not.

After Birth: Your Postpartum Playbook

The Most Common Complications After Delivery (and How to Spot the Signs of Each)

Once your baby is safely delivered, these are the possible postbirth complications you'll want to stay aware of in the days and weeks that follow:

- **Postpartum hemorrhage (PPH):** This is severe vaginal bleeding following childbirth. This can happen if the uterus fails to contract strongly enough after giving birth to compress the blood vessels where the placenta was attached to your uterine wall. It can also happen if parts of the placenta remain attached to the uterus, or if parts of your reproductive organs are damaged during delivery.

- **Perineal tears and episiotomy complications:** Tears in the area between the vagina and the anus (known as the perineum) can occur during childbirth and may be stitched closed after delivery. Episiotomy is a surgical incision the clinician delivering your baby may make to widen the vaginal opening to prevent tears; this is also stitched closed after your baby is born. Both tears and episiotomy can result in complications such as bleeding, infection, and prolonged pain and/or recovery time.

- **Postpartum infections:** These can occur in the uterus (endometritis), a C-section incision, and the breasts (mastitis).

- **Venous thromboembolism (VTE):** This happens when blood clots form in a deep vein, most commonly in the legs (deep vein thrombosis) or when part of that clot moves to the lungs (pulmonary embolism).

- **Emotional and psychological challenges:** Anxiety, depression, and difficulties coping with the intense demands of motherhood are very common and can last up to a year after giving birth. For a deeper dive into perinatal mood and anxiety disorders (PMADs), see page 191.

The U.S. Centers for Disease Control and Prevention (CDC) lists several urgent warning signs that could indicate a very serious medical complication after childbirth.[9] If you're experiencing any of the following, get medical care immediately.

- Severe headache that doesn't go away or gets worse over time
- Dizziness or fainting
- Thoughts about harming yourself or your baby
- Changes in your vision
- A fever of 100.4 degrees or higher
- Extreme swelling of your hands or face
- Trouble breathing
- Chest pain or fast-beating heart
- Severe nausea and throwing up (not like morning sickness)

- Severe belly pain that doesn't go away
- Heavy vaginal bleeding or leaking fluid
- Swelling, redness, or pain of your leg
- Overwhelming tiredness

Five Things Nobody Tells You About Your Postpartum Body

After childbirth, there's a good chance you'll hear a lot of platitudes about how the physical changes you're experiencing are normal and the importance of giving yourself time to heal. You'll also likely be reminded to love your postpartum body. Yet if we're to authentically revere our bodies for growing and bringing a baby into this world, we have to know what, exactly, is happening and why. Here are some of the changes too few of us talk about:

- **Your uterus may continue contracting.** After you deliver your baby and placenta, your uterus returns to its prepregnancy size—a process (called uterine involution) that can take about six weeks to complete. The contractions you feel are the result of the repeated squeezing and relaxing in your uterus muscle wall, which compresses the blood vessels to prevent bleeding. If you're breastfeeding or pumping, you may feel these postpartum contractions even more strongly: When your baby feeds, your body produces oxytocin, which causes uterine contractions.

- **Bleeding can last up to six weeks after giving birth.** Postpartum vaginal bleeding (aka lochia) happens after both vaginal deliveries and C-sections and is a sign your body is getting rid of tissue and blood in your uterus that helped your baby grow. While bleeding will likely be heaviest in the first three or so days after giving birth, it can continue for six weeks or longer. In the first week postpartum, the blood will likely be dark red and include blood clots (some of which may be as large as the size of a plum). As the weeks go on, bleeding should get lighter and the color will change to pink-brown, followed by a yellowish-white discharge.

- **You may have urinary incontinence.** Postpartum urinary incontinence is the involuntary leakage of urine that can occur after childbirth. You may experience this as stress incontinence (which happens when laughing, coughing, sneezing, or exercising puts pressure on your bladder and you can't control your urine flow). You may also experience urgency urinary incontinence (a sudden, strong urge to pee that's hard to stop). Or you can experience both—a condition called mixed incontinence.

- **Pooping can feel terrifying.** Given how sore you may feel in your perineal area, the first poop you have after giving birth can prompt a lot of fear. What's more, giving birth can irritate any hemorrhoids you developed during pregnancy, which can make that first poop after giving birth painful.

- **You may feel like you're in menopause.** During pregnancy, your estrogen and progesterone reach epic highs. After childbirth, these hormones plummet, similar to what happens during the menopause transition. This can lead to some of the same symptoms. For example, you might wake up in the middle of the night drenched in sweat. You may experience some mood swings. Your hair, which likely grew to its thickest, lushest state during pregnancy, may get thinner and shed. And your vulva may feel more dry than usual. The good news here is that, unlike in menopause, your body will eventually start cycling estrogen and progesterone again, and these symptoms should dissipate.

Beyond Kegels: How Pregnancy and Childbirth Can Impact Your Pelvic Floor, and What to Do for Optimal Pelvic Floor Health

Along with the other physical changes that come with pregnancy and childbirth, pelvic floor issues are common. Yet the symptoms that signal dysfunction in this important muscle group—think peeing a little when you laugh or run and pain with sex—are too frequently written off as "normal" (if annoying) aspects of giving birth. Then, if we do talk to our clinicians about our symptoms, the go-to advice is often to do Kegels, pelvic floor muscle strengthening exercises developed by gynecologist Arnold Kegel in 1948. But this advice doesn't always work and could even make your symptoms worse, because it doesn't take into account the complexity of this group of muscles and the many ways dysfunction can surface, says Carrie Pagliano, PT, DPT, doctor of physical therapy who specializes in women's pelvic floor health.

The pelvic floor is a group of muscles, ligaments, and connective tissues that sits at the bottom of your pelvis and plays a crucial role in supporting your bladder, uterus, and rectum. While this muscle group is often compared to a hammock, it's far more complex—more like a bowl with multiple hammocks made up of muscle, ligaments, and fascia supporting the structure. Here's what it looks like:

Top-down (aka Superior) View

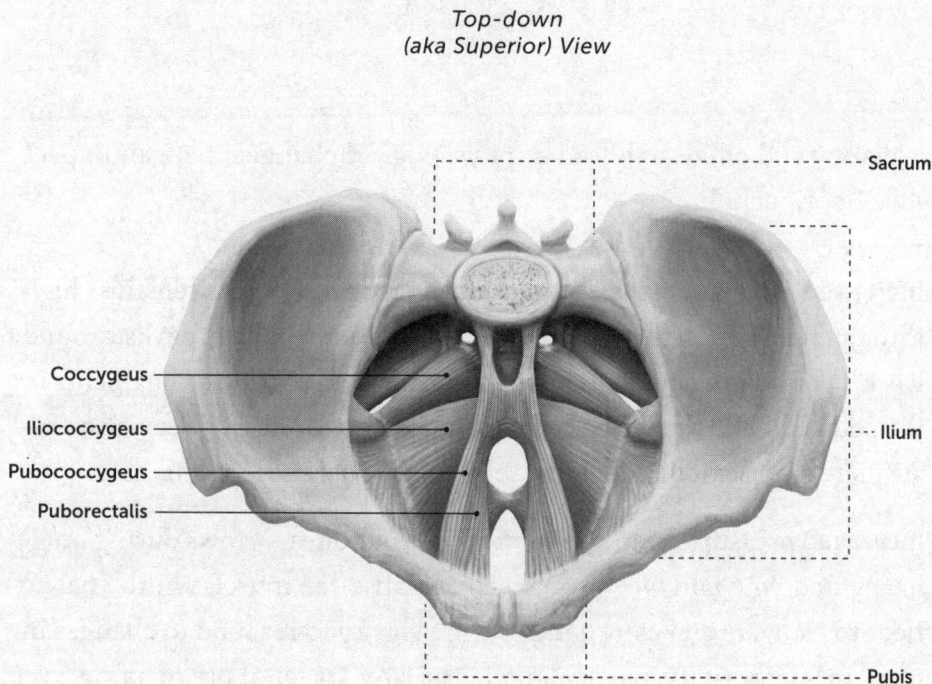

- Sacrum
- Coccygeus
- Iliococcygeus
- Pubococcygeus
- Puborectalis
- Ilium
- Pubis

Side View

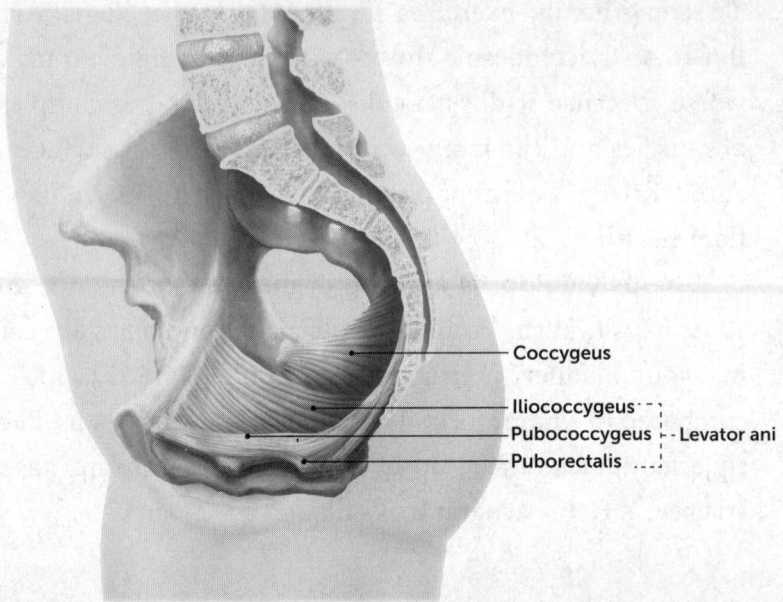

Coccygeus
Iliococcygeus
Pubococcygeus — Levator ani
Puborectalis

Pregnancy and childbirth lead to physiological changes that can impact the pelvic floor, including:

- **Increased levels of the hormones estrogen** (which remains high throughout your entire pregnancy) **and relaxin** (which peaks around week 14 of pregnancy), both of which increase laxity of the ligaments in the pelvis. While this helps prepare your body for birth, it can also create increased flexibility and instability in the pelvic floor muscles.

- **Increased pressure on the pelvic floor** as your uterus grows during pregnancy and you gain weight, which can cause the muscles in the pelvic floor to elongate and can change their capacity to respond to changes in pressure and activity, particularly in the later stages of pregnancy.

- **Changes in your posture** that can happen as your belly grows to accommodate your baby, which can affect the position of your pelvic floor muscles and potentially lead to symptoms like urine leakage and pelvic girdle pain.

- **Significant stretching of the pelvic floor muscles during vaginal delivery,** which enables your baby to pass through the birth canal but can lead to pelvic floor muscle tears or weakness. Having an episiotomy (a surgical incision made in the perineum to make the vaginal opening bigger) or spontaneous perineal tear during your delivery can also affect the integrity and function of your pelvic floor muscles, fascia, and ligaments—all of which support your pelvic organs.

There are a range of symptoms that can happen when your pelvic support structures—including the pelvic floor—aren't working optimally, including:

- **Leaking urine during activities** (stress incontinence) or having a sudden or strong urge to pee and an inability to control it (urge incontinence).

- **Leaking stool** or difficulty controlling your bowel movements (fecal incontinence or fecal smearing, which is having to wipe several times to get clean).

- **Difficulty fully emptying your bladder or bowels,** leading to a sense of incomplete peeing or pooping.

- **Pelvic organ prolapse,** which can involve a feeling of pressure or heaviness in your pelvic region or a visible protrusion of pelvic organs (the bladder, uterus, or rectum) into the vaginal canal.

- **Pelvic pain or pressure,** either intermittent or chronic, including during sex (dyspareunia).

- **Changes in sexual function or sensation,** including decreased sex drive and difficulty having an orgasm.

- **Back pain,** including the lower back, hips, or pelvis, that can be chronic or intermittent (often referred to as pelvic girdle pain).

Pelvic floor dysfunction tends to be one of two types of problems:

- **Pelvic floor hypertonicity,** which is high tone/activity in the pelvic floor muscles; or

- **Pelvic floor hypotonicity,** which is low tone/activity in the pelvic floor muscles

That's right: Despite what society tells us about tighter being better in this region, it's just not true. Like all muscles, your pelvic floor should be able to contract *and* relax. And while it may make logical sense that a weak pelvic floor can have a hard time contracting, a tight, nonrelaxing pelvic floor can have this same issue. If you have hypertonicity, your pelvic floor muscles may already be *so* tight that they can't contract any more. This scenario often results in a misdiagnosis of hypotonicity, because these muscles come across as weak to someone who isn't well trained in pelvic floor health.

"This is one reason why the blanket prescription to do Kegels is wrong," says Dr. Pagliano. "Telling a woman whose pelvic floor muscles are already too tight to work on strengthening them is not going to help her symptoms and could make them worse—and it leads to women feeling like they're broken, when actually they haven't received an accurate diagnosis."

How to Prioritize Your Pelvic Floor Health: An Action Plan

Here, Dr. Pagliano shares her top tips for optimizing the health of this important muscle group.

- **Get an assessment *before* you get pregnant.** If possible, schedule an appointment with a licensed physical therapist (PT) specializing in pelvic health when you're thinking of getting pregnant or soon after learning you're expecting. This can help you make sure your pelvic floor muscles are able to relax—something that's helpful if you give birth vaginally.

- **Remember that pregnancy and childbirth aren't the only factors that contribute to pelvic floor problems.** Dr. Pagliano asks her patients questions like *Did you ever have leakage as a kid when you jumped on the trampoline or giggled? Were you ever constipated as a child or did you wet the bed at night? Did you have pain with sex or when using tampons?* The answers to these questions can help a specialist understand if there was some pelvic floor dysfunction happening before pregnancy and what type.

- **Speak up about your symptoms whenever you have them.** You don't have to wait until your six-week postpartum checkup to talk about urinary leakage, constipation, or pelvic pain. Patients can be treated for such discomforts as early as two weeks after delivery, which not only helps you feel better but can also improve your long-term prognosis, preventing pelvic floor issues from recurring. That said, it's never too late to seek help—even if you're many years past having a baby.

"Perimenopause can prompt genitourinary symptoms that can be exacerbated by pelvic floor dysfunction that was never addressed," says Dr. Pagliano.

Perinatal Mood and Anxiety Disorders (PMADs), Explained

We're hearing more about postpartum depression (PPD) these days, which is great for awareness. After all, up to one in seven women will develop the condition, and for half of them, it'll be their first time experiencing depression.[10] Yet while the term *PPD* is used most frequently, there is actually a spectrum of disorders that can affect women and that can surface in pregnancy as well as the postpartum period. This is why there's a push to talk about mental health across the perinatal period, which includes pregnancy and the first year after a baby is born.

"There's so much stigma around these conditions because we still live in a society that doesn't embrace a new mom feeling not so great about being a new mom, and this prevents too many women from getting help that can make them feel better," says maternal mental health expert Karen Kleiman, MSW, LCSW. PMADs are more common than many of us realize, so it's important to be aware of them so you know when to seek help.

That said, we also need to normalize a new mother not feeling good about being a mother, adds Kleiman.

"The stress of motherhood can endure throughout motherhood, and while a mom may not meet the diagnostic criteria for a clinical mood and anxiety disorder, she may still need support and resources to help her feel like herself again."

PMADs—SYMPTOMS TO KEEP ON YOUR RADAR AND HOW MANY WOMEN THESE CONDITIONS IMPACT

PMAD	SYMPTOMS INCLUDE	IMPACT
Depression/anxiety during pregnancy	Persistent sad, anxious, or "empty" mood; feelings of hopelessness, irritability, guilt, worthlessness; being restless; difficulty concentrating, making decisions, sleeping; persistent doubts about your ability to care for the baby	15–21 percent of pregnant women
Postpartum depression (PPD)	Feelings of fear, anger, and/or guilt; lack of interest in the baby; difficulty making decisions and/or concentrating; appetite and sleep disturbances; thoughts of harming the baby or yourself	21 percent of women after giving birth
Perinatal obsessive-compulsive disorder (OCD)	Intrusive mental images and/or persistent thoughts related to the baby (obsessions); doing things over and over to reduce fears and obsessions (compulsions); having a sense of horror about the obsessions	Up to 11 percent of new moms
Postpartum post-traumatic stress disorder (PTSD)	A traumatic childbirth experience with dreams or thoughts that make you feel like you're reexperiencing the trauma; avoiding things associated with that traumatic event; persistent irritability and/or hypervigilance; experiencing an exaggerated startle response	9 percent of moms
Perinatal bipolar disorder	Symptoms associated with depression (low energy, worrying about the baby, worrying you're not a good mom); symptoms associated with mania (feeling on a high with lots of energy, talking and thinking quickly, strong feelings of self-worth that are out of character); psychotic symptoms (hallucinations, delusions, or disorganized thinking)	70 percent of women with bipolar disorder who stop taking their medication when they get pregnant
Postpartum psychosis	Strange beliefs (aka delusions) and/or hallucinations; decreased need for sleep; significant mood changes; poor decision-making; feeling very irritated; hyperactivity. The onset is usually sudden and most frequently occurs within the first four weeks postpartum.	About one to two of every one thousand deliveries

Source: Postpartum Support International[11]

PMADs Versus the "Baby Blues": How to Tell the Difference

If you're feeling physically and emotionally overwhelmed after giving birth and not like your usual self, you might chalk it up to the "baby blues," which is estimated to affect up to 80 percent of new moms[12] and includes symptoms such as:

- Crying often and not always for a specific reason
- Becoming easily annoyed or angry—and not understanding why
- Feeling exhausted, yet having trouble falling or staying asleep
- Having trouble thinking clearly
- Feeling very nervous around the baby

These are common symptoms during the first two to three weeks after giving birth and qualify as the "baby blues" if they happen within this time frame. If these symptoms or others persist after the first two to three weeks postpartum, it's a good idea to talk to a mental health professional—ideally someone who specializes in perinatal mental health.

Risk Factors for PMADs to Keep on Your Radar

While it's impossible to predict who will deal with a PMAD, certain situations increase your risk, including:

- A family or personal history of mood/anxiety disorder or depression
- A history of severe PMS
- Fertility treatments
- Thyroid changes during pregnancy
- Extreme lack of sleep
- Big life changes (like a new home or job or the loss of a loved one)
- Feeling isolated or lacking social or coparent support
- Childcare-related challenges

- A history of trauma, including domestic violence and systemic racism

- Substance abuse

- Financial stress

- Relationship issues

- Perfectionist tendencies or an anxious or highly sensitive personality

- Difficulty with transitions

- Unrealistic expectations of what motherhood should look like

- Having trouble breastfeeding

Ask an Expert

I'm having terrible, unwanted thoughts about my baby being harmed. Do I need to see a mental health professional immediately?

First, it's important to know that having unwanted, intrusive thoughts about your infant being harmed is extraordinarily common: Research shows as many as 91 percent of new moms (and 88 percent of new dads!) experience them, and as many as half of all new moms report thoughts about harming their baby on purpose.[13] These thoughts are almost always driven by anxiety and are not a sign of psychosis.

The most important question to ask yourself if you're dealing with unwanted thoughts is this: How much distress are the thoughts causing, and how much do they interfere with your ability to get through the day?

If the thoughts you're having are deeply disturbing and extremely anxiety-provoking, and feel inconsistent with who you are, these are ego dystonic thoughts. While these thoughts are highly distressing, they are not actually an emergency. Scary thoughts occur on a continuum from mild to severe—ranging from *What if my baby gets sick?* or *What if the bathwater is too hot?* to imagining details of your infant's violent, graphic death. Thoughts on the more extreme side of that continuum aren't more problematic than the others—they just feel scarier to you and therefore cause more distress. In other words, it's not the content of the thought that's the problem—it's your response and degree of distress and interference caused by the thought that needs attention. Once you can accept that intrusive thoughts are okay, even if bothersome, their power diminishes, and you'll feel less anxiety.

On the other hand, when scary thoughts of harm to your baby present as hallucinations or delusions, are out of touch with reality, and are associated with bizarre beliefs or paranoia, these thoughts are ego-syntonic and are symptoms of psychosis. Psychotic thoughts often present with little or no anxiety, and they are often experienced as acceptable—even though they are deeply disturbing to others. This is why psychotic episodes require aggressive intervention. If a mother does not perceive these thoughts as distressing, her well-being and her baby's well-being could be at risk. The presence of psychotic thoughts requires immediate medical attention and is very treatable.

Far too many women suffer in silence when they're having unwanted thoughts because they fear it makes them a terrible mom and someone is going to take their baby away. The more we talk about intrusive thoughts, the more we'll normalize how common they are and learn that perinatal intrusive thoughts feel scary because they involve our baby, but they are no different from negative thoughts at other times in our lives.

—Karen Kleiman, MSW, LCSW, maternal mental health expert, founder
of the Postpartum Stress Center, and author of *Good Moms Have Scary
Thoughts*

Preparing for Breastfeeding or Chestfeeding: Understanding the Mechanics and Sidestepping Struggles

More than 80 percent of new mothers attempt to breastfeed.[14] (Or, depending on your gender expression, *chestfeeding* may be the better term to describe how you'll feed your baby with milk from your chest as a new parent.) However, fewer than half are still exclusively breastfeeding after three months and only a quarter continue to exclusively breastfeed for six months, according to the CDC Breastfeeding Report Card 2022—and research shows the vast majority of new parents report having problems breastfeeding within days of giving birth.[15] That's because while breastfeeding may be natural, it's not easy, says breastfeeding specialist Linda Dahl, MD. "It's one of the most complicated things we do, and most of what you've been told—even by doctors—about how it works like magic every time is not true."

That said, if you understand how breastfeeding works and some of the most common challenges, it can go a long way toward helping you get the support you need as you explore the process.

A Brief Overview of Breastfeeding

This complex process involves multiple mechanisms to produce, release, and transfer milk from your breast to your baby.

- **Milk production.** During pregnancy, hormonal changes (particularly increases in estrogen, progesterone, and prolactin) stimulate the change from breast tissue to glandular tissue so your breasts are able to produce breast milk. The first milk produced by the breasts is colostrum, and it is incredibly nutrient dense. Two to five days postpartum, there's an abrupt decrease in estrogen and progesterone, which triggers a surge in prolactin, which in turn stimulates more milk production. During this time, the mammary glands begin to change from colostrum to transitional milk and then mature milk. Ten days postpartum—and as long as you are emptying milk from your breasts regularly and fully—prolactin levels remain elevated, which signals continued milk production. The more frequently and effectively milk is removed from the breasts (by either breastfeeding, pumping, or hand expression), the more prolactin levels will remain high and the more milk the breasts will produce.

- **Milk ejection (aka letdown).** Oxytocin is responsible for pushing milk out of milk-producing glands (alveoli) into the ducts and out of the nipple. This hormone is released in response to a baby's sucking or other stimuli associated with infant feeding. It is also released from pleasant touch (from any source), looking at pictures of your baby, and feeling connected. The "milk ejection reflex" that occurs when oxytocin is released causes the muscles around the alveoli to contract, squeezing milk into the ducts and toward the nipple. This reflex, called letdown, allows milk to flow freely for your baby to drink. It begins after thirty to forty-five seconds of pleasant nursing or nipple stimulation, lasts for several minutes, and can happen multiple times in each nursing or pumping session.

- **Infant latching and milk transfer.** Babies are born with reflexes that help them find and latch onto the breast for feeding. The rooting reflex prompts the infant to turn their head toward the breast, open their mouth, and find the nipple. Babies are hardwired to smell an oil around the nipple that helps them "find" the breast. Latching involves the infant unhinging their jaw, taking a large portion of the areola (the dark area surrounding the nipple) into their mouth, and maintaining a tight seal with their lips in order to create enough suction to be able to extract milk from the breast, explains Dr. Dahl. Once latched, infants use their tongue and jaw muscles to create a rhythmic sucking and swallowing motion, and a combination of suction and compression facilitates milk flow and allows effective milk transfer from the breast.

Most breastfeeding struggles stem from one of three issues, says Dr. Dahl:

1. Mom's ability to nurse. This mostly comes down to milk supply, which is her ability to make milk and how much she makes, and can vary depending on a number of factors, including:

- **Frequency and effectiveness of breastfeeding.** Infrequent feedings, short nursing sessions, or a shallow and ineffective latch and suckling can decrease milk supply.

- **Hormonal factors.** Women with higher baseline levels of prolactin or greater hormonal sensitivity may have higher milk production. On the flip side, hormonal fluctuations (whether related to illness, medications, stress, or other factors) can decrease milk supply. Certain medical disorders (like polycystic ovary disease or thyroid disorders) can cause an imbalance in hormones and result in a low or no milk supply.

- **Breast anatomy and physiology.** Factors such as glandular tissue composition and milk storage capacity vary among women and can influence milk production. (Women with more glandular tissue, regardless of breast size, may have higher milk-making ability and storage capacity, and potentially higher milk production as a result.)

- **Nutrition and hydration.** Eating a balanced diet and staying well hydrated supports milk supply and helps restore nutrients lost through breastmilk. Women who are well nourished and well hydrated are more likely to have optimal milk supply.

- **Breast surgery or trauma.** If you had a breast augmentation or reduction or experienced a breast injury or infection, you may have altered breast anatomy or compromised milk ducts, which can affect your supply.

2. Baby's ability to nurse. There are two main anatomical issues that can prevent babies from effectively transferring milk from the breast, says Dr. Dahl. These can happen alone or together:

- **Gape restriction.** When babies are born, they're supposed to have the ability to "gape"—which means to unhinge their jaw when they open their mouths wide to latch. When they unhinge their jaw, it is a relaxed position, so they can use their strength to form a seal and stay latched onto the breast comfortably enough to feed.

When there's a gape restriction, the baby can't unhinge their jaw, which typically results in the baby's mouth sliding down to the nipple and not being able to stay latched and transfer milk efficiently. In this case, breastfeeding often becomes painful for the mom, as the baby's inefficient latch causes friction on the nipple. It also makes it much harder and sometimes impossible for the baby to breastfeed. Gape restriction is a result of certain anatomical factors, such as a high palate (aka roof of the mouth) and set back jaw and can be treated with office-based interventions.

- **Tongue tie**. When babies are in the womb, their whole face and head forms as two pieces until somewhere between four and eight weeks, when it fuses together in the middle. The tongue starts out as two pieces of muscle, fuses together, and connects to the floor of the mouth via a stringy connective tissue called a lingual frenulum. That tissue is supposed to thin and recede in utero. When it doesn't, babies are born with tongue tie, which can restrict the movement of the tongue and make it difficult to latch and suck. It can also cause issues into adulthood, such as tightness in the jaw and quiet or slower speech due to limited tongue movement.

3. How you work together. Breastfeeding happens between two people, which means you have to take into consideration how well (or not) you and your baby are able to work together. There's a physical "fit" to consider. For example, your breast anatomy and/or milk supply may not work with your baby's anatomy: If you have flatter breasts and/or low milk supply, breastfeeding will likely be challenging if your baby has a high palate and recessed jaw. That same baby may breastfeed more easily if the mom has fuller breasts and an oversupply of milk.

The bottom line: If you really want to breastfeed but you're struggling, find a clinician who can help you diagnose and treat (if possible and if you want to treat) the root cause of why you're struggling as early as possible.

"This is where understanding the basics of breastfeeding and the anatomical issues that can happen is key, because otherwise it's impossible to know if the advice you're getting is correct or not," says Dr. Dahl.

It's also important to get honest about what you really *want* to do rather than listening to all of the *should*s when it comes to feeding your baby. If you don't want to continue breastfeeding or do an intervention to fix an anatomical issue that's preventing your baby from successfully breastfeeding, your baby will be fine—and you may be a happier parent for giving up this battle. Remember, there are other ways of feeding and bonding with your little one.

Your Game Plan: Tips to Help You Navigate the Major Transition of Becoming a Mother

Becoming a mom can feel both exhilaratingly expansive and unthinkably difficult at once, which is why it can be helpful to consider how you'll navigate the highs and lows of this time *before* you're riding the waves. Here, Nicole Pensak, PhD, a clinical psychologist who specializes in matrescence, shares her best advice.

Ditch your fantasies about what motherhood should look like. It's so easy to buy into what Dr. Pensak calls the myth of motherhood, which often includes expectations of bonding with our babies immediately, loving our new lives, and "bouncing back" after giving birth. The reality is that it's common to have a lot of conflicting feelings about your new role of mom.

Notice every time you think or say the words *should* or *must*—sure signs you're focused on society's expectations for how motherhood should be going for you rather than how it's *actually* feeling—and transform them into what Dr. Pensak calls "*and* statements." For example, "I shouldn't complain about being so sleep-deprived because I have a healthy, happy baby" becomes "I'm so grateful I have a healthy, happy baby *and* I hate the fact that I'm always so exhausted." Forgetting your old daydreams about what you thought new motherhood would or should look like and replacing them with the reality of the mixed bag it *actually* entails validates that you can have all of these mixed emotions—and still be a great mom.

Give yourself time. So often, we think of the six-week checkup as a benchmark that signals the end of the postpartum period. We get the go-ahead for sex and exercise and think, *Okay, I must be good to go*. But healing after giving birth, both physically and emotionally, is often a monthslong (or even yearslong) process, and the timeline is personal. So be gentle with yourself and remember that the healing and adjustment process your sister or best friend went through may look totally different from your own.

Tee up providers who'll care for your body and mind. Dr. Pensak tells all women who are thinking about starting a family to establish care with a perinatal or postpartum mental health specialist right after they pee on that stick and find out they're pregnant. During the perinatal period, your brain goes through a synaptic pruning process where old connections are eliminated to make way for new ones that help you take care of the tiny human you've just brought into the world. Working with a therapist during this time not only can help you troubleshoot the tough stuff that can surface during this major transition but also can fast-track your personal growth, thanks to your brain's newfound ability to reorganize itself.

"Motherhood is a normative trauma where you have to learn to rise to every relentless challenge," says Dr. Pensak. "With trauma can come the silver linings of newfound resilience, meaning, and purpose—and working with a professional can help highlight and even expedite the ways you're growing."

To find a maternal mental health specialist, search the Postpartum Support International database of providers. Nobody in your area? Inquire about virtual appointments with someone who looks like a good fit for you.

Share your (honest) story. The more we start talking about matrescence and sharing the truth about our postpartum journeys, the more we'll collectively start to destigmatize the challenges and, in turn, more fully celebrate the wins. The truth is that along with all of the opportunities for personal growth that can come with new-mom brain neuroplasticity, there are land mines as well.

"There's still this pervasive thought that the more you suffer, the better a mother you are, but that's BS," says Dr. Pensak. "The more we talk about all the things, the easier a time we'll have of showing ourselves some grace and compassion—and the more likely we'll be to get to a place where we feel like we're thriving."

· · · · ·

Thinking about how you'd like to approach the journey of labor and delivery, as well as what to expect during the postpartum period, can help you feel prepared for—and truly embrace—the physical, emotional, and even spiritual shifts that so often come along with *your* birth as a mother.

Chapter 8

The Endocrine System (aka Your Hormones)

What Hormones Are and
How to Optimize Yours to Feel Your Best

> *Culturally, women receive the message that hormones make them moody, volatile, and incompetent—while also receiving little to no real education about the impact of hormones on their bodies.*
>
> —Elizabeth Comen, MD, *All in Her Head: The Truth and Lies Early Medicine Taught Us About Women's Bodies and Why It Matters Today*

Y ou're so hormonal."

At some point in your life, there's a good chance this statement was or will be used to describe you. You may even use it to describe yourself.

Maybe you've been called (or have called yourself) moody—sad, mad, frustrated, or feeling some other emotion that's a little off from your usual demeanor. Perhaps you have your period, and the perception is that your fluctuating hormones are making you "crazy."

If you're dealing with premenstrual syndrome or in the menopause transition, there's a good chance you have indeed *felt* hormonal—that is to say, you understand symptoms like moodiness, brain fog, and hot flashes are a direct result of your changing hormones. The trope of the "hormonal" woman is so deeply ingrained in our culture that even many healthcare practitioners use it to downplay our (oftentimes life-altering) symptoms. The result? Our hormones are often overlooked and even used against us, when they should be at the center of the conversations we have about our health.

In this chapter, we'll learn . . .

- **What, exactly, a hormone is**—and how the fifty-plus known hormones of the human body send messages that regulate nearly all of your bodily processes.

- **The ins and outs of the endocrine system**, which is made up of various organs and glands that control the secretion of all of these little chemical messengers. This network is genius, complete with a built-in feedback system that monitors hormone levels in your body and secretes more or less as needed to keep your body functioning as it should— what scientists call homeostasis.

- **Which hormones you'll hear about the most over the course of your lifetime**. Yes, we'll cover the sex hormones we're collectively made to believe are the be-all and end-all when it comes to women's health. But we'll also take a look at the brain hormones, stress and sleep hormones, and metabolism hormones.

- **How hormones are supposed to work**, what prompts them to go out of whack, and how they change—every day, every month, and throughout our lives.

- **The symptoms you *can* blame on your hormones**, with explanations to help you understand why your hormones are wreaking such havoc and what you can do about each scenario.

Carrie Jones, ND, naturopathic physician and women's hormone expert

Angela DeRosa, DO, founder of the Hormone Health Institute and author of *A Woman's Hormonal Health Survival Guide*

Tasneem Bhatia, MD, board-certified integrative medicine physician and author of *The Hormone Shift: Balance Your Body and Thrive Through Midlife and Menopause*

Andrea C. Gore, PhD, professor of pharmacology at the University of Texas at Austin, who studies endocrine disruptors

The Endocrine System: Understanding the Processes That Make These Chemical Messengers Work

First, What Exactly Is a Hormone?

Hormones are chemicals that are produced by various glands in the body to function as messengers. As Carrie Jones, ND, explains, you can think of hormones like text messages that are sent from one area of the body to another with instructions on what the recipient needs to do.

"A hormone travels through the bloodstream to a specific cell to tell it to do something," says Dr. Jones. "Once it arrives at its intended location, the hormone then binds to specific receptors either on the surface or inside of the cells there, and this binding triggers a specific response."

Let's say you're super stressed. When your brain perceives this stress, your hypothalamus releases a hormone called corticotropin-releasing hormone (CRH), which then travels to the pituitary gland and tells it to secrete another hormone, called adrenocorticotropic hormone (ACTH). ACTH then hightails it to your adrenal glands with a message to start making and releasing cortisol, "the stress hormone." After cortisol is released into your bloodstream, it travels to cortisol receptors with instructions to do things to help you respond to stress—such as raise your blood glucose levels so you have more energy to run from a threat—and suppress functions that aren't necessary in a true emergency situation, like digestion, reproduction, and some facets of your immune system.

But it's not a one-way system: Hormone secretion is regulated by a feedback loop that helps your body maintain just the right amount of hormones. When a particular hormone reaches a certain level, this signals your body to stop the production of that hormone. (In the case of high levels of cortisol, the hypothalamus and pituitary gland get a signal to reduce the release of CRH and ACTH, which in turn lowers cortisol production.) When this feedback mechanism doesn't work, it can lead to hormone dysregulation—and result in different disorders, depending on the organ(s) involved.

The Organs and Glands That Secrete Hormones

To further understand how your hormones work, it helps to have a basic knowledge of the network of organs and glands that regulate many of the body's functions by secreting hormones. Here are the major players:

- **Hypothalamus:** Think of this as your endocrine system's team captain, which drives the endocrine system and keeps your body in a stable state (aka homeostasis). It acts as a link between your nervous system (the network of cells in charge of your body's thoughts and actions) and the endocrine system.

- **Pituitary gland:** This pea-sized gland located at the base of the brain makes several hormones and also tells other endocrine glands to release hormones.

- **Pineal gland:** This tiny gland located deep within the brain makes and releases the hormone melatonin, which plays a significant role in the sleep-wake cycle—also known as the circadian rhythm.

- **Thyroid gland:** Located at the front of your neck, this gland produces and releases hormones that are mostly related to your metabolism, which is how your body transforms the food you eat into energy.

- **Parathyroid glands:** Situated next to the thyroid are these four small glands that release parathyroid hormone (PTH), which stimulates the bones to release calcium into the blood when blood calcium levels are low to keep our muscles and nerves working well.

- **Thymus:** This gland is part of both the endocrine system and the lymphatic system. White blood cells called T cells travel to the thymus to mature and become specialized to fight infection and disease.

- **Pancreas:** This organ functions as a gland and is part of both the endocrine system and the digestive system. It makes hormones that control the amount of sugar in your bloodstream as well as enzymes that help with digestion.

- **Adrenal glands:** Situated on top of each kidney, these glands produce hormones that help regulate your body's response to stress, as well as blood pressure, metabolism, and the immune system.

- **Ovaries:** In those assigned female at birth, these glands produce and store eggs and make several hormones (particularly estrogen and progesterone) that control the menstrual cycle and pregnancy.

- **Testicles (aka testes):** In those assigned male at birth, these glands make sperm and sex hormones, particularly testosterone.

- **Bone, muscle, fat, and other tissues:** There are a number of other organs and body parts that release hormones or hormonelike substances. For example, fat cells make and release estrogen as well as the hormone leptin (which helps inhibit hunger). The gastrointestinal tract releases appetite-regulating hormones. Your liver, your kidneys, and even your heart also produce hormones that regulate various other body systems and functions. And if you get pregnant, the placenta produces hormones that help maintain a healthy pregnancy and prepare your body for labor and breastfeeding.

The Hormones You'll Hear About Most and What to Know About Each

By now, you're likely starting to see that your hormones work together in elegant—though complex—ways. Having a basic knowledge of some of the biggest hormonal "players" and what they do can help you better listen to your body and understand the signals it's sending, says Angela DeRosa, DO, who walks us through those hormones here.

The Sex Hormones

» ESTROGEN

Most people think of estrogen as one hormone. Yet there are actually three main types of estrogen, each of which plays an important but different role in our bodies.

- **Estradiol (E2)** is the most potent and prevalent form of estrogen during the reproductive years. It plays a crucial role in regulating the menstrual cycle and is also responsible for the development of a female's secondary sexual characteristics, including breast growth and a widening of the hips. Estradiol also plays a significant role in bone health, heart health, and brain function, and works as a powerful anti-inflammatory agent in the body.

- **Estrone (E1)** is the primary form of estrogen your body makes after menopause and can actually convert to estradiol when your body needs it. It's produced mostly in the adrenal glands and fat tissue, though the ovaries also produce some estrone. While it plays a role in reproductive health and sexual function, it isn't as powerful as other types of estrogen. And while estradiol helps reduce inflammation in the body, estrone is pro-inflammatory.

- **Estriol (E3)** is produced in big quantities during pregnancy, with levels rising steadily as pregnancy progresses. (While everyone makes estriol, levels are almost undetectable in those who aren't pregnant.) Estriol's main job is to help your uterus grow as your baby gets bigger, make your body more sensitive to other pregnancy hormones, and prepare your body for labor, delivery, and breastfeeding.

» PROGESTERONE

This hormone plays several key roles in people assigned female at birth, primarily when it comes to preparing your body to get and stay pregnant. It stimulates the growth of blood vessels in your uterine lining, creating a nutrient-rich environment for a potential fertilized egg to implant and grow. (If you don't get pregnant, progesterone levels fall, which prompts the shedding of the endometrial lining—aka menstruation.) Progesterone also modulates the immune response within the uterus, which helps to prevent the mother's immune system from rejecting the embryo thanks to its foreign DNA from the father.

If you don't become pregnant, progesterone still serves you well. It's known to have a calming effect and may help improve sleep. In the context of menopause hormone therapy, you'll hear about the importance of progesterone when it comes to cancer prevention. That's because in those with a uterus, supplementing with estrogen stimulates the growth of the lining of the uterus (endometrial lining). Taking progesterone is necessary to regulate that endometrial growth stimulated by estrogen; it prevents the uterine lining from becoming excessively thick and decreases the risk of excessive cell growth that can lead to endometrial cancer.

» TESTOSTERONE

Think of this as the "male" hormone? Turns out, women actually produce about three times as much testosterone as estrogen during our reproductive years. (As we go through the menopause transition, testosterone gradually declines.) That said, testosterone levels in women are about one-tenth (on average) of what they are in men around the same age. Yet this hormone has a number of key functions in the female body.

Testosterone contributes to libido, mood, and energy and plays a role in the menstrual cycle and fertility. It also impacts bone and muscle health, as well as glucose sensitivity: Testosterone promotes glucose uptake into muscle cells, and low testosterone is associated with higher blood sugar levels and risk of developing insulin resistance and diabetes. And while estrogen and progesterone fluctuate when we have our periods and drop precipitously after we reach menopause, testosterone takes a more gradual decline as we age.

» DIHYDROTESTOSTERONE (DHT)

This is a hormone that's present in women in much smaller amounts than in men. It's produced from testosterone—a conversion process that occurs mainly in the ovaries and skin—and is much more potent than testosterone.

» HUMAN CHORIONIC GONADOTROPIN (hCG)

This hormone is produced by the cells of the placenta when a woman becomes pregnant and triggers your body to make more estrogen and progesterone. It's often referred to as the pregnancy hormone and is the basis for most pregnancy tests. (That's because hCG can be detected in blood and urine around eleven days after conception.) This hormone helps thicken the uterine lining to support a growing embryo and also tells the body to stop menstruating.

The Brain Hormones

» OXYTOCIN

This hormone plays several crucial roles, particularly when it comes to reproduction, childbirth, breastfeeding, and bonding. It's released in large amounts during labor to stimulate the uterine muscles to contract and help you deliver your baby. This hormone continues to be important during lactation: After you give birth, oxytocin causes contractions in your milk ducts to move milk through your breasts, and when your baby sucks at your nipple, oxytocin prompts your milk to be released.

There's a reason oxytocin is also called the love hormone: It's released when we hug, kiss, hold hands, or have an orgasm and is thought to facilitate trust and bonding between individuals and promote relaxation and feelings of stability.

» FOLLICLE-STIMULATING HORMONE (FSH)

During the menstrual cycle, FSH is produced in the pituitary gland and stimulates the ovarian follicles to grow and prepare for potential ovulation. (Only one of the developing follicles forms a fully mature egg, usually around days 10 to 14 of the menstrual cycle.) As the follicles mature, they begin to release estrogen and a small amount of progesterone. In people assigned male at birth, FSH is essential for sperm production (aka spermatogenesis).

FSH levels vary throughout the menstrual cycle. During perimenopause, FSH levels tend to rise (it's your body's attempt to plead with your ovaries to make more estradiol), and they stay consistently higher after menopause, when the ovaries officially "retire."

» LUTEINIZING HORMONE (LH)

When FSH has done its job stimulating the ovarian follicles to mature and estradiol levels have peaked, it triggers the pituitary gland to start making LH. A big spike in LH prompts ovulation. (In fact, this "LH surge" is a key indicator of fertility.) Once a mature egg is released from the ovary, the ruptured follicle transforms into a corpus luteum, which secretes progesterone—and LH supports the formation and function of the corpus luteum. After ovulation, LH is released at a constant pace for the last two weeks of the menstrual cycle. (In men, LH stimulates cells in the testes to produce testosterone.)

During the menopause transition, estradiol may not hit that critical threshold point to prompt LH to surge, which can lead to delays in ovulation—and a longer follicular phase (aka the first part of your menstrual cycle) as a result. This can mean longer stretches between periods.

The Endocrine System (aka Your Hormones)

» GONADOTROPIN-RELEASING HORMONE (GNRH)

Produced by the hypothalamus, this hormone directs the production of FSH and LH in the pituitary gland. In women, this prompts the ovaries to make estrogen and progesterone; in men, FSH and LH cause the testicles to make testosterone.

» HUMAN GROWTH HORMONE (HGH)

Secreted by the pituitary gland, this hormone is responsible for growth in kids and regulates metabolism. It peaks in early adulthood and declines with age. The decrease in HGH is often associated with age-related conditions such as lower bone density, memory loss, sleep disruptions, weight gain, and heart disease.

» PROLACTIN

This hormone is released from the pituitary gland during pregnancy to promote the development of mammary glands within the breast tissues to support milk production. After childbirth, a drop in progesterone increases the number of prolactin receptors in the breast, enabling milk to be secreted through the nipples. Once you've delivered your baby, prolactin levels spike during periods of nipple stimulation (like when your baby is feeding). If you stop breastfeeding, prolactin decreases, and milk production goes down.

The Stress and Sleep Hormones

» CORTISOL

You've probably heard cortisol referred to as the stress hormone for good reason. The adrenal glands pump out this hormone to help the body manage and respond to stress. For example, cortisol increases blood sugar levels by releasing stored glucose. This way your body has a ready source of energy so you can fight or flee—even if you haven't eaten. Cortisol also helps to regulate blood pressure (by increasing the sensitivity of blood vessels to epinephrine and norepinephrine, which constrict blood vessels) and has anti-inflammatory properties that help suppress the immune system.

Cortisol levels naturally fluctuate throughout the day, peaking in the morning and gradually declining by bedtime. However, chronic stress can lead to prolonged periods of too-high cortisol levels, which can contribute to a range of health conditions including weight gain, digestive problems, sleep problems, memory issues, and mood disorders such as anxiety and depression.

» DEHYDROEPIANDROSTERONE (DHEA)

DHEA is produced mainly in the adrenal glands and is a precursor to estrogen and testosterone. It primarily aids in overall adrenal function, helping us manage stress, and also helps promote healthy sleep, muscle mass, energy, immunity, and mood.

» EPINEPHRINE (AKA ADRENALINE)

This hormone plays a crucial role in the body's fight-or-flight response. It's produced mainly by the adrenal glands, and its release is triggered by the nervous system in response to stressful or dangerous situations. Adrenaline is what gets the body ready to fight or flee from whatever danger is in front of us: It increases the heart rate, causes blood vessels in essential areas like the muscles and heart to expand in order to increase blood flow, and constricts blood vessels in nonessential areas; it relaxes the muscles in the airways to allow for improved airflow to the lungs; it boosts alertness, focus, and reaction time.

» NOREPINEPHRINE (AKA NORADRENALINE)

Like adrenaline, this hormone is part of your sympathetic nervous system and plays a big role in your fight-or-flight response. When released during times of stress, it travels to multiple areas of your body—including your eyes, heart, airways, and blood vessels—with a message to react until the stressor has passed. This norepinephrine "message" prompts your pupils to dilate (to let more light in and help you see), diverts blood to your muscles so you can run, makes your heart pump harder and faster to deliver more blood to your muscles (so they can react with strength and speed), and opens up your airways so your body gets more oxygen.

» MELATONIN

Given all of the sleep supplements containing melatonin on the market these days, you likely know this hormone plays an important role in the body's sleep-wake cycle. It's produced by the pineal gland in the brain, which releases the highest levels of melatonin when it's dark and decreases production when you're exposed to light. This helps to explain why melatonin levels typically rise in the evening, peak during the night, and decrease in the early morning—a pattern that keeps our circadian rhythm working optimally. Exposure to light, especially blue light from screens or artificial lighting, can suppress this natural melatonin production in the body and disrupt sleep-wake patterns. The pineal gland gradually produces less melatonin as we age, which contributes to the sleep issues (especially difficulty falling asleep, lighter sleep, and more frequent awakenings during the night) commonly seen in older adults. (For a lot more detail on sleep, see chapter 18.)

The Metabolism Hormones

» INSULIN

We know the food we eat becomes glucose and enters the bloodstream. When the pancreas (which you can think of like your body's glucose monitor) detects a rise of glucose in the blood, it releases the hormone insulin. Insulin's job is to regulate blood glucose by pushing it into the body's cells, where it can be turned into energy. This process is often described using a lock-and-key analogy:

- Think of your body's cells as having locks on their surfaces, which are the cells' insulin receptors.

- When insulin is released into the bloodstream, usually in response to rising blood sugar levels after you eat, it travels to the body's cells and acts like a key.

- When the insulin "key" reaches a cell, it should fit perfectly into the insulin receptor "lock," which triggers a reaction that allows the cell to open up and let glucose from the bloodstream in, where it can be used for energy or stored for future use.

- When insulin is able to get into the body's cells, it lowers the amount of glucose in the bloodstream and helps bring blood sugar levels back to a normal range.

The body regulates insulin production based on blood sugar levels: The more glucose in the bloodstream, the more insulin the pancreas releases in an attempt to lower blood glucose levels. When there's insulin resistance, the insulin receptors on cells—the locks—don't work properly. The result? When blood glucose levels rise and the pancreas produces insulin, there are plenty of keys but the locks are jammed—and glucose can't enter the cells. This leads to continually elevated blood sugar and insulin levels—a hallmark of type 2 diabetes.

» GLUCAGON

When blood glucose levels fall below a certain threshold (think between meals or during prolonged exercise), the pancreas releases glucagon into the bloodstream, which in turn signals the liver to convert stored glycogen into glucose—a process known as glycogenolysis. The newly produced glucose is then released into the bloodstream to raise blood sugar levels and provide energy to the body and prevent low blood sugar (aka hypoglycemia). Glucagon can also prevent your liver from taking in and storing glucose (so that more glucose remains circulating in your blood), and it can help your body make glucose from other sources, such as amino acids.

» INCRETINS

There's a good chance you've heard about this group of metabolic hormones, thanks to the growing popularity of semaglutide (a drug used for weight loss that is commonly known by its brand names, Ozempic and Wegovy) and tirzepatide (Mounjaro and Zepbound). The two main incretin hormones are glucagon-like peptide-1 (or GLP-1) and gastric inhibitory polypeptide (GIP), both of which are secreted from the intestine.

Incretin hormones are released after eating (especially after consuming glucose and fats) and increase insulin secretion from the pancreas to help regulate blood glucose levels after a meal. Incretins also help lower blood glucose by inhibiting glucagon secretion from pancreatic cells, slow gastric emptying (which delays the absorption of nutrients into the bloodstream and leads to a more gradual rise in blood glucose levels), and reduce appetite. Semaglutide drugs mimic the action of GLP-1, which is how they work to help treat diabetes and promote weight loss. (Skip ahead to page 557 for more information on semaglutide drugs.)

» THYROID HORMONES

These hormones—produced by the small, butterfly-shaped thyroid gland at the bottom of the front of your neck—influence almost every organ system in the body and are essential for metabolism, growth, and development. There are several key hormones produced by the thyroid gland and/or related to thyroid function:

- **Thyrotropin-releasing hormone (TRH)** is produced in the hypothalamus to stimulate the secretion of thyroid-stimulating hormone (TSH). It's primarily responsible for initiating the chain of events that control thyroid hormone production and secretion.

- **Thyroid-stimulating hormone (TSH)** is produced by the pituitary gland and triggers your thyroid to release T4 and (to a lesser degree) T3. It operates on a feedback loop: More TSH is released when levels of T4 and T3 are low, and secretion is suppressed when T4 and T3 levels are high.

- **Thyroxine (T4)** is a prohormone, which means it's an inactive molecule that needs to convert to its active form (T3) to trigger a response from the body's cells.

- **Triiodothyronine (T3)** is the active molecule that can impact the body's cells.

- **Reverse T3 (RT3)** is like a decoy molecule that can sit in the thyroid receptors in the body's cells and block the active T3 molecule from getting into the cell's receptors.

- **Calcitonin** is a hormone released by the thyroid gland to help regulate calcium levels in the blood.

When diagnosing thyroid disorders, all of these thyroid hormones should be tested, says Dr. DeRosa, who also recommends testing thyroid peroxidase antibodies (TPO), which develop when the immune system mistakenly attacks thyroid cells, leading to an autoimmune thyroid disease, such as Hashimoto's disease or Graves' disease.

Ask an Expert

It feels like so many women have thyroid disorders. Are they on the rise—and what can I do to keep my thyroid functioning optimally to prevent these conditions?

We are seeing an uptick in the number of women with thyroid conditions, which are already five to eight times more likely to develop in women than in men. There are a couple of reasons for this:

1. We're stressed. The thyroid and adrenal glands work in tandem, and when the adrenal glands produce a lot of cortisol (like they do in times of stress), it impacts thyroid gland production, leaving you with a sluggish thyroid and potentially a deficiency in thyroid hormones.

2. So much of our food is highly processed. This leaves us nutrient deficient, which impacts the thyroid gland.

There are several types of thyroid disorders to keep on your radar:

- **Hyperthyroidism (aka overactive thyroid).** This can be caused by inflammation, nodules on the thyroid, excess iodine intake, or a genetic predisposition. Most often, hyperthyroidism is caused by Graves' disease, an autoimmune disorder where the thyroid gland overproduces thyroid hormones.

  ### COMMON SYMPTOMS:

  - Unexplained weight loss
  - Lack of concentration
  - Muscle weakness
  - Feeling anxious
  - Rapid heartbeat
  - Feeling warm

- **Hypothyroidism (aka underactive thyroid).** This happens when your thyroid gland doesn't make enough thyroid hormones, which can happen during times of extreme stress, when you're pregnant, as a result of taking certain medications, or due to your genetics.

  ### COMMON SYMPTOMS:

  - Unexplained weight gain
  - Feeling tired or weak
  - Memory loss
  - Constipation
  - Always feeling cold and being unable to tolerate cold weather
  - Muscle cramps

- **Hashimoto's disease.** This autoimmune disease develops when your thyroid becomes inflamed and your immune system mistakenly attacks it. It's the primary cause of hypothyroidism and typically progresses slowly over time.

  ### COMMON SYMPTOMS:

  - Swelling at the front of the throat
  - A decline in thyroid hormone levels over time

- Fatigue
- Increased sensitivity to cold
- Dry skin
- Muscle aches, tenderness, stiffness, or weakness
- Constipation

- **Goiters, nodules, and thyroid cysts.** Inflammation in the thyroid gland doesn't always alter thyroid function. The thyroid gland can become enlarged (causing a swelling on the neck known as a goiter), and cysts or nodules can grow on the thyroid gland. All of these conditions should be watched over time to make sure they don't impact your thyroid health.

COMMON SYMPTOMS:

- A lump, swelling, or feeling of fullness or tightness in the neck
- Difficulty swallowing or breathing
- Coughing
- Hoarseness or other voice changes

To gauge the health of your thyroid gland, start with a blood test that checks all of your thyroid hormones as well as thyroid antibodies. As for what you can do to keep your thyroid working optimally, start by assessing your stress. If you notice you're on overdrive, make the time to do something you find relaxing—even if it's just a twenty-minute solo walk around your neighborhood. Also, try to eat foods with the following nutrients that have been shown to improve thyroid health: iron, selenium, magnesium, and iodine. Almonds, Brazil nuts, dark chocolate, iodized salt, leafy greens, red meat, and sea veggies like nori and kelp are all good sources of these thyroid-supporting nutrients.

—Tasneem Bhatia, MD, board-certified integrative medicine physician and author of *The Hormone Shift: Balance Your Body and Thrive Through Midlife and Menopause*

How Hormones Are Supposed to Work,
and Where (and Why) Things Go Wrong

In an ideal scenario, a hormone travels to its intended location with its specific message, the target cell then does what the hormone "told" it to do, and the hormone is then metabolized (the technical way to say the hormone is converted into an inactive form) and excreted by the body—a use-it-then-lose-it scenario that's often referred to as hormone metabolism. Sometimes it's referred to as hormone "detoxification," though that makes it sound like hormones are toxins—and they are not!

Here's the gist of how hormone metabolism works:

- After a hormone has delivered its message, it travels to the liver, where various enzymes modify hormones to make them inactive.

- The kidneys then filter these hormone metabolites out of the blood. Some are then excreted in our urine. Some are excreted into bile and eliminated in feces. Some are excreted through sweat or even exhaled in our breath—though this pathway isn't as common as the others.

- In the case of estrogens, some inactivated estrogens are eliminated by the kidneys via urine. Some head for the intestines, where an enzyme called beta-glucuronidase can actually reactivate estrogen so it can be reabsorbed into the bloodstream. (Interestingly, some of that reactivated estrogen sticks to the fiber in your stool, so it doesn't actually get reabsorbed.)

So What Prompts Hormones to Go Out of Whack?

Your hormones are choreographed to be released at a certain time and day every month. When this choreography is on point, it's like an orchestra playing in perfect balance and harmony. But if there's too much or too little of a certain sound—or in the case of the endocrine system, too much or too little of a particular hormone—that's when things start to feel a little funky and we get symptoms, says Dr. Jones.

Here's what can inspire one or more of your hormonal "players" to deviate from where it should be in the elaborate choreography that is your endocrine system:

Chronic stress. This is one of the most significant contributors to hormonal imbalances, because elevated cortisol prompts the body to focus on essential activities only—and can disrupt the production of other hormones (including your reproductive and thyroid hormones) as a result.

Poor diet and nutrition. Eating nutrient-dense foods is key when it comes to the normal production and regulation of hormones in your body. If a diet filled with excessive processed foods, sugar, and unhealthy fats has led to weight gain, excess body fat can disrupt your hormone balance— especially insulin, estrogens, and testosterone.

Drinking too much alcohol. Alcohol has a big impact on the liver. The body likes to get rid of it quickly, so it gets priority when it comes to what the liver processes. Drink excessive amounts of alcohol, and it'll be what your liver focuses on—and everything else (like hormone metabolites hitting your liver for processing and elimination, which needs to happen for your endocrine system to work optimally) won't be handled as efficiently as it should be, potentially causing problems.

Too much or too little exercise. Intense physical activity (especially for prolonged periods) can raise cortisol levels, which in turn can suppress the production of reproductive hormones like estrogen and progesterone and impact thyroid function. A lack of regular exercise can lead to decreased insulin sensitivity, increasing your risk of insulin resistance and, over time, metabolic conditions like type 2 diabetes.

Poor sleep. Not getting enough shut-eye can impact the production of several hormones, including insulin, leptin, and cortisol.

Acute or chronic disease. When the body is dealing with an illness— especially one that's severe—it can trigger a stress response, leading to an increase of cortisol and adrenaline that can disrupt other hormones. Chronic conditions can impact hormonal glands either directly (as in the case of an endocrine disorder, like diabetes or thyroid disorders) or indirectly via systemic inflammation.

Endocrine-disrupting chemicals. Commonly found in plastics, some personal care products, and pesticides, certain chemicals can actually mimic hormones when they enter your body, causing major confusion to your endocrine system.

The good news is that the endocrine system responds very well to the basics, says Dr. Jones.

"If you get more and better-quality sleep, eat good food, move your body, and spend time doing things and being with people that bring you joy, it's going to positively affect how you make hormones, how they communicate with each other, and how you detox them out of your body," she says.

What Are Endocrine Disruptors— and How Do They Work?

Endocrine disruptors are chemical substances that can mimic, block, or interfere with our hormones once they get into our bodies. This can have significant impacts on our overall health as a result.

"What's scary about endocrine disruptors is that they're ubiquitous," says Andrea C. Gore, PhD, a professor of pharmacology at the University of Texas at Austin who studies endocrine disruptors. You've probably heard about them in plastics (chemicals like bisphenol A, or BPA), but they're also in pesticides used on our foods, in our personal care products, and in industrial pollutants that taint the air—and they've been linked to a range of health issues, including early puberty, developmental disorders, immune system disruption, neurological issues, and an increased risk of cancers (particularly breast, prostate, and thyroid cancers). And they can be especially harmful during prenatal development.

"The old-fashioned view is that a fetus is completely protected from the environment—nothing gets to the fetus other than nutrients from the mom—but we know that endocrine disruptors can get through the placenta and then act like hormones in the fetus's body, influencing the processes normal hormones would prompt," says

Dr. Gore. The result? They can affect growth and development and even lead to health issues that pop up later in life. This is referred to as developmental programming: changes that happen in utero that set the stage for subsequent health events later in life. So what can we do about these chemicals around us and in us?

- **Avoid certain plastics.** Are you one of those people who buy plastic water bottles for convenience? They usually contain both BPA and phthalates, as do many plastic food containers. Don't be fooled by the label "BPA-free." BPA has been found in some of these products despite the label saying otherwise, as well as BPA replacements that are also endocrine disruptors. (You'll see recycling codes 3 and 7 on items made with these chemicals; plastics with codes 1, 2, 4, 5, or 6 are generally safer.) Your best bet is to invest in nonplastic reusable water bottles and food storage containers.

- **Don't microwave food in plastic.** There will be times you just can't avoid eating food packaged in plastic. But heating or reheating that food in plastic can cause chemicals to leach into your food. Instead, use glass or ceramic containers or dishes.

- **Wash your produce.** Pesticides and herbicides commonly used to grow nonorganic food can be removed by washing fruits and vegetables before you eat or prepare them. If it's in your budget, opt for organic produce, which can reduce your exposure.

- **Choose fresh over processed foods.** Many foods—even those that are good for us—can be exposed to chemicals during processing and packaging. Take spinach, for example. Even if it was grown organically and then frozen, it's chopped up, goes into a plastic package, and during that process can easily be exposed to chemicals, Dr. Gore points out.

- **Read labels on personal care and household products.** Many conventional products contain phthalates and parabens, which can act as endocrine disruptors. If it's tough to decipher what's free of these chemicals and what's not, visit the Environmental Working Group's (EWG's) Skin Deep database, which lets you search for products by name, ingredient, and company and will point you to safe picks. EWG also has a database for cleaning products that are free of endocrine disruptors.

Ten Signs Your Hormones May Be Out of Whack

As women, our fluctuating hormones are often blamed for everything that ails us—from mood swings to musculoskeletal pain. And while broadly pointing the finger at the cyclical swings of these chemical messengers is misguided, the fact is that some of the symptoms we experience *can* be blamed on hormones that aren't working optimally. Knowing what health woes are tied to which specific hormones can help you have an informed conversation with your healthcare provider and get to the root cause of your issues. Here, Dr. DeRosa explains some of the most common symptoms of hormone dysfunction and the possible hormone connections for each.

THE SYMPTOM	THE POSSIBLE HORMONE CONNECTION
Acne (especially on the jaw, chin, and neck)	Fluctuations in hormones like testosterone, estrogen, and progesterone can increase the amount of oil your skin produces, ultimately blocking your skin's pores and leading to what we see as acne (like whiteheads, blackheads, and cysts).
Hair loss	Without enough of the thyroid hormones T4 and T3, or with dysfunction in TSH, individual hair follicles don't have the support they need to grow, which can result in hair loss or thinning. Declining levels of estrogen and progesterone during the menopause transition can also trigger hair loss. And testosterone excess can be problematic as well. Some women are also predisposed to hair loss if they have a genetic condition that involves an overconversion of testosterone to DHT, the more potent androgen.
Brain fog	When brain fog feels gradual at first and then becomes chronic, it could mean low progesterone. If your fogginess easily turns into depression, it may be associated with high estrogen. This can also occur with estrogen and/or testosterone deficiency.
Fatigue	When exhaustion won't let up, even when you're getting plenty of sleep and incorporating your go-to stress-busting activities into your daily routine, it could be a sign of testosterone deficiency. Both underactive and overactive thyroid can also lead to tiredness and fatigue.
Bloating, constipation, and irritable bowel	Gut dysfunction and hormone issues may go hand in hand. For example, fluctuating estrogen and progesterone during the menstrual cycle can affect gut motility (the movement of food through the GI tract) and high cortisol can lead to bloating, constipation, diarrhea, or other digestive issues.
Irregular and/or heavy menstrual cycles	Estradiol deficiency is a prime driver of irregular cycles. Low progesterone can mean the lining of your uterus isn't able to shed fully each month and can make your flow more intense the following month. Thyroid, insulin, and cortisol dysfunction can also lead to irregular cycles and heavier bleeding when you do get your period.
Joint pain and/or muscle loss	Estrogen helps to protect joints and reduces inflammation in females, and a dip in this hormone can cause joint pain. Thyroid hormones regulate metabolism, which impacts muscle mass, meaning thyroid dysfunction can lead to muscle weakness and, eventually, muscle loss (sarcopenia). Testosterone deficiency may also cause muscle and joint pain.
Low sex drive	Deficiencies in testosterone, progesterone, and/or estrogen can all impact your libido.
Mood changes	Anxiety, anger, crying spells, depression, and irritability can all be signs your hormones are off. For example, if estrogen is too high or too low, depression tends to be the dominant syndrome. If you have too much testosterone, you can feel angry, on edge, and ready to blow; too little testosterone can dampen your sex drive and prompt fatigue, depression, and indecisiveness. Your thyroid hormones also impact mood: Too much and you may experience fear, worry, and anxiety; too little is more likely to induce sadness and depression.
Weight gain	When your thyroid is underactive, it doesn't produce enough of the hormones that regulate how efficiently your body uses fuel for energy, leading to a metabolism slowdown that can lead to weight gain. Low testosterone is another culprit, as it affects glucose metabolism directly and can lead to insulin resistance, which can in turn prompt weight gain.

Your Game Plan:
How to Keep Your Hormones Working Optimally

If the endocrine system is an orchestra in which all the players hit the right notes and are in tune with one another, your body functions smoothly. But as we've seen, if one or more of your hormones are too high or too low, it can disrupt the harmony, leading to various health issues. So how do we get these hormone "players" working in concert with one another to help you feel your best? Integrative medicine physician Tasneem Bhatia, MD, explains where to start.

Assess your gut health—and take steps to improve it if needed. One of the most important jobs of your gut microbiome—the millions of bugs that live in your digestive tract—is to metabolize and distribute hormones throughout your body. Certain bacteria in the gut have enzymes that modify hormones, either activating, deactivating, or altering their form. If your gut microbiome is thriving, this enzyme activity works effectively, helping you maintain optimal hormonal function and health. When your gut health is off, your gut bugs can't modify, stimulate, and interact with all of your hormones as intended, and hormone dysfunction becomes more likely.

For a quick DIY assessment of your gut health, Dr. Bhatia recommends asking yourself a few questions: Do you go to the bathroom regularly, and does your poop look healthy? This is a sign you're digesting your foods well. (For more on what your poop should look like, flip to page 425.) Do you eat a wide range of foods, especially fiber-rich fruits and veggies? This tees you up to have a diverse, thriving microbiome.

"I've seen countless patients turn around hormone dysfunction just by improving their gut health and making no other changes," says Dr. Bhatia.

Make sure you're eating enough healthy fats. The steroid hormones produced in the body (these include cortisol, estrogen, progesterone, and testosterone) require a crucial starting material, often referred to as a precursor: cholesterol. That's right, this substance so many of us try to keep as low as possible because of its role in the development of heart disease is essential for our hormone health.

Now, that's not to say you should let your cholesterol get sky-high in the name of your hormones. However, it is an argument for making sure you're eating enough healthy fats—like olive oil, avocado, nuts, seeds, wild-caught fatty fish, and grass-finished beef—which will help ensure you're producing enough cholesterol to help your body manufacture the hormones it needs.

Sleep according to your circadian rhythm. Among the many benefits of getting enough good quality shut-eye is hormone health. Sleep influences the secretion, regulation, and function of a number of important hormones, and it turns out *when* you sleep is especially important: Listening to your biological clock (aka circadian rhythm) and sleeping from about 10:00 p.m. until about 6:00 a.m. every day optimizes your melatonin production (which regulates your sleep-wake cycles to keep you on this ideal sleep schedule) as well as regulating your stress hormones, hunger hormones, and reproductive hormones.

Of course, the catch is that during times of big hormonal transitions, sleep is often elusive. The wild hormonal swings of puberty can change the timing and secretion of melatonin and sex hormones, which can make falling asleep more difficult. The major drop in hormones during the postpartum period (coupled with a newborn's wonky sleep schedule) can also lead to frequent nighttime awakenings, fragmented sleep, and less sleep overall. For many women, sleep woes go hand in hand with the perimenopause transition, thanks to hormone changes impacting the sleep-wake cycle, symptoms like night sweats causing frequent awakenings, and even changes in body composition prompting sleep-related breathing disorders (like sleep apnea), which can impact the quality of your shut-eye.

If you're dealing with sleep issues, talk to a specialist who can help assess the root cause of why you're not sleeping well and help you come up with strategies that can help.

Widen your emotional bandwidth. As women, our emotions are often blamed on our hormones in a derogatory way. But the truth is that there *is* a connection between our hormones and how we feel, and recognizing where we are on the emotional ladder can help us clue in to what our emotions might be telling us about our hormonal health, says Dr. Bhatia. For example, if you're feeling lower on the emotional vibration scale—worried, angry, or like you can't kick that negative outlook—there's a good chance you're in a state of hormone depletion. Rather than ignore this lower mood or brush it off as no big deal, can you get curious about why it might be happening?

Where are you in your cycle? Which hormones might be out of sync, given your symptoms? You may not have the answers to these questions, but the inquiry can help you start to see patterns, says Dr. Bhatia.

"This is a great starting point for a conversation with your clinician, who can then help guide you toward the best treatment plan to address your specific hormone issues."

· · · · ·

With this information about the endocrine system and how it works, we can have more informed conversations with our healthcare providers and one another about how our hormones may be impacting how we feel. We'll be better able to recognize when our hormones are being used to explain away our symptoms. Best of all, we'll be able to more deeply appreciate our hormones for the amazing work they do to keep us healthy, happy, and feeling like we're operating at the top of our game.

Chapter 9

The Menopause Transition

Navigating the Big M with a

Sense of Empowerment and Possibility

> *Here's what I really want my patients who are going through this transition to know: It can actually be an incredible time. If you know what to expect and have a doctor who can help you treat your symptoms, you don't have to suffer. And that can put you in a great position to treat perimenopause like the empowering transition it has the potential to be.*
>
> —Mary Jane Minkin, MD, gynecologist and clinical professor in the Department of Obstetrics, Gynecology, and Reproductive Sciences at the Yale University School of Medicine

When it comes to the major hormonal and emotional transitions in a woman's life, puberty, pregnancy, and motherhood tend to get all the attention. That's not a bad thing. Women should feel supported through these important changes, and access to great healthcare, solid information, and support from our circle are essential to helping us move through these big life changes with more ease.

Yet when it comes to the menopause transition—another major hormonal upheaval with long-term health implications—we often talk in whispers, if we talk about it at all. The result? Many of us feel blindsided when those symptoms surface. So we suffer in silence. Or we frantically Google our sudden sleep issues, achy joints, brain fog, and heart palpitations—and freak out. Even those of us who go to our doctors have a good chance of having our concerns dismissed. After all, a whopping 20 percent of medical school residents surveyed said they hadn't had a single lecture on the subject of menopause, and just 7 percent said they felt adequately prepared to care for women experiencing menopause.[1] Astounding for something that roughly half the population will experience.

Which is why the information and advice you'll find in this chapter are so crucial. They'll help you both recognize and understand the changes that can happen during the menopause transition so you can speak up if they start happening to you and get the treatment you need to feel better.

In this chapter, we'll learn . . .

- **The difference between perimenopause and menopause**—terms that are often used interchangeably but refer to decidedly different things—as well as what's happening hormonally during this transition.

- **Some of the health conditions women are at increased risk of developing after menopause** and how to lower your risk of each.

- **The many symptoms of the menopause transition** so you can track what you're experiencing and talk to your healthcare provider.

- **What menopause hormone therapy (MHT)** is, why it was considered controversial for so many years, and the facts every woman needs to know to combat the rampant misinformation that still exists on the topic.

- **How to feel empowered during this transition** so you can create a game plan to treat your symptoms and emerge from this time of your life as a happier, healthier version of you.

Meet the Experts

Mary Jane Minkin, MD, gynecologist and clinical professor in the Department of Obstetrics, Gynecology, and Reproductive Sciences at the Yale University School of Medicine

Cynthia Stuenkel, MD, clinical professor of medicine at the University of California San Diego School of Medicine and a founding member and past president of the Menopause Society

Heather Bartos, MD, ob-gyn and menopause specialist in Frisco, Texas, host of *The Sex Podcast*, and author of *Quickies: One Hundred Little Lessons for Living Sexily Ever After in Midlife*

Vonda Wright, MD, orthopedic surgeon, sports medicine specialist, and author of *Unbreakable: A Woman's Guide to Aging with Power*

Heather Quaile, DNP, women's health nurse practitioner and specialist in menopause and sexual health

Lauren F. Streicher, MD, professor of obstetrics and gynecology at Northwestern University Feinberg School of Medicine and author of *Hot Flash Hell: A Gynecologist's Guide to Turning Down the Heat*

Tanmeet Sethi, MD, integrative family medicine physician and author of *Joy Is My Justice: Reclaim What Is Yours*

Pelin Batur, MD, professor of ob-gyn and reproductive biology at Cleveland Clinic Lerner College of Medicine of Case Western Reserve University and physician lead of the Cleveland Clinic Women's Comprehensive Health and Research Center

Understanding Menopause: What It Is, When It Happens, and the Health Changes It Can Prompt

When you hear the word *menopause*, what comes to mind? Wild mood swings that rival the ones you experienced during puberty? Hot flashes and night sweats? Weight gain and brain fog? While all of these symptoms are associated with menopause, they can also surface during *peri*menopause—the time leading up to your last period. For some women, perimenopause starts as early as the mid-thirties; for others, it can be as late as the mid-fifties. For the majority of women, menopause happens around age fifty-one or fifty-two.

There's a lot to understand about this transition—and a lot of different terms that get tossed around during this important phase of a woman's life. Here, Cynthia Stuenkel, MD, outlines some helpful definitions.

Perimenopause Versus Menopause: What's the Difference?

Menopause is the final menstrual period, which can be confirmed when you've gone a full twelve months with no period. (Keep in mind that if you go six or even eight months with no cycle and then you get your period again for even just one month, the clock gets reset and you'll have to go a full twelve months before you're technically in menopause.)

The menopause transition is the period of time leading up to your final menstrual period and can last months or years. Just as you got your period before or after some of your friends and had no way of knowing when it was going to arrive, there's no telling when exactly you'll enter the menopause transition—or how long it'll last. To get a sense of when it might happen for you, ask your grandma(s), mom, aunt(s), or older sister(s) when they started experiencing the symptoms associated with perimenopause.

The menopause transition is marked by an "early" phase, when you might experience subtle changes in menstrual cycles, and a "late" phase, which is when you may go two or three months without a period and experience other symptoms, such as hot flashes or mood changes.

Perimenopause is technically defined as the menopause transition plus one year after the final menstrual period. This word is often used interchangeably with "the menopause transition," and that's okay, says Dr. Stuenkel. "Technically, perimenopause is just a little longer than the menopause transition," she says.

Once it's been a year since your final menstrual period, you're considered **postmenopausal**, which is the status you'll be in for the rest of your life.

If your final period happens between ages forty and forty-five, it's considered **early menopause**. If your final period happens before age forty, it's called **premature menopause**, and it's often due to primary ovarian insufficiency. If your final period happens after age fifty-five, it's considered **late-onset menopause**. When menopause occurs because your ovaries are surgically removed (bilateral oophorectomy), it's called **surgical menopause**. When it occurs due to a medical treatment like chemotherapy, radiation, or medication, it's known as **induced menopause**.

It's also important to note that if you've had a hysterectomy without oophorectomy (read: when your uterus, cervix, and/or uterine tubes are removed but your ovaries are left in place) you'll likely go through menopause just as you would've if you hadn't had a hysterectomy—although some research shows menopause might happen one to two years earlier than it would've if you didn't have a hysterectomy. That said, once you lose that external cue of your menstrual cycle, it can be tough to know when you're in menopause. This is one of the few cases where hormone testing to diagnose menopause status may be indicated, says Dr. Stuenkel.

"However, keep in mind that hormone testing during this time always comes with a qualification that if levels come back normal, it doesn't mean you're not going through the menopause transition," she says. "It just means we caught you in a place of hormonal normalcy during this jagged-edge road you're on for years." (For more on why hormone testing to gauge menopause status isn't typically recommended, see page 237.)

Factors That Impact When You'll Go Through Menopause

So when will *you* hit menopause? The answer mostly comes down to genetics. If your mom, aunt, or older sister still got their period in their mid-fifties, there's a good chance you will, too. If they reached menopause in their forties, that's more likely to be what happens for you as well. However, there are a few physical and lifestyle factors that are associated with earlier or later menopause.

SOME OF THE FACTORS ASSOCIATED WITH EARLY MENOPAUSE
(BEFORE AGE FORTY-FIVE)

- **Being a woman of color.** Some studies show African American and Latina women are likely to experience natural menopause two years earlier than their white and Asian counterparts. Researchers say one reason for this could be the daily stresses of racism and systemic marginalization, known as weathering, which accelerates health declines.[2] Black women also have the highest rates of surgical menopause (when menopause happens immediately due to the removal of the ovaries).[3]

- **Smoking.** Women who smoke may reach menopause two years before nonsmokers, according to research.[4]

- **Night-shift work.** Some research suggests working rotating night work for ten or more years is associated with a higher risk of reaching menopause under age forty-five.[5]

- **A diet high in refined carbohydrates.** One large study tracked thirty-five thousand women for four years as they entered menopause and found that those with diets high in processed carbohydrates (like pasta and rice) experienced menopause 1.5 years earlier than women whose diet was rich in fish and legumes.[6]

- **Being underweight.** Research shows being considered underweight for your height puts you at a significantly higher risk of early menopause.[7]

SOME OF THE FACTORS ASSOCIATED WITH A LATE-ONSET MENOPAUSE
(AFTER AGE FIFTY-FIVE)

- **Pregnancy and breastfeeding.** Research shows that compared with those who've never been pregnant, women who had one full-term pregnancy lowered the risk of early menopause by 8 percent, two pregnancies by 16 percent, and three pregnancies by 22 percent. If you breastfed your babies, you may have an even smaller risk of early menopause.[8] Experts believe it's because pregnancy and breastfeeding temporarily halt the menstrual cycle, which may slow egg loss and delay menopause.

- **Being overweight**. In most studies, obesity is associated with a later onset of menopause.[9] One explanation: Fat tissue produces a type of estrogen called estrone, which may lead to higher circulating levels of estrogen and delayed menopause (which is prompted by estrogen deficiency) as a result.

Hormonal Changes During the Menopause Transition— and What They Feel Like

Perimenopause is often referred to as puberty in reverse due to the hormonal chaos that goes on during this phase. Here, menopause specialist Heather Bartos, MD, gives us a snapshot of the big hormonal players during the menopause transition, how they change, and what those changes can feel like during perimenopause and beyond.

- **Estrogen** production declines as your ovaries decrease production toward the end of your reproductive years. However, it's not a slow, steady decline. It's often more erratic.

- **Progesterone**, which is produced by your ovaries after ovulation, also fluctuates. During cycles where ovulation doesn't happen (anovulatory cycles), which become increasingly common the closer you get to menopause, your body produces significantly less progesterone than when you do ovulate.

- **Follicle-stimulating hormone (FSH)** skyrockets. As estrogen declines, the pituitary gland and hypothalamus (regions in the brain that are like a control center for hormone production) stimulate production of FSH. You can think of it like a desperate attempt to get the ovaries to get to work again and produce estrogen.

- **Sex hormone–binding globulin (SHBG)** typically drops. SHBG is a protein produced by the liver that binds to sex hormones (like estrogen and testosterone) and reduces their bioavailability, controlling how much of each hormone is free and active in the bloodstream. As estrogen declines, the body recognizes that not as much SHBG is needed, and levels decline.

- **Testosterone** declines with age. After testosterone hits its peak (which usually happens when you're in your twenties) it gradually decreases. By the time you reach menopause, your testosterone levels may be half of what they once were—but it's important to note that there's typically no sharp drop in testosterone during the menopause transition.

- **Cortisol** (the hormone primarily responsible for your stress response) tends to rise, especially during the later part of the menopause transition, which may increase your risk of cardiovascular disease, vasomotor symptoms (like hot flashes and night sweats), and even mood and cognition changes as well as bone loss.

- **Insulin** (the hormone produced by your pancreas in response to glucose in the food you eat) becomes dysregulated, largely thanks to the drop in estrogen, which puts you at increased risk of developing insulin resistance and its related diseases (read: prediabetes and diabetes).

- **Oxytocin** (the feel-good hormone that plays a key role in reproduction and social bonding) declines.

» WHAT THESE HORMONE CHANGES CAN FEEL LIKE IN PERIMENOPAUSE

During the early stages of perimenopause, your menstrual cycle may still be mostly regular, but those erratic changes in estrogen and progesterone levels can lead to annoying symptoms like hot flashes (also known as night sweats when they happen during sleep), fatigue, weight gain, brain fog, mood changes, and many other (we're talking a hundred or more) symptoms. As you progress through perimenopause, your usual twenty-eight-ish day cycle might get a little shorter or longer, and then you'll start skipping cycles.

» WHAT THESE HORMONE CHANGES CAN FEEL LIKE AFTER MENOPAUSE

As the hormonal fluctuations of the perimenopause years start to subside, there's a good chance all those symptoms you experienced will get better—and even go away. And if you ever dealt with painful gynecologic conditions like fibroids or endometriosis, the symptoms of these conditions often improve or even resolve completely, because both fibroids and endometrial tissue need estrogen to grow. Just keep in mind this can take some time after that final period.

Ask an Expert

Should I get my hormones tested during perimenopause?

Your doctor can check your estrogen and FSH levels with a blood test to get a basic sense of what's happening, but the results will only give you a moment-in-time snapshot of your ever-shifting and wildly unpredictable hormones. Sometimes estradiol and FSH levels will be normal because we drew the blood on a day when a perimenopausal woman's ovaries were working. But that doesn't predict what those same hormones will look like tomorrow, when her ovaries may not be working.

This is why hormone tests don't provide a clear picture of where you might be in the menopause transition. Plus, these tests can be expensive. A better indicator of what your hormones may be doing is how you *feel*. What symptoms are you experiencing? When did they start? What is your menstrual cycle like now, and how (if at all) has it changed?

Perimenopause is a retrospective diagnosis, meaning we officially know you went through it once you're past it. That said, good symptom tracking and a detailed conversation with your practitioner should help you get a good sense of whether or not you're in peri-menopause.

—Mary Jane Minkin, MD, gynecologist and clinical professor in the Department of Obstetrics, Gynecology, and Reproductive Sciences at the Yale University School of Medicine

Health Conditions You're at Greater Risk of Getting After Menopause

As if the many changes happening to you physically during perimenopause and in the first few years after menopause weren't intense enough, the hormonal shifts causing your symptoms also increase your risk for certain health conditions. Knowing what they are—and what you can do to lower your risk—can help you take charge of your health.

» HEART DISEASE

Estrogen is like a miracle worker when it comes to maintaining your heart health. It helps keep your blood vessels flexible so they contract and expand as needed to optimize blood flow. Estrogen also promotes a healthy balance of good and bad cholesterol. This may explain why before age fifty-five, women generally have a lower risk of heart disease than men—and why after menopause, when estrogen levels in women go way down, your risk of heart disease rises.

Lower your risk: In addition to following a heart-healthy lifestyle (for more details on this, see chapter 14), it becomes crucial to "know your numbers" in your postmenopausal years—including your cholesterol, blood pressure, and blood sugar levels, all of which can impact your cardiovascular disease risk. Talk to your physician about your heart and, if possible, schedule a preventive appointment with a cardiologist, a heart-health specialist who can look at your specific risk factors for heart disease and work with you on setting a course for optimal heart health.

» STROKE

After age fifty-five, your risk for stroke doubles every decade—and for women who go through menopause before age forty, the stroke risk is slightly higher.[10] Researchers believe lower levels of estrogen may prompt blood vessels to harden and cholesterol to build up on artery walls, which can increase the risk of both heart disease and stroke.

Lower your risk: In addition to the go-tos proven to reduce stroke risk (keeping blood pressure, blood sugar, and cholesterol in the normal range; quitting smoking; limiting alcohol; treating heart disease if you have it; and staying at a healthy weight), it's important to know the signs of a stroke so you can get medical help immediately.

The American Stroke Association recommends learning the acronym FAST:

> **F**—**Face drooping**. Does one side of your face droop, or is it numb?
>
> **A**—**Arm weakness**. Is one arm weak or numb? If you try to raise both arms, does one drift downward?
>
> **S**—**Speech difficulty**. Is your speech slurred, or are you unable to speak? Can you repeat a simple sentence? Is it difficult for others to understand what you're saying?
>
> **T**—**Time to call 911**. If you or someone you love experiences any of these symptoms (even if they go away!), call 911 immediately.

» OSTEOPOROSIS

Throughout your life, bone breaks down and re-forms continuously, and estrogen acts as a signaling molecule for building bone. As estrogen levels drop, bone loss speeds up—and it puts you at greater risk for developing osteoporosis, which happens when the creation of new bone doesn't keep up with the loss of old bone. The result? Bones become weak, brittle, and more prone to breaking.

Lower your risk: The first step when it comes to taking care of your bones is noticing them, explains orthopedic surgeon Vonda Wright, MD.

"Most of us never think about our bones until they fracture," she says, "which is a shame—especially for women. Because when a woman falls and breaks her hip, 50 percent of the time she won't return to pre-fall function and up to 30 percent of the time a woman will die in that first year after a fracture."

To keep your skeletal system in optimal health, focus on lifestyle habits, such as exercise (including lifting weights, jumping, and agility training), eating an anti-inflammatory diet, avoiding tobacco, and drinking in moderation (if at all). Menopause hormone therapy (MHT) can also help prevent bone loss. You can gauge your bone density by getting a dual-energy X-ray absorptiometry (DXA) scan, which measures the strength of your bones. Your results will help your clinician determine whether your bone health is normal or if you have osteoporosis or its precursor, osteopenia. Talk to your clinician to decide on the best timing for your first DXA scan based on your risk factors for osteoporosis.

» URINARY TRACT INFECTIONS (UTIs), URINARY INCONTINENCE, AND OVERACTIVE BLADDER

After menopause, a drop in estrogen can lead to changes in the lining of the bladder and lower levels of lactobacilli (helpful bacteria you can think of as your body's natural defense mechanism against UTIs), which creates an environment that's more vulnerable to infection. Urinary incontinence (the loss of bladder control and resulting accidental loss of urine) and overactive bladder syndrome (the presence of urgency to pee, with or without urinary incontinence) are also more common in postmenopausal women due to decreased estrogen levels weakening the bladder and urethra.

Lower your risk: Low-dose vaginal estrogen is safe and effective at both treating and preventing these conditions. (For more information on how vaginal estrogen works to help prevent and treat UTIs, flip back to page 115.)

Understanding the Many Symptoms of the Menopause Transition: What to Track and Talk to Your Healthcare Provider About

In an ideal world, your healthcare provider would run through a list of symptoms that can happen when you hit perimenopause. In reality, the onus will likely be on you to know the range of what you might experience and bring up what you're dealing with to your doctor so you can talk about treatment options.

Here are some of the most common symptoms that happen throughout the menopause transition:

- **Menstrual cycle changes.** As ovulation becomes more unpredictable, changes in both the timing of your period and your experience of it can change. When estrogen and progesterone stop working reliably during perimenopause, the length of time between periods can get shorter or longer, your flow can get heavier or lighter, and you may even skip some periods. That said, it's important to talk to your clinician about abnormal bleeding and not just assume it's a menopause symptom, as it could be a sign of another health condition.

- **Hot flashes and night sweats.** Also known as vasomotor symptoms, up to 80 percent of women experience them at some point.[11] They are characterized by a sudden feeling of warmth or heat in the upper body (usually the chest, neck, and face) that can cause sweating, a rapid heartbeat, and feelings of anxiety or irritability. Night sweats are hot flashes that occur during the night. (For more on why they happen during perimenopause, see "Anatomy of a Hot Flash" on page 244.)

- **Genitourinary syndrome of menopause (GSM, formerly known as vaginal atrophy).** As estrogen levels go down, the tissues that make up the labia, clitoris, vagina, vaginal opening, urethra, and bladder lose lubrication and elasticity, prompting thinning, drying, or even inflammation that can cause a range of symptoms. These include dryness, burning, and/or irritation in the vulvar area; lack of lubrication, discomfort, and/or pain during sex; difficulty achieving orgasm; bleeding after sex; loss of libido; and urinary symptoms including painful urination, urinary incontinence, urinary urgency, and/or recurrent UTIs.

- **Mood disorders**. Research shows a woman is four times more likely to develop depression during the menopause transition than when she was premenopausal.[12] And women with a history of depression are up to five times more likely to be diagnosed with major depressive disorder during perimenopause than those without a prior history of depression.[13] Fluctuating hormone levels during this time can affect the production and function of neurotransmitters that impact mood, such as serotonin. What's more, the physical symptoms that often come with perimenopause can make you feel like a different person—and inspire thoughts that spiral downward, fast. (*I'll never sleep soundly again! My sex life won't ever be the same! I'm worried I have dementia!*)

- **Sleep disturbances**. Difficulty falling or staying asleep may be due to night sweats, depression, and the stuff of life that often surfaces just as we're going through the menopause transition (caring for aging parents, supporting kids as they launch into adulthood). Fluctuating hormone levels can also mess with your circadian rhythm, prompting you to be more alert during the night and sleepier during the day. The catch, of course, is that not getting quality sleep can make any other symptoms you're experiencing worse. (For a lot more on sleep and tips to improve the quantity and quality of your shut-eye, skip ahead to chapter 18.)

- **Cognitive issues (aka brain fog)**. Experts used to think estrogen affected mostly reproduction. Now we know the brain is full of estrogen receptors, which means this sex hormone impacts the way we remember, concentrate, and think. As estrogen becomes more variable during perimenopause, we may experience more forgetfulness than usual. Other symptoms lumped into the term *brain fog*—including decreased verbal fluency and attention, fuzzy thinking, and more—can also surface. In addition to variations in estrogen, other factors like stress, poor sleep, a poor diet, and lack of exercise can also contribute to cognitive issues during perimenopause.

Other Common Signs and Symptoms of Menopause

COGNITIVE ISSUES AND MOOD DISTURBANCES

- Inability to concentrate
- Inability to remember why you walked into a room
- Anxiety
- Depression
- Fatigue
- Mood swings and irritability
- Low or no libido

SKIN ISSUES

- Dry, itchy skin everywhere (even in places you don't expect, like inside your ears)
- A feeling of insects crawling on skin (formication)
- Thinning hair and other hair changes
- Wrinkles

OTHER ISSUES

- Weight gain
- Breast pain
- Joint pain
- Heart palpitations
- Panic attacks
- Constipation
- Dizziness
- High blood pressure
- High cholesterol
- Dry eyes
- Dry mouth
- Burning tongue and gums
- Lightheadedness
- Headaches or migraines

There are so many wide-ranging symptoms that can surface during the menopause transition. How can I tell if what I'm experiencing is due to perimenopause—or something else?

In my practice, I treat your symptoms. If we try a low-dose estrogen patch, for example, and track you over the course of four to eight weeks and see that your symptoms improve, well, that points to your symptoms being part of the menopause transition. If your symptoms persist, then we'll look at other diagnostic testing to see what's going on.

What women in midlife most need is a healthcare provider who really listens to their story and understands how to provide the nuanced care the menopause transition demands. Unfortunately, what happens more often than not is that women go to their clinician with symptoms of perimenopause—not just the obvious hot flashes and night sweats but heart palpitations, joint pain, brain fog, and itchy skin, eyes, and ears—and they're told that they're just anxious or depressed or, worse, that nothing's wrong with them. This often leads that patient to feel like she's crazy or what she's experiencing is all in her head. What needs to happen is for healthcare providers to really listen to women and believe them, and to understand that even if a patient is in her thirties, she's not too young to be dealing with perimenopause.

—Heather Quaile, DNP, women's health nurse practitioner and specialist in menopause and sexual health

Anatomy of a Hot Flash: Why They Happen—and How They Can Impact Your Overall Health

Experiencing a hot flash—a sudden flush of heat that spreads over your face and upper body, accompanied by a flushed feeling in your skin, increased heart rate, and sweating—can be miserable, and it's incredibly common. As many as 80 percent of women experience hot flashes and night sweats (vasomotor symptoms) during the menopause transition, and research shows they can continue happening for an average of 7.4 years, usually beginning several years before a woman's final period and continuing for an average of 4.5 years afterward. Women who experience hot flashes earlier in perimenopause tend to deal with them longer—a span of 11.8 years on average.[14] Research also shows significant racial differences in hot flashes, with Black women more likely to experience more frequent and intense flashes that go on for more years than women of other races.

» WHY DO HOT FLASHES HAPPEN?

Like so many symptoms of the menopause transition, declining estrogen is a culprit. That's because estrogen helps regulate the "thermoregulatory zone" in your brain's hypothalamus.

As estrogen levels fluctuate during the menopause transition, this zone gets very sensitive to even the smallest changes in core body temperature. This can mistakenly trigger a cooling response when the body isn't actually overheated, explains Lauren F. Streicher, MD, professor of obstetrics and gynecology. Here's what happens:

- Your hypothalamus receives signals from temperature receptors located throughout your body that you are too hot (even if you're not).

- Your hypothalamus then sends a signal to your blood vessels to widen (dilate), which allows more blood to flow to the surface of your skin, where it can dissipate heat.

- Your hypothalamus also triggers sweating, which further helps dissipate heat from the body. (As the sweat evaporates, it helps lower your body temp—sometimes so much so that you'll actually get the chills after a flash.)

If you're experiencing vasomotor symptoms, it's important to know this: They are not harmless and not something to chalk up to "the change" and tough out, says Dr. Streicher. "Hot flashes aren't just about that sudden sensation of heat you feel. They trigger an inflammatory response that impacts every part of your body." In fact, a growing body of research points to links between hot flashes and multiple health conditions, including:

- **Cardiovascular disease.** One study found that women who had at least four hot flashes a day tended to have more signs of cardiovascular disease (CVD).[15]

- **Breast cancer.** Women with persistent hot flashes are more likely to be diagnosed with breast cancer than those who never experienced vasomotor symptoms, according to the large-scale Women's Health Initiative (WHI), which looked at more than twenty-five thousand women and found that those with vasomotor symptoms lasting ten or more years had a higher incidence of breast cancer.[16]

- **Cognitive decline.** Scientists are increasingly interested in the association between hot flashes and cognitive issues such as dementia and Alzheimer's disease. One study found a strong correlation between the number of night sweats a woman has and damage to tiny blood vessels in the brain.[17] But here's the catch: The researchers can't say whether the hot flashes were causing the damage or the changes in the vessels due to lower levels of estrogen during the menopause transition were causing the hot flashes.[18]

» OKAY, SO WHAT CAN WE DO ABOUT HOT FLASHES?

Many women consider hot flashes an inevitable part of the menopause transition and suffer through them silently. However, there are some treatment options that can help—beyond dressing in layers and keeping the bedroom cool while you sleep.

- **Menopause hormone therapy (MHT).** Supplementing with estrogen during a time when it's dwindling can help the hypothalamus (the part of the brain that controls your body temperature) better regulate your internal temp, ultimately reducing the frequency and severity of hot flashes. "Estrogen has the added benefit of treating more than just hot flashes and can help other symptoms of the menopause transition," says Dr. Streicher.

- **Antidepressants and other prescription medications.** The selective serotonin reuptake inhibitor (SSRI) paroxetine (Brisdelle) is a nonhormonal treatment approved by the FDA to treat hot flashes. Other nonhormonal drugs include fezolinetant (Veozah) and elinzanetant, which have been shown to reduce the severity of hot flashes.

- **Cognitive behavioral therapy.** This type of psychotherapy aims to help patients recognize negative behaviors and thought patterns and reevaluate them so it's easier to cope with them. And while this common treatment approach is well known for helping people manage mental health conditions, research shows it may help women manage vasomotor symptoms during menopause, likely by helping you calm the stress response you may have to a hot flash, which can exacerbate your symptoms and make your hot flash last longer and feel more intense.[19]

Caring for Yourself During This Transition: How to Find the Right Support and Emerge Feeling Better Than Ever

How to Find a Menopause Specialist

When you're going through this big transition, feeling like you can talk to your healthcare practitioner about your symptoms—and having confidence that they will take your complaints seriously and talk to you about treatment options, rather than shoo you out of the exam room—is crucial. Yet for many of us, that's harder to find than it should be.

Thankfully, we're starting to see some progress. Menopause clinics are popping up at major university hospitals around the U.S., and a growing number of practitioners are specializing in menopause, going through additional training and getting special certifications to treat this demographic. If you live near one of these institutions or the gynecologist you've been seeing for years has undergone menopause-specific training, you've hit the jackpot. If that's not the case, you'll need to do some legwork. Here's where to start, says Dr. Bartos:

1. Search for a specialist near you. The Menopause Society (menopause .org) maintains a database of healthcare providers who have expertise in menopause care. Use their online tools to plug in your zip code, and you should be able to find a healthcare practitioner in your area who's completed specialized training in menopause care.

2. Ask your doctors and friends for referrals. Talk to your primary care physician, gynecologist, or other healthcare specialists about whether they can recommend a practitioner who specializes in menopause care. Some of the best referrals may also come from friends and family members who've had a great experience with a practitioner. Also, it's important to remember that you might benefit from having a team of clinicians who can help you manage the many symptoms that may surface during perimenopause, including a psychologist for mood issues, a dietitian for concerns about weight gain and even fatigue, as well as gastroenterologists, rheumatologists, and other specialists depending on your specific issues.

3. Clue in to how you feel during your first appointment. Once you've identified a potential menopause specialist, schedule an appointment and ask lots of questions. Inquire about the practitioner's training, menopause certifications, experience, and approach to care. Talk about things like how the practitioner diagnoses and treats menopause-related symptoms and what services they offer. You might even share some of the symptoms you're experiencing and discuss possible treatments.

After your appointment, ask *yourself* some questions: Did you like what you heard? Is the provider experienced in treating women going through perimenopause? Did she feel like someone you can talk to about all of your symptoms (including ones that feel super private or even embarrassing)? Is it someone with whom you feel comfortable advocating for yourself, and who you feel will advocate for you? If the answer to most of these questions is no, keep looking.

The Upsides of Menopause and Why They're Important to Embrace

Far too often, the conversations about menopause we have with our healthcare providers and one another focus on the big bummers that come along with this transition. It's understandable. The changes happening to our bodies and minds—not to mention the way we start to notice society looking at us differently—can feel completely disorienting. It's a natural reaction to grieve for what we once had, worry about what's coming, and resist *the change*.

"Yet there is an open field of possibility in the stark change that menopause ushers in," says integrative family medicine physician Tanmeet Sethi, MD. "It can be a big emotional and spiritual transition—a time to reinvent ourselves and claim what we really want and need."

It sure sounds better than focusing solely on the hot flashes, insomnia, and itchy ears—but where do we start when it comes to seeing the potential to feel vibrant and empowered during our postmenopausal years?

- **See change as possibility**. Think back to other big changes in your life, whether it was a career pivot, a big move, or a breakup. When you were in the thick of the tough emotions those transitions prompted, it was probably difficult or maybe even impossible to see all the ways you were growing. Now, with some perspective, you can likely see how your most challenging moments helped you become the person you are today. Dr. Sethi says recalling those times can help you remember the possibility this change holds as well. "It can help us stay tender about our human tendency to only grieve what we once had by also honoring the potential of what's coming," she adds.

- **Focus on the ways your body's changes are a *good* thing**. No more periods or worrying about birth control are at the top of the list for many women, but the changes go far beyond that. There are also physical changes that happen in your brain that can lead to more emotional control, which often translates to feeling more self-confident and less reactive and being able to move through life with more empathy and emotional stability—all of which correlates with more contentment.

- **Slow down.** In order to figure out what we want to usher into our lives in this new, postmenopausal era, we have to give ourselves some time and space to let the truth bubble to the surface. "We must create space for what needs to arise—and oftentimes this involves taking an intentional pause," says Dr. Sethi. Maybe that means a solo trip or retreat to celebrate this new phase of your life and set intentions. Perhaps it involves simply slowing down a little each morning or evening, giving yourself some time to really think about your day. "These pauses help us step into a more sacred way of being," she says. "They help us learn to honor the menopause transition as an extraordinary part of life."

- **Notice what's happening *inside* your body.** During this phase of life, it can be especially tempting to figuratively step out of our bodies because we don't like what's happening. After all, it's uncomfortable to not be sleeping as well as you once did, or to feel some extra fat around your belly that never used to be there. However, being embodied—cultivating a connection and coherence between our bodies and minds—is how we step into our power. It's how we listen to our bodies' wisdom. It's how we see the symptoms we may be dealing with not as terrible pathologies but rather as part of a *transition*. And it's how we listen to what this change is telling us we really want—and go after it.

The Truth About Menopause Hormone Therapy

Mention menopause hormone therapy (MHT)—or hormone replacement therapy (HRT), as it's still widely called—and there's a good chance you'll see cringes and heads shaking "no." Even some healthcare practitioners are hesitant to prescribe MHT, a science-backed treatment for many of the symptoms of the menopause transition. One large survey found fear of hormones and side effects were the main reasons women didn't want to consider MHT as a treatment for their symptoms. That same survey found a staggering 62 percent of those women said their decision to avoid taking MHT was supported by their physician.[20]

This hesitation on the part of women and their healthcare providers alike has persisted despite years of menopause experts trying to give MHT a much-needed perception makeover. So why does this proven treatment for menopause symptoms still get such a bad rap—and what misinformation about the treatment should you avoid?

» FIRST, WHAT EXACTLY IS MHT AND HOW DOES IT WORK?

MHT involves the use of medications containing estrogen, progesterone, or a combination of both to supplement the hormones that decline during the menopause transition. These therapies are used to alleviate some of the symptoms of the menopause transition and may also help improve bone density and reduce your risk of fractures.

How MHT works depends on the specific hormones you receive. In general, estrogen therapy works to supplement declining estrogen levels in the body. Progesterone is always added to systemic estrogen therapy if you still have a uterus, as progesterone protects the uterine lining (endometrium) from overgrowth, which reduces the risk of endometrial cancer. What's more, there are a number of different ways MHT can be administered—from pills and patches to gels, creams, and vaginal suppositories.

» A BRIEF HISTORY OF MHT: WHAT WE GOT WRONG

Doctors used to routinely prescribe MHT to women dealing with the uncomfortable symptoms of perimenopause. Then, in 2002, its use plummeted thanks to results of a large clinical trial that found that women who received MHT had an increased risk of breast cancer and heart disease.

That trial was one arm of the Women's Health Initiative (WHI), which studied health outcomes for more than 160,000 women, including about 68,000 postmenopausal women between the ages of fifty and seventy-nine. Back in 2002, scientists stopped the arm of that trial in which women were given a combo of estrogen and progestin (a synthetic form of progesterone) because the adverse effects were outweighing and outnumbering the benefits.

The trial's investigators found the risk of heart attacks increased by 29 percent, risk of strokes increased by 41 percent, and risk of breast cancer increased by 26 percent.[21]

These scary stats made news headlines around the world—and understandably prompted hundreds of thousands of women taking MHT to ditch their prescriptions. The use of MHT declined by 46 percent in the U.S. and 28 percent in Canada,[22] and similar data were observed in Europe.[23]

Yet here's the thing: The average age of the women in the WHI study was sixty-three years old, a population that's significantly older than the average age of menopause (fifty-one) *and* a population that's already at an increased risk of breast cancer, cardiovascular disease, and other health issues. In fact, when scientists reanalyzed the WHI findings and stratified the results by age, they found MHT use among women in early postmenopause had a beneficial effect on the heart. As for that 26 percent increased risk of breast cancer? Experts say that stat was not statistically significant. In fact, the risk amounts to one additional case of breast cancer for every thousand women treated with MHT per year—and no increase in the risk of dying of breast cancer.

In the years since the WHI study, experts have continued to look at the data. What has emerged is much more reassuring. The biggest takeaway? The timing of when a woman starts taking MHT is key. Research shows that starting MHT younger than age sixty or within ten years of menopause has a beneficial effect, reducing coronary heart disease and risk of all-cause mortality.[24]

» THE FACTS ABOUT MHT EVERY WOMAN NEEDS TO KNOW

Now that you know what MHT is and the backstory on why it has such a sullied reputation, let's dive into the facts menopause experts want you to know—*and* talk to every woman in your life about—so we can collectively start to rebrand MHT as the helpful, effective treatment it's been scientifically proven to be.

Fact No. 1: MHT isn't intended to replace hormones to premenopause levels.
This is one reason why menopause and midlife women's health specialists are pushing for the term *hormone replacement therapy* (HRT) to be phased

out when referring to hormone therapy prescribed during the menopause transition and after menopause.

"For a woman who is thirty-five and had her ovaries removed due to endometriosis—meaning she's in menopause years before she otherwise would've reached it on her own—we're replacing the level of hormones her ovaries would've made," says Dr. Stuenkel. "That's a scenario when the term *hormone replacement therapy* is appropriate."

On the other hand, if you've recently gone into menopause and you're experiencing symptoms, the hormone therapy you take isn't aiming to fully replace your hormones to premenopausal levels. The goal is to supplement with just enough to ease symptoms and protect your bone health.

Fact No. 2: The estrogen used in the birth control pill (ethinyl estradiol) is much more potent than the estradiol in MHT.

This fact shocks many women, who never thought twice about going on the pill but don't want to take hormone therapy because the perception is that it's a stronger, more potent dose of hormones. This common belief is factually wrong, says Dr. Streicher. "The estrogen in the pill is far more potent than what's in MHT because it has to suppress the hormones that prompt you to ovulate—that's how the pill works," she says. "MHT doesn't need to be that strong because you're not trying to suppress ovulation; you're simply trying to supplement your body with some estrogen."

Fact No. 3: You don't have to wait until you're officially in menopause to see if you're a candidate for MHT.

If you're dealing with hot flashes and night sweats and/or mood disorders during perimenopause—or you're at a high risk for bone loss—you may be a candidate for MHT even if it hasn't been a year since your last menstrual cycle, says Dr. Stuenkel. Also, keep in mind that hormonal birth control like the pill and the noncopper IUD can also be used to help alleviate symptoms like heavy bleeding, mood issues, hot flashes, night sweats, and more.

Fact No. 4: Timing matters when it comes to when you start MHT.

If you're younger than sixty and within ten years of menopause, *and* you have no contraindications (more on those in a few), MHT is considered the most effective treatment for menopause symptoms. If you start MHT more than ten years after menopause—or you're sixty or older—your benefit-risk ratio of taking MHT is less favorable and your risks of coronary heart disease, stroke, and dementia are higher.

Fact No. 5: There are some women who aren't good candidates for MHT.
Just as some women aren't good candidates for birth control pills (like smokers), MHT can also pose risks for women who are at an increased risk of side effects. Your clinician may decide MHT isn't right for you if you have a history of:

- uterine or estrogen-positive breast cancers
- heart attack, stroke, or a life-threatening blood clot
- any hormone-induced blood clots that happened when you were on birth control pills
- MHT- or pregnancy-induced deep vein thrombosis
- unexplained vaginal bleeding that happened while taking MHT

"You really want to give your clinician an accurate, extensive medical history when discussing if hormone therapy is right for you," says Heather Quaile, DNP, specialist in menopause and sexual health.

Fact No. 6: Even if you're not a candidate for systemic hormones, you may be able to use vaginal estrogen.
Current guidelines suggest that those who can't take systemic estrogen *can* be on vaginal estrogen. Why? "Because it's such a small dose of estrogen it's not absorbed systemically," says Dr. Quaile.

However, keep in mind that systemic and vaginal estrogen treat different symptoms. Systemic estrogen helps with symptoms like hot flashes and protects your bones over the long term. Vaginal estrogen eases the symptoms of genitourinary syndrome of menopause, such as vaginal dryness, itching, or burning; pain during sex; urinary incontinence or urgency; frequent UTIs; and painful urination.

Fact No. 7: "Bioidentical" hormones aren't necessarily safer or better than synthetic hormones.

In the wake of the WHI study, many women were hesitant to try traditionally prescribed formulations of MHT but eager to find something else to help treat their symptoms. Enter marketing pros, who started offering up "bioidentical" hormones as a supposedly safer option to the big-pharma options the women in the WHI study were taking. Unfortunately, there's still a lot of confusion about whether bioidentical hormones are a safer option than synthetic hormones.

The fact is that the FDA has approved both bioidentical and synthetic hormones, and one is not necessarily safer than the other, says Dr. Pelin Batur. A bioidentical hormone means the biochemical structure of that molecule is identical to the hormone molecule the body makes. A synthetic hormone means the biochemical structure isn't identical to a hormone—but it still has to be similar enough to fit into its receptor, so it works like a hormone in the body.

"All bioidentical hormones come from the same few places in the world, whether you get that bioidentical hormone from a compounded pharmacy or it's an FDA approved pharmacy," says Dr. Batur. "The benefit is that when it's FDA approved, the FDA is overseeing everything and making sure safety measures aren't being skirted."

You might hear some people talk about compounded bioidentical hormones being safer because they're more "natural," but science has not consistently supported this, says Dr. Batur.

"In fact, a synthetic form of estrogen called Premarin, which is a brand that comes from horse urine, is the only form that's been shown to reduce the rates of breast cancer, as well as the risk of dying from breast cancer," possibly because some of the components of Premarin break down into some of the components found in breast cancer preventive treatments like tamoxifen. "We don't have that same breast safety data for the bioidentical form of estrogen."

Fact No. 8: MHT from a compounding pharmacy isn't necessarily better or more personalized than a prescription you fill at your go-to pharmacy.

In fact, while many compounded estrogens are readily absorbed through the skin, many compounded progesterones aren't as readily absorbed, which can leave you vulnerable to uterine cancer. (Remember, if you're taking systemic estrogen and you still have a uterus, taking progesterone is essential. Estrogen alone can increase the risk of uterine cancer by stimulating the growth of the lining of the uterus.) That said, there are some cases where a compounded hormone prepared at a special pharmacy may be necessary, says Dr. Batur.

"We prescribe compounded hormones when there's not an FDA approved version available and appropriate for the patient," she says. "But it's crucial that compounded hormones are made by a pharmacy where they know what they're doing. The progestogen hormones need to absorb well enough into your circulation to get to protective levels in the uterus, not just treat your symptoms. The good news is that these days, we have multiple FDA approved bioidentical options that come in multiple forms—gels, patches, vaginal rings, and pills."

Fact No. 9: There isn't a testosterone product approved by the FDA for use in women, but many doctors prescribe it off label.

Testosterone gradually declines as we age, and a growing number of menopause specialists are speaking up about testosterone having the potential to treat some menopause-related symptoms.

As of this writing, the FDA has approved testosterone use in men only. However, you may be able to get testosterone from a doctor prescribing it for off-label use. Because testosterone formulations are indicated for use only in men, women are typically prescribed one-tenth the dose. Transdermal formulations are also the preferred method of delivery: Many clinicians will prescribe a gel formulation, which comes in a little sachet (about the size of a ketchup packet) that patients have to divide into ten doses. Pellets and injections are typically avoided, says Dr. Batur, as both may expose you to too-high levels of testosterone.

Finally, keep in mind that while you'll likely hear a lot of claims about what symptoms testosterone can help treat (like muscle strength, fatigue, and general well-being), the only good data we have on using testosterone in women is for libido and sexual function, says Dr. Batur, who adds that it should be prescribed only after a thorough evaluation and consideration of other possible causes of a patient's sexual concerns.

Given the complexities of assessing what type of MHT might be right for you given your symptoms, age, stage of the menopause transition, and health history, it's crucial to find a healthcare practitioner who can work with you on individualizing your plan. You also want to make sure your clinician reevaluates what you're taking every year.

Your Game Plan: How to Feel Empowered Throughout This Big Transition

Navigating perimenopause can be seriously daunting. It's a time that generates a lot of confusion, thanks to countless symptoms and no real way to predict which ones will hit or when. Add to that the fact that most doctors haven't been adequately trained to treat menopause symptoms—not to mention all of the misinformation out there about this transition and its treatments—and it's no wonder so many of us feel like we're floundering during this time.

But it doesn't have to be this way, says Dr. Bartos.

"You don't have to apologize for symptoms, play them down as no big deal, or feel like you're complaining when you talk about debilitating—and, might I add, *treatable*—symptoms," she says. Here's what you can do to feel more prepared for this time in your life and not settle until you get the professional help you deserve.

Keep track of your symptoms, starting sooner than you think you need to. If your periods are still regular, you might think there's no need to keep track of the night sweats, mood swings, or other symptoms you might experience every so often. Yet the best time to start keeping track of the signs perimenopause may be approaching is *before* you're in the thick of symptoms, says Dr. Bartos. You'll want to track your period with as many details as possible: timing, how heavy your flow is, and any PMS symptoms. It's also a good idea to track mood swings, weight gain, hair loss or hair sprouting in new places, changes in your sex drive—even things you might write off as normal signs of getting older or consider no big deal should get written down.

"This is data," says Dr. Bartos. "When you bring this kind of data to your healthcare provider, it's like bringing in a story that will help her help you."

Find a doctor you actually want to talk to about the tough stuff. Finding a healthcare provider who feels like the right fit is important for your health across the board. Yet considering how life-altering the symptoms of perimenopause can be—and how many women feel ignored or minimized when they bring up those symptoms to their doctors—it's especially important to feel like you have an ally. In fact, it's so important that you might consider teeing yourself up with a menopause specialist *before* you hit perimenopause, says Dr. Bartos, so you've got someone in place who can help you when those first symptoms hit.

Share all the gory details with your friends. For many women making their way through the many symptoms that perimenopause can prompt—as well as the changes the postmenopausal years usher in—the best support system is probably going to be peers who are going through (or have been through) similar changes.

"If you're like most women, you did not get 'the talk' from your mom or grandma about what to expect during perimenopause," says Dr. Bartos. "The women who came before you likely suffered in silence—which means they probably didn't feel equipped to give you the tsunami warning they should've."

But this doesn't mean we should follow their lead and stay quiet about what we're experiencing. In fact, sharing all the details with our peers (and daughters!) can help normalize this transition, clue us in to treatments our doctors may not have mentioned, and collectively ditch the stigma that still exists around this natural transition half the human population will experience.

"Whatever you do, don't think you have to be all Pollyanna about it," says Dr. Bartos. "There are parts of perimenopause that absolutely suck. But knowing you're not alone—and leaning on your friends for help—can make it suck a little less."

Change your mindset so you see menopause as a new beginning. There's no denying menopause can be a time of change—not all of it for the better. Yet making our way through the menopause transition gives each of us an opportunity to redefine this time in our lives, says Dr. Bartos.

"In traditional Chinese medicine, menopause is also known as the second spring," she says. "We need to start thinking of menopause like the Chinese do!" Consider the many ways this time in our lives is liberating. No more periods or worrying about birth control. No more PMS, cramps, or surprise cycles.

"The hormonal hell so many women go through during perimenopause is like being in a raft riding down white-water rapids," says Dr. Bartos. "But after menopause, you've made your way down the canyon and you get to the lake, where it's placid and beautiful. This makes it a great time to reassess and recalibrate." Are you as healthy as you'd like to be? Are you on target when it comes to your personal goals? Menopause is a time to actually *pause*—to take stock and make sure you're where you want to be.

"It really can be a freeing, beautiful time—especially if you go into it thinking it can be," she says.

· · · · ·

Thankfully, we're now starting to talk more—and a little more freely and loudly—about menopause. Movies, TV shows, and books are also focusing on menopause, helping us reframe this transition in a more powerful way. Researchers are (finally!) studying this time in our lives in a more substantial way. Even better, we're collectively starting to see that while this transition may be tumultuous, it also holds the possibility of positive changes that can set you up for a healthier and happier future.

Chapter 10

Breast Health

From Lumps to Cancer,

What You Need to Know to Keep Your Girls Healthy

> *Take it from someone who's around breasts all day, every day, and has been known to dream of them at night—women can have very emotional associations with their breasts . . . Our feelings about our breasts run the gamut from pride in their shape and size, to awe over their milk-producing and life-affirming function, to trepidation and dread that someday they may give us cancer.*
>
> —Kristi Funk, MD, *Breasts: The Owner's Manual*

For an area of the female body that gets a lot of attention from the outside world, it's wild how little we're taught about our breasts and how to keep them healthy.

Sure, our breasts inspire awe when we consider their ability to feed our babies and bring us sexual pleasure. But they also inspire immense fear when we wait for the results of a diagnostic test after finding a lump or if we hear the dreaded diagnosis of breast cancer. Our relationship to our breasts is often complex, and it often evolves over the course of our lives.

Yet there's far more to breast health than most of us realize, which is why in this chapter, we'll learn . . .

- **The anatomical basics about your breasts,** including what they're made of and why the major hormonal transitions in your life can lead to big changes in how your breasts look and feel.

- **The different kinds of lumps that *aren't* cancer.** Yes, finding a lump may (understandably!) cause panic. However, almost 80 percent of all breast lumps *aren't* cancer[1]—and knowing what the most common benign breast conditions are, why they form, and what to do about them can help you stay calm as you go down the screening and testing path.

- **Breast cancer screening options,** including the information you need to make a shared decision with your healthcare provider about the right screening plan for you based on your individual risk.

- **How, exactly, breast cancer is diagnosed,** to help demystify the experience of getting a core needle biopsy.

- **The different types of breast cancer** and how it's "staged," so you have a clearer understanding of what every type of breast cancer diagnosis means.

- **Gene mutations associated with breast cancer** beyond BRCA1 and BRCA2, and the information you need to decide if genetic testing is right for you.

- **The importance of accurately assessing your risk of breast cancer, and the tools to do it yourself.** This way, you can bring your results to your next checkup and start the conversation with your provider about *your* risk and the screenings you need.

Meet the Experts

Jeannie Shen, MD, breast surgical oncologist and medical director of the Huntington Hospital Breast Program at Cedars-Sinai Cancer Center

Lisa Larkin, MD, board-certified internal medicine and women's health expert, founder and CEO of Ms. Medicine, and founder and executive director of HERmedicine, a nonprofit committed to advancing free, evidence-based women's health education for women and the clinicians caring for them

Elizabeth Comen, MD, medical oncologist specializing in breast cancer, associate professor of medicine at NYU Langone, and author of *All in Her Head: The Truth and Lies Early Medicine Taught Us About Women's Bodies and Why It Matters Today*

Dorraya El-Ashry, PhD, chief scientific officer at the Breast Cancer Research Foundation

Sabrina Sahni, MD, breast medicine and menopause specialist and assistant professor of medicine at the Jacoby Center for Breast Health at the Mayo Clinic

Healthy Breast Basics, Plus the Changes That Can Happen That Aren't Cancer

Breast Anatomy: What Are Breasts Made of, Anyway?

Female breasts are a remarkable and complex part of the body. Understanding the basics can help you stay in tune with your body, recognize the early warning signs of potential issues, and take charge of your breast health.

Fatty tissue: The amount of fatty tissue varies among individuals and can affect the size of the breast; the more fatty tissue, the larger the breast.

Connective tissue: This helps to support the breast structure and gives it shape.

Lobes and lobules: Lobes are found in the fatty tissue and connective tissue (each breast has around fifteen to twenty lobes). Each lobe contains smaller structures called lobules, which contain groups of tiny, grapelike sacs known as alveoli. Alveoli are responsible for producing milk in response to hormonal signals after giving birth.

Ducts: Milk produced in the alveoli is transported to the nipple through a network of tiny tubes called ducts. Each breast has about ten duct systems that open at the nipple.

Nipple: This is the raised part in the center of the breast.

Areola: This is the darker pigmented area of skin surrounding the nipple. It releases small amounts of fluid during breastfeeding to help to lubricate the nipple.

Blood vessels and arteries: These supply the breast tissue with oxygenated blood and carry away waste.

Nerves: The breasts are filled with nerves, which provide the sense of touch, pain, and temperature. Nipples have hundreds of nerve endings, making them extremely sensitive to touch.

Lymphatic system: There's a network of lymph vessels and lymph nodes—near the breasts, in clusters in the armpit, above the collarbone, and in the neck and chest—which is part of your immune system and helps drain away waste, fluid, or substances like bacteria or damaged cells.

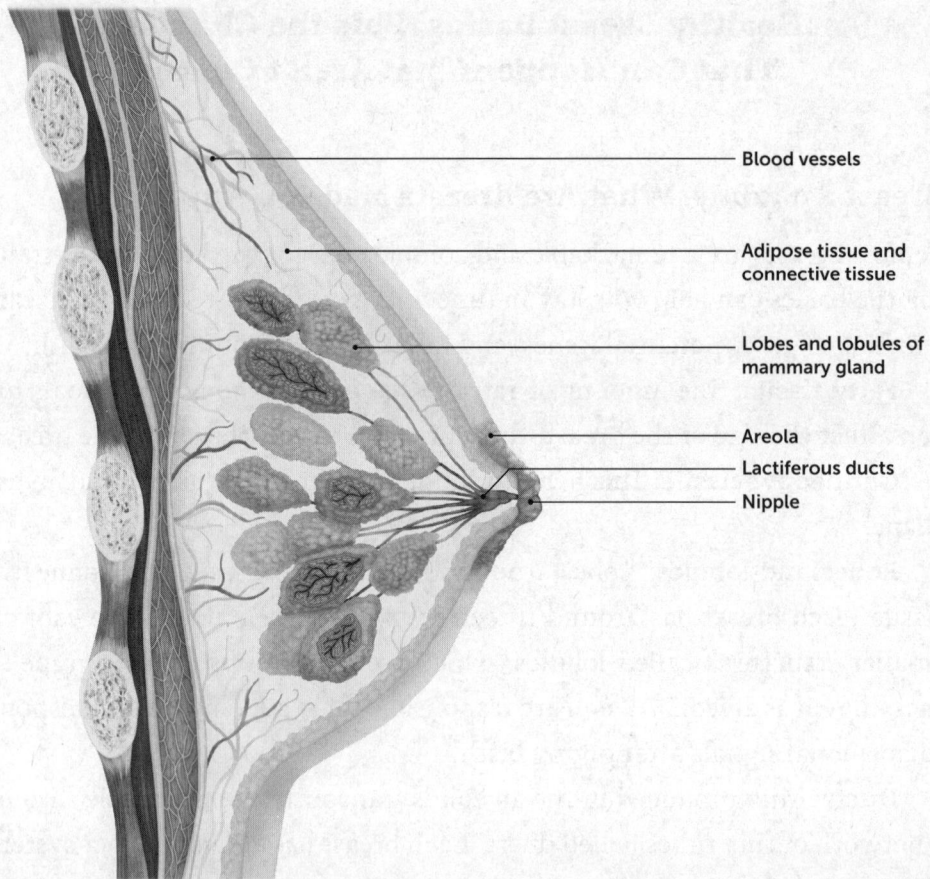

Labels:
- Blood vessels
- Adipose tissue and connective tissue
- Lobes and lobules of mammary gland
- Areola
- Lactiferous ducts
- Nipple

Your Boobs: A Timeline

Breasts go through several changes throughout a woman's life, all of which are primarily influenced by hormonal shifts. It's important to know about these changes and clue in to how your breasts feel at different times. Why? This knowledge will help you know what's normal for you—and make it more likely you'll notice any sudden or unusual changes that could indicate a situation that needs medical attention. These are some of the key changes in breast tissue across a woman's life:

- **Puberty.** As estrogen rises during this major hormonal transition, fat starts to accumulate in the connective tissue, which prompts breasts to grow in size. The breast's duct system also starts to grow. The areola gets larger as well and can become raised, forming a second mound above the rest of the breast along with the nipple. In the final stage of breast development, breasts become more rounded and only the nipple is raised.

- **Your period.** Once menstruation begins, fluctuations in two key hormones (estrogen and progesterone) can lead to changes in your breasts including tenderness, swelling, and lumpiness. During the first half of your cycle, estrogen is predominant and stimulates the growth of milk ducts. In the second half of the cycle, progesterone levels rise, which stimulates the formation of the milk glands. During your period, the glands in your breasts enlarge to get ready for a possible pregnancy, which can lead to a feeling of lumpiness.

- **Pregnancy.** This is a time when breasts undergo considerable changes in preparation for breastfeeding. Breasts often become larger, the areola may swell and get darker, and the small glands on the areola that help to lubricate the nipple during breastfeeding may become bigger and more noticeable. Most people also feel breast soreness during pregnancy and a tingling in the nipples, which is usually due to the growth of the milk duct system and the formation of many more lobules.

- **Breastfeeding.** During lactation, the alveoli (the sacs that produce and store milk) are activated, which can lead to breasts feeling full or engorged. Your breasts may leak (especially at first), and your nipples may be sore as they adjust to your baby's sucking. Your breasts will likely continue to stay large as long as you're nursing, though you may notice they feel smaller after you've fed your baby.

- **After breastfeeding**. When lactation is complete, your breasts should decrease in size—a process that can take about forty days. They may return to their prepregnancy shape, remain slightly larger, or even become slightly smaller than before pregnancy and breastfeeding. Drooping is common.

- **The menopause transition**. There can be a lot of changes in how our breasts look and feel as we move through perimenopause and beyond. For some, breasts get bigger—in fact, about one in five of us needs a new (larger) bra size after menopause.[2] Thanks to the hormonal ups and downs of the perimenopause years, breasts may also feel lumpier, more tender, and even painful at times. After menopause, the glandular tissue in our breasts shrinks and loses shape, and breast tissue can become less dense and more fatty—changes that can make your breasts feel softer. That said, taking menopause hormone therapy is associated with an increase in breast density,[3] which can make breast cancer harder to detect via mammogram (and may mean you need additional screenings).

Lumps That Aren't Cancer: Why They Form and What to Do About Them

At some point in your life, the odds are high that you will see or feel a lump in your breast. When that happens, there's also a very good chance your mind will travel down a worst-case-scenario spiral, and you'll convince yourself it's breast cancer. Here is the number one thing to remember in this moment, says breast surgeon oncologist Jeannie Shen, MD: A whopping 60 to 80 percent of breast lumps aren't cancer or even precancer.[4] In fact, they're so often nothing to worry about that the standard recommendation is to take note of where you are in your cycle when you first noticed the lump, then wait until you finish your *next* period and see if the lump is still there or not.

"If the lump goes away, it's not cancer," says Dr. Shen. "Cancer doesn't play peekaboo—it doesn't come and go." Benign lumps can fluctuate in size and even go away completely without your doing anything. That's because they are naturally responsive to hormones, explains Dr. Shen, and even normal fluctuations in estrogen and progesterone can make breast lumps grow or shrink.

However, the advice is different for women after menopause, who aren't going through the same hormonal fluctuations as younger women and whose risk of breast cancer is already higher. So if you find a breast lump after menopause, get it checked out right away, says Dr. Shen.

The Most Common Noncancerous Lumps

» CYSTS

Many breast lumps turn out to be fibrous tissue (fibrosis) and/or cysts, which are often referred to as fibrocystic changes in breast tissue. Cysts are fluid-filled sacs inside the breast, and they're very common. While experts don't know exactly what causes breast cysts, they do know they are naturally responsive to hormones, which is why they're more common in women under age fifty and in postmenopausal women who take hormone therapy.

Signs and Symptoms

Cysts typically feel like a smooth, movable lump and may be tender or even painful to the touch. You may notice an increase in their size just before your period and a decrease in size after your period.

Treatment Options

An ultrasound can confirm that what you're feeling is a cyst. If you're experiencing pain, your doctor may recommend aspirating the cyst—a quick and simple procedure to drain the fluid inside the cyst. This isn't necessarily a long-term fix, as cysts have a tendency to grow back. However, if you do opt for aspiration, make sure it's done with imaging guidance, suggests Dr. Shen.

"The standard of care is to aspirate under ultrasound, which helps us make sure the cyst completely collapses and makes it less likely to grow back. The ultrasound can also show us if there's anything inside the cyst—junky cells that have shed into it called debris." If your cyst has debris inside, your doctor will do a core needle biopsy to test it for cancer. Cancerous "debris" inside a cyst is rare, occurring in less than 1 percent of cysts in premenopausal women and less than 5 percent of those in postmenopausal women, adds Dr. Shen.

» FIBROADENOMA

This is a solid breast lump that isn't cancer and is most common between the ages of fifteen and thirty-five, though this type of lump can be found at any age in women who are still getting their periods. As with breast cysts, experts haven't pinpointed exactly what causes them to form. They do know fibroadenomas are sensitive to estrogen and tend to grow during pregnancy and shrink during menopause. Females who take oral contraceptives before age twenty also tend to get these breast lumps at higher rates than the general population.[5]

Signs and Symptoms

Fibroadenomas usually feel firm, smooth, and rubbery; they've been described as having a consistency similar to a handball. They're also easily moved and can change in size during big hormonal transitions like adolescence, pregnancy, or menopause, or during hormonal treatment (like menopause hormone therapy).

Treatment

If a fibroadenoma is small and asymptomatic and the diagnosis is certain, your doctor will likely recommend observation with periodic checkups. In some cases, your doctor will confirm the diagnosis by performing a biopsy, which involves taking a small sample of tissue from the lump and testing it for cancer. In cases where a fibroadenoma is large, causing pain, or growing, surgery to remove the lump is an option. Cryoablation (a nonsurgical treatment where a thin probe is used to freeze and destroy the fibroadenoma) is also an option for some fibroadenomas.

» ABSCESS

A breast abscess is a painful collection of pus that forms in the breast due to an infection, often caused by bacteria that enter the breast tissue through a damaged or cracked nipple. This condition is more common in women who are breastfeeding.

Signs and Symptoms

An abscess usually causes tenderness or pain in the area of the breast in which it develops and can be detected as a visible lump or swelling, redness, and even warmth over the skin of the affected area. You might even experience fever and flu-like symptoms—signs your immune system is hard at work fighting the infection that caused the abscess.

Treatment

If you suspect a breast abscess, make an appointment with your healthcare provider as soon as possible, as delaying treatment can lead to complications, including the infection spreading to other parts of your body. Treatment usually involves antibiotics to help fight the infection; in some cases, an abscess may need to be drained with a needle. In more severe cases, surgery may be needed to remove the abscess.

» CALCIFICATIONS

These are small deposits of calcium that show up on a mammogram as a bright white speck on the soft tissue of the breasts. They're especially common after age fifty and are usually noncancerous. However, certain patterns of calcifications may indicate breast cancer or precancerous changes, which means you'll likely be called back for more imagery if your initial mammogram shows calcifications.

Signs and Symptoms

You won't know you have calcifications until you get a mammogram.

Treatment

If the radiologist reading your mammogram spots calcifications, they will look closely to see if the spots have any features suggestive of an underlying cancer. The size, the appearance, and how the calcifications are distributed in the breast tissue can signal to doctors if they're more likely to be benign or associated with cancer.

» INTRADUCTAL PAPILLOMAS

These are benign tumors that grow in the milk ducts. There can be one (a solitary papilloma), which usually grows in the large milk ducts near the nipple, or there can be several (multiple papillomas) that are found in small ducts farther from the nipple.

Signs and Symptoms

Papillomas can cause symptoms (such as clear or bloody nipple discharge or a breast lump), or they can show up as abnormal areas on imaging tests.

Treatment

Depending partly on the size of the papilloma(s), they may or may not need to be treated. Your clinician may recommend monitoring small solitary papillomas if you don't have symptoms, but most need to be removed.

Breast Changes That Aren't a Lump—but Could Be a Sign of Cancer

While most of us are trained to call our doctors if we feel a breast lump, there's a chance you might feel or see another type of an abnormality—which is important to get checked out, too. Keep these signs in mind and schedule an appointment with your healthcare practitioner if you notice any of them.

- Thickening or swelling of part of the breast

- Dimpling or irritation of the breast skin

- Changes in the look or texture of the skin covering your breast, such as redness or flaky skin that may look like a rash

- A pulling in of the nipple (retraction), pain in the nipple, and/or nipple discharge other than breast milk

- Any change in the shape or size of the breast

- Pain in any area of the breast[6]

You've Just Been Told You Have Dense Breasts. Now What?

Breast density is a measure of the amount of fibrous and glandular tissue compared with fatty tissue in the breasts, and it's assessed via mammography—not by feel. Having dense breasts means you have more fibrous and glandular tissue and less fat.

Radiologists classify breast density in four categories:[7]

A: Breasts are almost all fatty tissue.

B: There are scattered areas of dense glandular and fibrous tissue.

C: More of the breast is made of dense glandular and fibrous tissue (aka heterogeneously dense).

D: Breasts are extremely dense.

The categorization is essentially a score by the radiologist who reads your mammogram. Sometimes your score might be on the fence between two categories, so over the course of a few years you might see one report that says you have extremely dense breast tissue and another report that says you have heterogeneously dense breast tissue, says Lisa Larkin, MD.

Having dense breasts is normal and is especially common in young women. And while having dense breasts doesn't usually cause any symptoms and isn't considered a medical condition, it does increase your risk of breast cancer—and the greater the amount of dense tissue, the higher your risk.[8] What's more, dense breasts make it harder for doctors to see breast cancers on mammograms. (Fatty tissue is translucent, which makes it easier to spot cancer cells on imaging.) That said, having dense breasts also makes you more likely to receive a false positive result, which is when a screening mammogram shows an abnormal finding that could be cancer when, in fact, there's no cancer in the breast.

If you have extremely dense breasts, you'll want to make sure the imaging center that does your mammograms has 3D mammography. You might also talk to your healthcare provider about your breast density and ask them to help you understand your individual risk for developing breast cancer, because there are specific guidelines for additional breast cancer screenings, such as breast ultrasound or breast MRI, for those considered to be high risk.[9]

Detecting Breast Cancer: Understanding Your Risk and Your Screening Options

Historically, multiple medical associations put out different guidelines on breast cancer screening. The result? Many of us were left confused about how to stay on top of our breast health. Today, most guidelines recommend starting to screen for breast cancer with a mammogram at age forty, yet there's still disagreement on how regularly this screening should occur, with some guidelines recommending annual mammograms and others saying every two years is fine.

What we know for sure is that early detection of breast cancer (combined with advances in treatments if breast cancer is diagnosed) saves lives: The mortality rate for women with breast cancer fell 58 percent from 1975 to 2019 in the U.S., according to research.[10] However, according to a CDC report, about 25 percent of women ages fifty to seventy-four don't get the screenings they need. The report also found the more health-related social needs a woman is dealing with (things like food insecurity, lack of transportation, and feeling socially isolated), the less likely she is to get a mammogram.[11]

"We have definitely ping-ponged women and confused them about the guidelines for breast cancer screening," says medical oncologist Elizabeth Comen, MD. Here's what Dr. Comen recommends:

- **Have a conversation with your healthcare provider about your risk of breast cancer,** which is a discussion that'll incorporate your personal risk factors and family history.

- **Begin breast cancer screening with a yearly mammogram at age forty** if you are at average risk for breast cancer.

- **Talk to your clinician about whether you need an additional ultrasound or MRI to help detect breast cancer if you have dense breasts.** (All mammogram reports must include a statement about breast density and indicate if your breasts are "dense" or "not dense.")

- **Consider screening earlier than age forty and also with breast MRI if you have a greater than 20 percent lifetime increased risk of breast cancer.** (Flip to pages 290–291 for more information on the online tools that can help you determine your lifetime risk.)

Screening Techniques—and What to Know About Each

- **Clinical breast exam:** This is likely the first screening you'll get, well before the recommended guidelines to start mammography screenings at age forty. It usually involves your healthcare provider feeling and looking at your breasts, under your arms, and around your collarbone for any abnormalities or changes.

- **Mammography:** This is an imaging technique—essentially an X-ray machine designed specifically for the breasts—that's used both as a routine screening tool (to detect tumors that are too small to be felt or that are in the earliest stages, before symptoms develop) and as a diagnostic tool (to investigate suspicious breast changes, such as a lump, pain, or skin changes, or if a potential abnormality was found during a previous screening). There are a few different types of mammography, though digital breast tomosynthesis (aka DBT or 3D mammography) is now widely considered the preferred choice because it identifies breast cancer at higher rates and earlier stages than 2D mammography. Contrast-enhanced digital mammography (CEDM) uses an intravenous (IV) contrast agent in combination with more X-ray images of the breast than a standard mammogram. The dye makes it easier to find the new blood vessels that develop when cancers grow.

Once the mammogram images are taken, a radiologist (a medical doctor specially trained in diagnosing and treating health conditions using imaging equipment) will examine them for any abnormalities in the breast tissue and compare the new images with any previous ones to look for changes over time. Increasingly, artificial intelligence (AI) is being studied for its ability to accurately identify cancer.

- **Breast ultrasound:** This imaging technique uses sound waves to create a real-time picture of the internal structure of the breast and is usually used to determine whether a lump detected on a mammogram or felt during a physical exam is filled with fluid (a cyst) or solid (possible tumor). It's also used to help guide a needle biopsy if a suspicious area is detected or to monitor an abnormality if one has been detected.

- **Breast magnetic resonance imaging (MRI):** This is a very sensitive tool for finding abnormalities in the breast. Before the MRI, a contrast agent is injected into a vein to help highlight certain areas of the breast tissue, making any abnormalities easier to see. While a breast MRI doesn't replace a mammogram, it may be recommended for women at high risk for breast cancer (such as those with a strong family history of breast cancer or a known gene mutation). A newer, abbreviated breast MRI (aka fast breast MRI) is a lower-cost option that captures fewer images but still can be effective when it comes to detecting potential cancers. If you can't get insurance coverage for a full breast MRI, talk to your healthcare provider about this newer option, which is still typically self-pay and usually costs between $250 and $500.

- **Thermography:** Breast thermography uses infrared imaging to measure the temperature of breast skin. The thinking is that when cancer cells proliferate, they require an increased blood supply, leading to an elevated temperature in that area of the breast. However, there is no evidence proving thermography can detect breast cancer early, when it's most treatable, and it is not a substitute for a mammogram.

- **Liquid biopsy:** There's been ongoing research in the development of blood tests (aka liquid biopsy) to screen for breast cancer. These tests aim to detect signs of cancer in the blood by looking for circulating tumor cells, DNA from tumors, and other cancer-related biomarkers. While liquid biopsy is not yet part of standard screening practices, many experts are hopeful this will offer early, noninvasive screening.

Ask an Expert

Are breast self-exams worth doing?

I am a firm believer in breast self-exams. There has been some controversy about this, with some saying it's not necessary and doesn't save lives. But treating breast cancer isn't just about saving lives. When you catch a cancer earlier, it often means less invasive, less toxic, and less disfiguring treatment and surgeries.

While breast self-exams are critical for all women at every age, they're especially important for women under age forty. That's because 80 percent of women under age forty find their own breast cancers themselves. Given the rise in breast cancer among young women, it's crucial to know your breasts at every age.

Here's how to do a breast self-exam: Once or twice a month, stand in front of a mirror, clasp your hands behind your head, and look at your breasts. Notice if there's been any changes in size, shape, or symmetry, or if anything looks different on your skin (like dimpling, redness, or thickening) or nipples (like discharge or retraction). Then, using circular motions, press into your skin—starting at your neck, then moving into your armpit and working toward your nipple—to feel for any lumps, swelling, or areas that

Breast Health

feel thicker, tender, or painful. Ideally, aim to do this after your period, as your breasts are more likely to be lumpy and painful before your period.

The bottom line: Breast self-exams are about knowing your body so you're better able to detect when something is new or different. I want women to be accustomed to touching their body and to feel comfortable doing so. When you have an awareness of your body and a general sense of how your breasts look and feel, you'll be more likely to trust your instincts and seek out help if you're concerned about something.

—Elizabeth Comen, MD, medical oncologist specializing in breast cancer, associate professor of medicine at NYU Langone, and author of *All in Her Head: The Truth and Lies Early Medicine Taught Us About Women's Bodies and Why It Matters Today*

Breast Cancer Risk Factors You Can't Change— and Ones You Can

All of us (including men) have a chance of developing breast cancer, though some of us are at a higher risk than others. Here are some of the risk factors you can't change:

- **Being born female.** That's because a woman's breast cells are exposed to estrogen and progesterone, hormones (especially estrogen) linked with breast cancer.

- **Age.** The risk of breast cancer increases as you get older.

- **Genetic mutations.** About 5 to 10 percent of breast cancer cases are thought to result from genetic mutations passed on from a parent.

- **Family history.** Having a first-degree relative (mother, sister, daughter) with breast cancer doubles your risk, and the risk increases if multiple family members have been diagnosed. If your father or brother has had breast cancer, this also puts you at higher risk. (That said, it's important to know that most women who get breast cancer *don't* have a family history of the disease.)

- **Personal history of breast cancer.** If you're diagnosed with cancer in one breast, you have a higher risk of developing a new cancer in another part of the same breast or the other breast. This is especially true if you were young when you were first diagnosed with breast cancer.

- **Breast density.** Women with dense breasts have a higher risk of breast cancer. Dense breasts also make mammograms less effective in spotting cancers.

- **Race and ethnicity.** Some types of breast cancer are more common in Black women and those with Ashkenazi Jewish heritage. Black women are also more likely to have breast cancer diagnosed early (before age forty) and are more likely to die of the disease.[12]

- **Menstrual history.** Getting your period early (especially before age twelve) and going through menopause late (typically after age fifty-five) can increase breast cancer risk slightly, likely due to more exposure to estrogen and progesterone in your lifetime.

- **History of radiation to your chest.** Women who received radiation treatments to the chest area for another cancer (such as Hodgkin's or non-Hodgkin's lymphoma) have a significantly increased risk of breast cancer.

Here are some of the things you *can* do to reduce your risk:

- **Avoid or limit alcohol.** Studies show women who have one alcoholic drink a day have about a 7 to 10 percent increased risk of breast cancer compared with those who don't drink. If you have two to three drinks a day, that risk jumps to 20 percent.[13]

- **Get regular physical exercise.** Aim for at least 150 to 300 minutes of moderate-intensity exercise or 75 to 150 minutes of high-intensity exercise every week or a combination of these.

- **Consider genetic counseling and testing.** This is especially important for women with a family history of breast or ovarian cancer and can guide decisions about other preventive measures.

- **Preventive surgery.** In women at very high risk of breast cancer, preventive procedures like mastectomy (removal of healthy breasts) may be an option.

- **Chemoprevention medications.** Drugs like tamoxifen and raloxifene are approved for breast cancer risk reduction in high-risk women. These medications block estrogen's ability to reach estrogen receptors in breast cancer cells, which starves those cancer cells and prevents them from growing. Aromatase inhibitors are another type of drug that reduces estrogen levels to potentially keep cancerous cells from growing and spreading.

Source: American Cancer Society[14]

Breast Cancer in Young Women Is on the Rise. What's Driving It?

If you're hearing stories about more young women getting diagnosed with breast cancer, it's not a coincidence. While the median age at breast cancer diagnosis is sixty-two, rates of the disease among those aged twenty to forty-nine are on the rise.[15] And because regular breast cancer screening doesn't start until around age forty, younger women tend to be diagnosed with more advanced breast cancer that's tougher to treat.

Unfortunately, experts don't have clear-cut answers to explain this alarming trend, but they do have a few theories, explains Dr. Comen. Obesity is a known risk factor. We also know that alcohol is a carcinogen, and consumption is associated with an increased risk of breast cancer—a risk that increases with the amount of alcohol consumed. Girls are also getting their periods earlier, and women are having fewer children or opting to skip motherhood—all scenarios that mean a woman has more menstrual cycles, which correlates to a higher lifetime risk of breast cancer. Experts are also investigating environmental toxins and other endocrine disruptors that women are increasingly being exposed to at early ages through foods and personal care products.

Now, before you get too anxious, it's important to understand that breast cancer rates in young women are still relatively low, occurring in about forty-nine women under age fifty per hundred thousand, according to the Breast Cancer Research Foundation.[16] That said, it's crucial to understand your lifetime risk of breast cancer starting in your twenties (or at least long before age forty, when most guidelines recommend a first breast cancer screening), talk to your healthcare provider about early screening if you have a strong predisposition to the disease, and know the steps you can take to decrease your risk.

Diagnosing Breast Cancer: What You Need to Know About What's Involved

If imaging tests such as mammography, ultrasound, or MRI suggest that an area of your breast may have cancer, your doctor will order a biopsy.

"That's because a breast cancer diagnosis requires tissue," says Dr. Shen. "We can have a very high level of suspicion with imaging and a physical exam, but I need a biopsy to tell you with 100 percent confidence that it's cancer."

Here, Dr. Shen answers some of the most common questions about this diagnostic procedure.

How Is the Biopsy Done?

The standard of care is a core needle biopsy, a procedure in which your doctor (typically a surgeon or radiologist) will numb the area and then insert a thin, hollow needle through your skin and into the suspicious area. Using ultrasound imaging to ensure the tissue sample is taken from inside the potential tumor and not on the periphery of it, your doctor will then use the needle to cut a small cylinder or "core" of tissue. After the tissue samples have been taken, a tiny biopsy "clip" made of titanium or stainless steel is deployed through the center of the biopsy needle and left in place. While you're unlikely to notice it's there (it's so small, it won't even set off a metal detector if you walk through one), the clip serves as a helpful marker.

If the tissue from your core needle biopsy comes back from pathology with a cancer diagnosis, the clip can help guide the surgeon to the exact location of the biopsy if surgery is required.

"In some aggressive breast cancer cases where we prescribe chemotherapy or other medications to try to shrink a tumor before surgery, that biopsy clip marking a tumor can also help us see if the treatments are working to shrink or kill the cancer," says Dr. Shen. During breast surgery, the clip—along with the surrounding tissue—will be removed. Even if you get good news and you don't have cancer, the clip can be helpful in future mammograms or other imaging tests, showing that the area has already been biopsied. (And it can safely remain in your breast.)

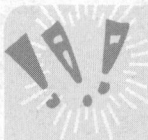

CORE NEEDLE BIOPSY VS. FINE NEEDLE ASPIRATION (FNA)

Doctors used to evaluate suspicious areas in breast tissue using FNA, which involves using a very thin needle to draw out (aka aspirate) a small amount of fluid and tissue from a breast lump. However, core needle biopsy is now the standard of care because it removes a larger sample of tissue, allowing for a more accurate diagnosis.

"In training, we joked that FNA stood for 'find nothing again,' because they are not reliable," says Dr. Shen.

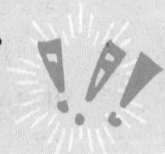

Can a Core Needle Biopsy Cause Cancer to Spread?

Years ago, when experts first started doing core needle biopsies, they worried that inserting a needle into a cancerous lump might cause the cancer to spread by "seeding" cancerous cells along the path of the needle.

"The thought was that you could be dragging cancer cells through healthy breast tissue," says Dr. Shen. In fact, doctors even removed tissue along the needle "track" to be sure this didn't happen. However, the consensus based on many years of research is that the risk of cancer spreading due to biopsy is very small—and the benefit of getting a clear and accurate diagnosis far outweighs this minimal risk.

"Plus, if it *is* cancer, follow-up surgery, radiation, and medications eradicate the cancer anyway," adds Dr. Shen.

If You're 99 Percent Sure I Have Cancer, Why Biopsy? Why Not Go Straight to Surgery?

Even if imaging like mammogram, MRI, and/or ultrasound suggests the presence of cancer, a core needle biopsy is still a crucial step in both confirming the diagnosis and planning the best course of treatment. "A core needle biopsy gives us clarity on your diagnosis so we can do any additional workups—like more imaging or even genetic testing if it's indicated—before surgery," says Dr. Shen. "It's what allows your breast surgeon to do her homework so she has the best plan in place to get all the cancer out during your surgery."

What's more, some types of breast cancer benefit from a "medication first, surgery later" approach, adds Dr. Shen—and a core needle biopsy is crucial in determining what type of cancer you have, which will dictate what type of treatment you receive.

At What Point Will You Determine If Cancer Has Spread to the Lymph Nodes?

Assessing lymph node involvement is a critical part of a breast cancer diagnosis (it can indicate that the cancer is more likely to have spread to other parts of the body) and will help determine your treatment plan. Lymph node activity can be tested in a few ways:

- **Physical exam:** Swelling of the lymph nodes in the underarm area or around the collarbone may indicate that cancer has spread.

- **Imaging tests:** Mammogram, MRI, or ultrasound can show if lymph nodes appear enlarged or abnormal, suggesting potential spread of the cancer and necessitating further investigation.

- **Biopsy:** If a lymph node feels or looks abnormal, a biopsy may be done.

While enlarged lymph nodes can signal cancer, they can also mean your lymph nodes are responding to an infection, or even a traumatic, invasive procedure to the breast tissue—such as a core needle biopsy. This is why radiologists and oncologists aren't as interested in the size of a lymph node as its architecture, and why it's important for patients to avoid freaking out if they feel swollen lymph nodes after a biopsy.

If your doctor suspects cancer has spread to the lymph nodes, they can ask the radiologist to do a core needle biopsy under ultrasound guidance. This can be helpful in delineating the clinical stage of the cancer and helping determine the best first course of action, such as surgery or medication. For patients diagnosed with invasive breast cancer whose lymph nodes feel and look normal before surgery, they'll do what's called a sentinel node biopsy, which can often be done at the same time as the initial breast cancer surgery.

Dr. Shen describes sentinel lymph nodes like military guards on the front line, the gateway to the rest of the lymph node "troops." Sentinel nodes—there will be one to three of these, with a median of two—are the first nodes to which cancer would likely spread from the primary tumor. During a sentinel node biopsy, a dye is injected near the tumor and follows the lymphatic pathways. The nodes the dye travels to first are the sentinel nodes, which are then removed and checked for cancer cells. If no cancer is found there, it's unlikely the cancer has spread to other lymph nodes, and no further surgery is needed. If cancer is found in the sentinel lymph nodes, the standard of care used to be to automatically remove and test additional lymph nodes (typically an additional ten to twenty nodes in the armpit, which is where breast cancer tends to spread first) in a procedure called axillary lymph node dissection (ALND). However, new research shows that even if your sentinel nodes are positive, you don't necessarily need ALND.

"Removing more lymph nodes has never been proven to improve survival," says Dr. Shen, "but it does come with immediate and potentially long-term side effects." Initial pain and numbness, scar tissue that causes tightness of the shoulder, and a condition called lymphedema—swelling caused by a blockage in the lymphatic system—are all common. A surgical drain (a tube placed at the site of the surgery to help remove fluid that accumulates in the area after the procedure) is also more likely to be necessary in cases where more lymph nodes are removed.

Here's why experts feel confident that removing the sentinel nodes alone works well: If your cancer has spread to your sentinel node, the treatments that follow (such as radiation and medications) can help address any possible additional microscopic cancer cells in the remaining nodes.

The bottom line: There's been a big shift in lymph node diagnosis and treatment, with the new, less invasive approach showing no difference in treatment success rates and fewer short- and long-term side effects. "Treatment success rates have only gone up over time, and breast cancer survivorship continues to rise," says Dr. Shen. "This is one example of a significant shift that is helping us achieve our goal of making sure women are cancer free and living without long-term effects of surgery and treatment."

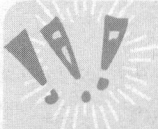

QUALITY OF PATHOLOGY IS EVERYTHING

If you are diagnosed with breast cancer, you have a right to request that a sample of the tissue biopsied be sent to another pathologist for a second opinion. Quality of pathology is the foundation of all cancer care, and this is an easy place to make a mistake if a less experienced center is looking at a breast cancer tumor—or any type of cancer, for that matter—especially if it's not a common type. "Pathology is an underappreciated part of cancer care and an aspect too few of us realize we have some control over in the diagnosis process," says Dr. Shen.

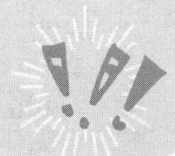

Types of Breast Cancer: What You Need to Know About the Most Common Types, Subtypes, and Stages

As if a breast cancer diagnosis wasn't already daunting, confusion often sets in when it comes to the many different types of the disease and different terms used to describe each. Here, Dorraya El-Ashry, PhD, chief scientific officer at the Breast Cancer Research Foundation, offers a helpful framework to understand the most common types of breast cancer and what you most need to know about each.

Noninvasive Breast Cancers

These are also known as stage 0, or carcinomas in situ—which is Latin for "in the original place"—and could become invasive if left untreated. There are two main types:

Ductal carcinoma in situ (DCIS) starts in the cells lining the breast's milk ducts but stays in place (in situ) and has not spread through the ducts into surrounding breast tissue, lymph nodes, or the bloodstream.

Lobular carcinoma in situ (LCIS) starts in the cells lining the glands that make milk (lobules) and is not likely to spread to surrounding tissues. However, it does increase a person's risk of developing invasive cancer in either breast in the future.

"You can think of these noninvasive breast cancers almost like a colon polyp that's removed during a colonoscopy and puts your doctors on higher alert for possible colon cancer," says Dr. El-Ashry. "They are precancers that haven't spread into the surrounding breast tissue or beyond, making them highly treatable if caught early."

DCIS is typically found during screening mammography—not a self or clinical breast exam—making it crucial to stay on top of breast cancer screenings. LCIS usually doesn't show up on mammograms and is most often discovered after a breast biopsy done for another reason, such as a suspicious breast lump.

Invasive Breast Cancers

These are cancers that haven't stayed put in the ducts or lobules and have left their place of origin and invaded nearby breast tissue, lymph nodes, and/or possibly even other organs in the body. There are two main types:

Invasive ductal carcinoma (IDC) starts in the ducts of the breast and then spreads into other breast tissue and possibly other body parts through the lymph system or bloodstream. There are multiple subtypes of IDC, based on whether or not the tumor is fed by the hormones estrogen or progesterone and based on a specific protein called HER2. (More on that next.) IDC is by far the most common type of breast cancer: About eight out of ten invasive breast cancer diagnoses will be IDC.

Invasive lobular carcinoma (ILC) starts in the lobules and typically grows in lines in the breast, rather than lumps. It accounts for approximately one in ten invasive breast cancer diagnoses.

Subtypes of Invasive Breast Cancers Based on Hormone and HER2 Receptor Status

After an invasive breast cancer diagnosis, you'll hear terms like *HR positive*, *HER2 positive*, *HER2 negative*, and *triple negative*. Essentially, these classifications are used to differentiate what's driving the cancer growth and customize a treatment plan based on that information. Here are the main categories to know:

Hormone receptor positive (HR positive): Breast cancer tumors that have receptors for either estrogen or progesterone (or both) are known as HR-positive breast cancers. This means the cancer cells pick up estrogen and/or progesterone signals that promote cell growth. HR-positive is the most common form of invasive breast cancer and tends to have a favorable prognosis, especially when diagnosed early, thanks to several available hormone therapies that either suppress estrogen's level in the body or prevent it from attaching to estrogen receptors.

HER2 positive: There's a protein in normal breast cells called human epidermal growth factor receptor 2 (aka HER2), which helps those cells grow and repair. In some breast cancer cases, cancer cells have extra copies of the gene that makes the HER2 protein. If a breast cancer tumor is found to have an overexpression of the HER2 protein, it's classified as HER2-positive breast cancer, which accounts for an estimated 25 to 30 percent of diagnoses. While this subtype of breast cancer tends to be aggressive, new HER2-targeted therapies have improved the prognosis for these patients.

Triple-negative breast cancer (TNBC): This is diagnosed when a breast cancer tumor tests negative for estrogen receptors (ER), progesterone receptors (PR), and human epidermal growth factor receptor 2 (HER2)—hence why it's called triple negative. While this subtype accounts for about 10 to 15 percent of breast cancer diagnoses, it's more common in younger women; Black, Hispanic, and Native American women; and those with a BRCA1 gene mutation.[17] Triple-negative breast cancers tend to be more advanced when diagnosed and more aggressive than ER- and/or PR-positive cancers.

Metastatic breast cancer: Also referred to as stage 4 breast cancer or advanced breast cancer, this is diagnosed when breast cancer cells have traveled from the original site in the breast or lymph nodes to other areas of the body, most commonly the bones, brain, liver, and lungs. While it's the form of breast cancer that is most deadly, there are more treatments than ever before and a growing body of research that's drastically improving patient prognosis and quality of life.

How Is Breast Cancer "Staged"?

When breast cancer is diagnosed, the healthcare team will determine how big the tumor is and whether it has spread within the breast or to other parts of the body—a process called staging. Here's the breakdown:

Stage 0: Abnormal cells are present but remain "in situ," meaning they have not spread to nearby tissue.

Stage 1: The tumor is less than two centimeters (cm) and is located in breast tissue, nearby lymph nodes, or both.

Stage 2: The tumor is slightly bigger (between two and five centimeters) and/or the cancer has spread to fewer than four lymph nodes.

Stage 3: The tumor is larger and has spread to lymph nodes or nearby tissues, such as the skin or the muscle of the breast.

Stage 4: Cancer that has spread beyond the breast to other parts of the body (metastatic breast cancer).

Stages 1 and 2 are divided into two additional subcategories (A and B), and stage 3 is divided into three additional subcategories (A, B, and C). Cancer pathologists use multiple pieces of information to determine breast cancer staging, from tumor size and lymph node involvement to hormone receptor and HER2 status, as well as how similar (or not) cancer cells look to normal cells. If you're diagnosed with breast cancer, it's important to know your exact stage, as it will influence your treatment plan.[18]

Other Rare Types of Breast Cancer

While these account for less than 5 percent of invasive breast cancers, they are important to know about.

Inflammatory breast cancer: This is a rare but aggressive form of breast cancer. It's more likely to be diagnosed in women under forty, and Black women have a higher risk of this subtype of the disease than white women. It occurs when cancer cells block lymph vessels in the skin, causing inflammation that typically presents as breast swelling, skin dimpling, and/or discoloration on the breast that can look like a rash.

Paget's disease: This type of breast cancer involves the skin of the nipple and areola. Approximately 1 to 4 percent of all breast cancers also involve Paget disease of the breast, according to the National Cancer Institute.[19]

Male breast cancer: Yes, men are also at risk for breast cancer—however, it's much more rare. (According to the American Cancer Society, the average lifetime risk of getting breast cancer is about 1 in 726 for men,[20] compared with 1 in 8 for women.[21]) Unfortunately, due to lack of awareness that breast cancer is a possibility in men, they are often unaware of changes in their breast tissue, so diagnoses tend to happen at a later stage.

Genetic Testing for Breast Cancer: The Gene Mutations Associated with Breast Cancer and How to Decide If Testing Is Right for You

There are two genes that likely come to mind when you think about breast cancer: BRCA1 and BRCA2. Yet while these are the most common genes associated with hereditary breast cancer, it's important to know this: Only about 7 to 10 percent of all breast cancers are associated with a genetic mutation, says breast medicine and menopause specialist Sabrina Sahni, MD.

"I see patients all the time who assume that they must have a genetic mutation if they have a family history of breast cancer, when in fact this isn't true," says Dr. Sahni. "Breast cancer is multifactorial—and a third of breast cancers can be altered by lifestyle factors."

When it comes to the genes associated with breast cancer, there are others beyond BRCA1 and BRCA2 that can increase your risk. Here, Dr. Sahni walks us through which ones to know about. "Remember, having a mutation in one or more of these genes doesn't mean you'll go on to develop breast cancer," she says. "But it does put you at increased risk, which makes it crucial to talk to your healthcare provider about screening recommendations and other preventive measures you should take."

THE GENES ASSOCIATED WITH BREAST CANCER

THE GENE	WHAT IT DOES	ESTIMATED LIFETIME BREAST CANCER RISK
BRCA1 and BRCA2	Every time a cell divides, there's an "editing" that happens to keep cells healthy. When there is a mutation in these BRCA genes, DNA repair is less precise and cells are more likely to grow out of control (read: become cancerous). Both men and women can have a mutation in one of these genes, which puts them at increased risk of developing breast cancer (and ovarian cancer in women) compared with the general population. (BRCA mutations are also associated with other cancers, such as pancreatic, prostate, and ovarian cancers.)	BRCA1: 60 to 72 percent BRCA2: 55 to 69 percent
PALB2	This gene acts as both a partner and a localizer for the BRCA2 gene to repair damaged DNA.	32 to 53 percent
PTEN	This gene helps regulate cell growth. A mutation in this gene is associated with a spectrum of disorders known as PTEN Hamartoma Tumor Syndrome (PHTS). Within this spectrum is Cowden syndrome, a rare condition associated with both benign and malignant breast tumors, as well as growths in the digestive tract, thyroid, uterus, and ovaries.	40 to 60 percent
TP53	This gene gives your body instructions to make a protein that helps stop tumor growth. An abnormal TP53 gene causes Li–Fraumeni syndrome, a disorder that causes various soft-tissue cancers occurring at a young age and continuing throughout the lifespan.	>60 percent
ATM	Like the BRCA genes, ATM helps repair damaged DNA. ATM mutation has been linked to an increased rate of breast, colon, and pancreatic cancers.	21 to 24 percent
CDH1	This gene makes a protein that helps cells bind together to form various tissues in your body. A CDH1 mutation can increase your risk of invasive lobular breast cancer, as well as a rare type of stomach cancer (hereditary diffuse gastric cancer) at an early age.	39 to 52 percent
CHEK2	This gene gives your body instructions to make a protein that stops tumor growth. A CHEK2 mutation can increase the risk of breast, colorectal, and prostate cancer.	20 to 40 percent
STK11	This gene helps regulate cellular growth and metabolism. A mutation in this gene is associated with Peutz–Jeghers syndrome (PJS) and may raise the risk of gastric and breast cancers, as well as non-epithelial ovarian tumors.	32 to 54 percent
NF1	This gene gives the body instructions for making a protein that regulates cell growth and suppresses tumors. A mutation is associated with an increased risk of neurologic tumors, gastric cancers, and can increase the risk of developing breast cancer before fifty.	20 to 40 percent
BARD1	This is a tumor suppressor gene that plays a role in DNA repair and cell regulation. Mutations in this gene can increase the risk of breast cancer.	17 to 30 percent
RAD51C and RAD51D	These are genes that aid in DNA repair. Mutations in these genes increase the risk of both breast and ovarian cancers.	RAD51C: 20 percent RAD51D: 20 percent

Who Should Get Genetic Testing?

The answer depends on your personal risk of breast cancer, as well as your personal and family health history and other risk factors you have. It's likely you'll be a good candidate for genetic testing if you have a family history of certain breast, ovarian, pancreatic, or prostate cancers. And if you've been diagnosed with breast cancer before age fifty, genetic testing is usually recommended. Knowing if your cancer is related to a known genetic mutation can aid in both treatment and management of the disease, says Dr. Sahni.

What Do I Do with the Results?

While a negative result can be reassuring, it doesn't eradicate your breast cancer risk. On the other hand, testing positive for one or more gene mutations doesn't mean a future breast cancer diagnosis is inevitable. To understand your test results and the steps you should take next, schedule a follow-up appointment with a genetic counselor or healthcare provider who can help you interpret the results and talk about what they mean in the context of your personal and family history.

Also, keep in mind that genetic knowledge and testing are continuously evolving. Talk to your healthcare provider about any genetic testing you've had in the past, as well as more updated panels you might be tested for now.

Your Game Plan:
How to Assess Your Risk of Breast Cancer

When we hear the phrase *breast health*, many of us think about breast cancer almost immediately and focus on getting our annual mammogram. Mammograms are an essential part of our fight, helping to detect breast cancer. But the key word there is *detect*, says Dr. Larkin.

"Mammograms do nothing to *prevent* breast cancer, which should be the real goal of our efforts," she says. "To prevent breast cancer, identifying women at high risk is the critical first step. We must educate and inform women about their individual, personal risk of developing breast cancer, and identify women at increased risk."

Unfortunately, Dr. Larkin says, individual breast cancer risk assessment isn't common in clinical practice and the majority of women at high risk are unaware of their risk and that they should be getting screenings beyond mammograms. "We must do better," she says.

Until that happens, Dr. Larkin recommends taking these steps:

Calculate your own risk. There are two evidence-based risk-assessment tools, both of which you can complete online:

1. The Tyrer-Cuzick Model (magview.com/ibis-risk-calculator/)

Also known as the International Breast Cancer Intervention Study (IBIS), this detailed questionnaire assesses a woman's likelihood of developing breast cancer within the next ten years and throughout her lifetime. It takes into account age, three generations of family history, genetic factors (such as a known BRCA1 or BRCA2 gene mutation), menstrual history, reproductive history (like age at first live birth and hormone therapy use), personal medical history (such as prior breast biopsies), as well as breast density, BMI, height, and weight.

2. The Gail Model (bcrisktool.cancer.gov)

Also known as the Breast Cancer Risk Assessment Tool, this is a shorter questionnaire that calculates a woman's risk of developing breast cancer within the next five years and within her lifetime (up to age ninety). It considers several factors, including age, race/ethnicity, reproductive history, first-degree family history of breast cancer, personal history of breast biopsies, and breast density.

Bring your results to your next doctor visit and start the conversation about what they mean and how they'll inform your screening plan. You can tell your doctor, "I learned about these risk assessments. Here are my scores on each, and I'd like your help interpreting them because I'd like to know if I need a breast MRI in addition to my annual mammogram." Dr. Larkin likens the scenario to when Viagra first came out in the 1990s for male erectile dysfunction, and the drug manufacturers assumed urologists would be the only ones prescribing it—until men asked their primary care physicians about the drug in record numbers, which forced them to start prescribing it, too. "This has to happen when it comes to breast cancer risk calculations," says Dr. Larkin.

• • • • •

Talking about our breasts with our healthcare providers and one another often doesn't happen until we face challenges. Concerns about breast size, breastfeeding difficulties, and breast cancer scares and diagnoses tend to get the conversation started. Yet having a basic understanding of your breast health and the steps you can take to prevent and detect breast cancer is a great way to optimize your breast health now and throughout the rest of your life.

Part II

The Specialties

*Staying Informed
and Attuned*

Chapter 11

Your Immune System

The Genius Way Your Body Keeps You Healthy—
and Why Women Are at Greater Risk of
Autoimmune Disease

> *Billions of immune cells die, transform, and are born every second,*
> *and that means we have daily (even hourly!) opportunities to trans-*
> *form the integrity and resilience of our immune health.*
>
> —Heather Moday, MD, *The Immunotype Breakthrough: Your Person-*
> *alized Plan to Balance Your Immune System, Optimize Health, and*
> *Build Lifelong Resilience*

Considering the *millions* of bacteria, viruses, parasites, fungi, and other bugs we're exposed to every day, it's a miracle that any of us can survive what life throws our way. But we can, thanks in large part to our always-alert immune system—the army of organs, cells, proteins, and chemicals in our body that monitors threats and fights foreign invaders to keep us healthy.

It's a complex job. After all, there are bacteria in the world around us *and* in our bodies, and your immune system needs to know how to distinguish the nefarious (like a virus that could make you really sick) from the no-big-deal (like the mix of bugs that make up your microbiome). It also has to know how to fine-tune any necessary attacks so it does its job of taking out the bad guys without wreaking havoc on all of the good stuff happening in your body.

The way your immune system does all of this is downright awe-inspiring. For women, this is especially true, given the different ways our immune system must adapt to things like pregnancy (not attacking a fetus due to its foreign DNA in our bodies) and the monthly swings and postmenopausal dip of our sex hormones (which play a role in immune function). Understanding the basics of how this amazing system operates can help you make sure *yours* is working optimally.

In this chapter, we'll learn . . .

- **What, exactly, the immune system is and how it works.** We'll also outline the anatomy of an immune response, which can help you understand what your body's up to after you come in contact with a bug—whether you know it (and have a bad head cold or worse to prove it) or not.

- **How a woman's immune system is different from a man's.** From hormonal transitions like puberty, pregnancy, and perimenopause to differences in how the immune system responds in women versus men, there are key points of differentiation that we can benefit from knowing.

- **The many factors that can disrupt the immune system** and cause it to become dysregulated. From an ever-growing list of chemicals experts are now referring to as immune-disrupting chemicals (IDCs) to less talked-about triggers, such as trauma, knowing what can throw your system out of whack can help you prevent dysregulation from happening in the first place.

- **What you need to know about autoimmune diseases**, including what they are, why women are at a significantly higher risk for these conditions than men are, and the signs and symptoms of the most common autoimmune conditions in women.

- **How vaccines work—and the answers to some of the most common questions about them.** Vaccine misinformation and disinformation are on the rise around the world, which makes it more important than ever to know the unbiased facts about how vaccines work on our immune systems and how they're studied.

- **An action plan** to optimize your immune health, including the straightforward steps you can take to improve your immunity.

Meet the Experts

Heather Moday, MD, allergist and immunologist and author of *The Immunotype Breakthrough: Your Personalized Plan to Balance Your Immune System, Optimize Health, and Build Lifelong Resilience*

Shilpa Ravella, MD, gastroenterologist and author of *A Silent Fire: The Story of Inflammation, Diet & Disease*

Aly Cohen, MD, integrative rheumatologist, environmental health expert, and author of *Detoxify: The Everyday Toxins Harming Your Immune System and How to Defend Against Them*

Zahida Maskatia, MD, allergist, immunologist, and medical director of Latitude Food Allergy Care

Boghuma K. Titanji, MD, PhD, assistant professor of medicine in the division of infectious diseases at Emory University School of Medicine

Meet Your Immune System: How Your Body Defends Itself

You've likely heard your immune system referred to as an army, an analogy that's used for good reason: Like a military force, your immune system has specialized components that work together to defend your body against threats and fight off illness.

There are two main branches to your immune system: the innate immune system and the adaptive immune system.

The Innate Immune System

This is the immune system you're born with, your body's first line of defense against infections and pathogens. It's called a nonspecific system because it responds the same way to all antigens, which are proteins on the surface of most foreign invaders (like bacteria, viruses, and parasites) that your immune system recognizes as bad guys.

You know your innate immune system is at work when you cough (which helps us get rid of invaders in our respiratory tract) or start making more mucus than usual (which traps those invaders so we can cough them up or blow them out of our nose). Immune cells in your skin, enzymes in your tears, and your stomach acid are also part of the innate immune system's genius way of getting rid of what may infect or irritate us.

A few different types of cells and proteins make up the innate immune system. Here are some of the most important:

- **Mast cells**: These cells are strategically located in tissues throughout the body, particularly in areas that interface with the outside world (think skin, respiratory passages, and gastrointestinal tract). When mast cells detect bad guys, they activate and release inflammatory chemicals that recruit other immune cells to the site of infection or injury in an effort to heal it. For example, that swelling or redness you see after you cut your finger are mast cells hard at work.

- **Phagocytes**: These cells are like Pac-Man, engulfing and digesting foreign invaders (a process called phagocytosis).

- **Natural killer cells (aka NK cells)**: NK cells detect and destroy infected or abnormal cells (think virus-infected cells or cancer cells). They also release proteins called cytokines.

- **Cytokines**: These proteins act as messengers between immune cells to regulate immune responses and inflammation. Cytokines can be pro-inflammatory (triggering or heightening inflammation) or anti-inflammatory (lessening inflammation to prevent an excessive immune response).

The Adaptive Immune System

This branch of your immune system provides specific, targeted defense against pathogens and foreign antigens. You can think of it like a special-ops army: While the innate immune system is the general, frontline response, the components of your adaptive immune system are the highly trained specialists who come in when more precise, long-term support is needed. The adaptive immune system is also able to "remember" germs so that the next time you face a germ it's already met, you can fight it faster.

While you're born with your innate immune system in place, your adaptive immune system develops over time and continues to change and adapt throughout the rest of your life, storing information in its "memory bank" in response to exposure to antigens and environmental stimuli, infections you contract, and vaccines you receive. This helps explain why you get some "natural immunity" after a bout of COVID-19, and you'll have some protection against future infections of the variant your immune system just faced. It's also why getting a vaccine is like training your immune system so it's able to mount a fast, effective attack if you're exposed to that virus in the real world. (For more on how vaccines work, flip to page 321.)

The Immune System in Action: Anatomy of an Immune Response

Given the immune system's mind-blowing intricacies, it can be tough to wrap your head around how it works in real time. To help you do that, let's look at how it fights a pathogen that causes the common cold.

- A pathogen (in this case, a strain of virus that causes the common cold) enters your body. Maybe it got in through a crack in the skin on your hands, or you breathed it in because it was lurking in droplets in the air after someone who was infected sneezed or coughed. No matter how this virus got into your body, your immune system recognizes it as an invader.

- Your mast cells detect the pathogen and release chemicals that recruit a specific type of white blood cell called lymphocytes to the site of the virus or infection.

- Your mast cells also release cytokines, which act as chemical messengers in your immune system to let the rest of your body know it's in for a fight. This initial immune response is all part of your innate immune system, which has one main job: to launch an inflammatory response.

- This inflammatory response is trying to clear that virus out of your body, and it has a number of strategies. For example, it can raise your body temperature, which you experience as a fever, in an attempt to stop the virus from replicating. Inflammatory cells also flood your nose and accumulate, prompting you to blow your nose in an effort to clear the virus from your body. As much as inflammatory responses like these can feel like no fun for you, the symptoms are a sign your immune system is hard at work.

- If the virus you've been exposed to is mild and your immune system does an A+ job fighting it, those white blood cells die off and clear out—and you start to feel like yourself again.

- If you're still feeling sick after three or four days, odds are you're dealing with a gnarlier germ—and those white blood cells need backup. They essentially start screaming at your lymph nodes, "Hey! We need some backup—we can't clear this infection!"

- This is when your adaptive immune response kicks in. Those immune cells that initially jumped into action recruit *more* white blood cells from your lymph nodes, which respond by spitting out B cells (which make antibodies that "mark" pathogens to be killed) and T cells to finish the fight. This lymph node action is why it may feel like you've got two gigantic marbles under your jaw.

- Those antibodies make copies of themselves, which get stored in your immune system's memory—aka your immunological memory. Every time you're exposed to this particular virus again, it'll kick your adaptive immune response into gear so you're better able to fight it the next time.

- Once the virus is vanquished, your inflammatory response will wind down and you'll start to feel like yourself again.

- Sometimes, however, even when your immune system did everything it was supposed to do, your body's inflammatory response doesn't turn off as it's supposed to. When this happens, it's often because your innate immune response continues to flood your body with cytokines (something called a cytokine storm) even though your adaptive immune response has those powerful T cells and B cells on the front lines of the war. Unfortunately, that cytokine storm does more harm than good and prompts your T cells and B cells to work on overdrive—and they get tired as a result. This is what immunologists call "T cell exhaustion," and it means your immune system's killer cells aren't able to fight as they should. The result? Continued inflammation in your body—and more symptoms that continue to make you feel sick.

The XX Immune System: Some of the Ways the Female Surveillance System Is Different from a Male's

While there is still a lot of research that must be done to understand all the ways the female and male immune systems differ, there are some key distinctions we do know that influence how we respond to infections, vaccinations, and autoimmune disease triggers.

- **Estrogen enhances the female immune response.** Estrogens influence adaptive immunity by increasing levels of antibodies circulating throughout the body. This may be why research shows that women tend to mount a stronger response to infections and vaccines.[1] However, this is also thought to influence a woman's fourfold higher risk of autoimmune disease:[2] Higher levels of antibodies (molecules that mark foreign substances in the body to be attacked and killed) and autoantibodies (which attack the body's own cells) may cause this increased prevalence of autoimmune disease in women.

- **Women generally mount higher innate and adaptive immune responses than men**. And we produce more signaling molecules involved in initiating an inflammatory response and recruiting immune cells to fight pathogens. This speedy innate immune response, combined with the influence of sex hormones, may be another factor in our susceptibility to autoimmune diseases, as our heightened immune response can lead to an overactive immune system—which starts mistakenly attacking the body's own tissue.

- **Vaccines are more effective in women.**[3] Our higher antibody production and better protection against infectious disease after receiving vaccinations is thought to be due in part to the influence of sex hormones on the immune system. It may also help explain why women are more likely to report adverse reactions after getting a vaccine.

Hormonal Transitions That Impact the Female Immune System

The major hormonal upheavals women go through have a big impact on our immune system. That's because many of our hormones modulate the immune system to keep it working optimally. Major fluctuations in hormones can prompt immune system dysregulation. Here's a closer look at the big ones.

» PUBERTY

The years of puberty mark a major remodeling of the immune system. It's a time when your immune cells mature, helping you develop a more robust immune system that's capable of mounting an effective response to various pathogens. It's also a time when significantly higher levels of sex hormones start coursing through your body—and your immune system has to recognize this major hormonal upheaval as normal and not think your body is under attack and jump into overdrive.

When it does this successfully, it's yet another example of your body's self-regulating genius. If it misses the mark, immune dysfunction can result. This explains why puberty can trigger the onset of several autoimmune diseases. (More on how autoimmunity develops on pages 314–317.)

» YOUR PERIOD

If you ever feel sick during your menstrual cycle—a phenomenon commonly referred to as the period flu—there's a reason: Your immune system is responding to the normal inflammation that's happening in your uterus as it prepares to shed its lining. Those body aches, that general feeling of *blahness*, and even the low-grade fever you can get before or during your period are the outward signs of that internal inflammation.

Additionally, during the first half of your cycle (the follicular phase), estrogen is on the rise, which, in turn, leads to an increase in inflammatory responses and may help you ward off germs. During the second half of your cycle (the luteal phase), estrogen drops and progesterone rises, which can result in a suppression of the immune system and a higher chance of your getting sick. In theory, this is all your immune system's effort to help you get pregnant: During the first half of your cycle, the immune system is upregulated in order to fight off invaders so you stay healthy enough to get pregnant; during the second half of your cycle, your immune system downregulates so that if you are pregnant, your body won't reject your fertilized egg.

» PREGNANCY

Along with the many changes your body goes through if you get pregnant, your immune system experiences significant shifts. Once an embryo implants and starts to develop, the immune system has to make serious alterations in how it works so that it doesn't attack your fetus. Your body does this in a number of ways, including expanding the production of anti-inflammatory molecules and altering the activity of your killer cells to prevent excessive immune responses. Hormones produced by the placenta (like human chorionic gonadotropin, or hCG, and progesterone) also boost immune tolerance to support your baby's development. Progesterone is also an immunosuppressant when present in high levels, as it is during pregnancy.

As your pregnancy proceeds, your immune system also does remarkable work on behalf of your growing baby's budding immune system: A small number of your immune cells actually slip across the placenta, enter your baby's body, and provide some passive immunity. This transfer of immune cells helps your developing baby's immune system learn to tell the difference between foreign substances and self. This immune system "education" you're giving your baby in utero is helping to tune their immune system early on. And if you breastfeed, your baby's immune system continues to benefit. Breast milk is filled with antibodies and cytokines that provide your newborn with "passive immunity" that acts as short-term help while your baby's immune system has a chance to finish developing and start working.

» PERIMENOPAUSE AND POSTMENOPAUSE

As we age, our immune system becomes slower to respond—a phenomenon you may experience as slower wound healing, more intense inflammatory responses (hello, aches and pains), less effective protection after getting vaccines, and increased risk of everything from the common cold to chronic diseases. For women, a decline in estrogen during the menopause transition may weaken the immune system even more.

Ask an Expert

What do you do to prevent getting sick—or to support your immune system when you get a cold or upper respiratory infection?

It starts with the basics: I wash my hands frequently, avoid alcohol and high-intensity exercise, and make sure I'm getting good-quality sleep. In fact, I try to get even more sleep than usual. As women, we tend to power through our schedules and to-do lists even if we're feeling under the weather. But anything that puts a stress on your body takes energy away from your immune system's ability to do its job.

I try to get more vitamin C, zinc, and vitamin D—all of which have compelling data showing they are powerful in supporting the immune system—either in my diet or via supplements. Elderberry syrup, which I like to use in the initial stages of cold or flu, has antiviral properties and a safe track record. And I also use propolis, which is found in honeybee hives and has pretty good evidence showing that its use in a spray form in the throat can help kill viruses we breathe in. These are all good things to have on hand and to use either preventively or when you feel like something is coming on.

—Heather Moday, MD, allergist and immunologist and author of *The Immunotype Breakthrough: Your Personalized Plan to Balance Your Immune System, Optimize Health, and Build Lifelong Resilience*

Understanding Inflammation: How It Works, Why It's Amazing, and How Such a Good Thing Can Sometimes Turn Bad

The human body is constantly working in remarkable ways to keep us healthy. Our inflammatory response is a perfect example of this. Inflammation is one of the body's most powerful forces—a protective process that helps defend us against injury and foreign pathogens.

There are two main types of inflammation: acute inflammation and chronic inflammation.

Acute inflammation is what happens immediately after exposure to a pathogen like a bacteria or virus or as the result of an injury: Think about the last time you burned yourself after touching a hot pan or stubbed your toe. That redness, swelling, and pain you saw and felt were the result of inflammation happening inside the body. While this type of inflammation may hurt, it's actually helping you heal.

However, the immune system doesn't wage this helpful pro-inflammatory war only when you have an injury or infection that's obvious to you. It quietly does the same thing inside your body when it perceives that something is off. For example, an inflammatory response can happen if your body doesn't tolerate certain components of bread, allowing little pieces of the bread to migrate out of your gut and prompting your immune system to fight the foreign bits of food. It also happens if plaque builds up on the walls of the arteries around your heart, creating inflammation in your blood vessels because that plaque isn't supposed to be there.

The response is brilliant—up to a point. When your inflammatory response handles what it set out to do and helps your body heal, you're good to go. But when inflammation rages on and on—which can happen when the insults don't let up, or when a fault in the system turns the immune system on healthy cells—you get inflammation that shifts into perpetual high gear. When this happens, your immune soldiers start releasing inflammatory chemicals that *damage* your body's tissues instead of healing them.

This is the kind of inflammation that's more likely when you have chronic inflammation, and it can create some pretty big problems. That's because these unhelpful inflammatory soldiers travel around your body via your circulatory system, often making their way to specific organs—like your heart, brain, or gut—and can do real damage there over time, causing cardiovascular diseases like heart disease and high blood pressure, gastrointestinal conditions such as inflammatory bowel disease, lung diseases like asthma, neurodegenerative conditions such as Alzheimer's and Parkinson's, and a host of other health conditions.

Are There Ways to Tell If I Have Chronic Inflammation?

While acute inflammation is often easy to see and feel, chronic inflammation is often slow to build and silent—undetectable for months or even years. However, there are a few known triggers that ignite chronic inflammation, says gastroenterologist Shilpa Ravella, MD, and knowing what they are can help you assess your situation.

- **You have excess belly fat**. Fat cells are metabolically active: They can spit out molecules that ramp up inflammation, and the plumper they get, the more they do this with gusto. Carrying excess fat around your middle could be a sign that you also have visceral fat—the term for the kind of fat that wraps around your abdominal organs and is known to be the most inflammatory type of fat.

- **You've been diagnosed with insulin resistance or diabetes**. These conditions are both associated with higher levels of cytokines, which essentially tell your pro-inflammatory immune soldiers to stay on the front lines rather than retreat.

- **Your C-reactive protein (CRP) levels are high**. CRP is produced by the liver in response to systemic inflammation, and your level can be tested via a simple blood test. CRP is considered a general marker of inflammation somewhere in your body; the test can't help you home in on the exact location or cause. (A high-sensitivity C-reactive protein, or hs-CRP, test is more specific and can help determine your risk for heart disease.) When CRP is elevated, it can correlate to inflammation in your body.

What Are the Best Ways to Decrease Chronic Inflammation?

Two of the most important things you can do are to make some changes to your diet and to exercise regularly, says Dr. Ravella.

One dietary change that has a big impact is boosting your fiber intake. The recommended dietary allowance (RDA) of fiber each day is twenty-five grams, but most American adults only get about ten to fifteen grams. Ideally, we'd all get more than the recommended twenty-five grams per day.

"We are a nation with a fiber deficiency—95 percent of American adults aren't getting enough," says Dr. Ravella. "Yet it's a critical anti-inflammatory agent." That's because fiber manipulates the immune system through our gut bugs. When our gut bacteria digest soluble fiber (found in foods like oats, beans, apples, carrots, and citrus fruits), they make short-chain fatty acids, which can calm chronic inflammation throughout the body.

Another smart move when it comes to decreasing chronic inflammation is to incorporate some type of movement into most days. Exercise is anti-inflammatory. Regularly moving your body has also been shown to improve the diversity of the microbes in your gut, which, similar to eating plenty of fiber, can ease chronic inflammation.

The Chemicals That Mess with Our Immune System (Plus, What to Do About Them)

You've likely heard of endocrine-disrupting chemicals (EDCs) and how they are ubiquitous and essentially unavoidable in modern life. These synthetic substances, such as bisphenol A (BPA), phthalates, and polychlorinated bi-phenyls (PCBs), are found in everything from our food and personal care products to the clothing we wear, the furniture in our homes, and the water we drink.

We've long known that EDCs interfere with our endocrine system, thanks to their ability to mimic, block, or alter the function of hormones in the body. Now emerging evidence shows that these chemicals wreak havoc on the immune system as well—so much so that they are increasingly re-ferred to as immune-disrupting chemicals (IDCs), which play a key role in the development and management of immune system disorders.

Integrative rheumatologist Aly Cohen, MD, explains a few ways this happens.

- **IDCs trigger inflammation.** When the innate immune system's surveil-lance team first encounters one of these chemicals, it recognizes it as an enemy and initiates an immune response, which typically starts with the production of inflammatory chemicals to help your body put up a fight. With repeated exposure to these chemicals over time, this inflammatory response isn't able to calm down as it was designed to. Over time, this can lead to immune system dysregulation and is a risk factor for numerous diseases.

- **IDCs increase our sensitivity to allergens.** Continuous IDC exposure can lead to the development of new allergic reactions or the exacerbation of existing allergic diseases, such as asthma and food allergies.

- **IDCs make us more prone to autoimmune diseases.** There are proteins in most IDCs that look similar to proteins our own bodies make, which can confuse our immune system and prompt it to start to see its own healthy tissue as "enemy" and attack it—the definition of autoimmunity.

- **IDCs manipulate our immune system's killer cells**, making them less effective. Research shows that these chemicals can influence the function and activity of certain T cells and NK cells, both of which play crucial roles in our bodies to defend against pathogens and eliminate infected or abnormal cells.

- **IDCs mess with our cells' apoptosis, or ability to self-destruct**—which, counterintuitive as it may sound, is a crucial process that eliminates damaged or abnormal cells and keeps the body in homeostasis. When IDCs are absorbed by the body, they mimic, block, or interfere with the action of hormones like estrogen, thyroid, and glucocorticoids, all of which play important roles in regulating apoptosis in various cell types and tissues.

So what can we do to minimize our exposure to IDCs? Dr. Cohen recommends starting here:

» NO. 1: TAKE A QUICK SURVEY OF WHAT YOU'RE EATING AND THE PRODUCTS YOU'RE USING

Every day, we're exposed to hundreds of natural and synthetic compounds in the food we eat, our personal care products, the cleansers we use in our homes, and even the air we breathe, says Dr. Cohen. "There are more than ninety thousand chemicals approved and registered for use in all our products in the U.S.," she says. "The food industry alone uses more than three thousand food additive chemicals in their products, and the average American consumes five pounds of these in a year."

To help you get a sense of the IDCs *you* may be exposed to, make a list of all the products you use in a typical week: Write down what you put on, in, and around your body. Then scan the list and do a quick assessment: Are you eating or using a lot of things that contain IDCs? You'll find great resources on the Environmental Working Group (EWG) website that can help you answer that question.

» NO. 2: CONSIDER MAKING CHANGES IN THE AREAS THAT CAN HAVE THE BIGGEST IMPACT

Dr. Cohen says this includes things like the water you use to drink and cook with (reverse-osmosis filtration is ideal, and you want to avoid using plastic water bottles, which can leach IDCs), the food you eat (the less processed the better, and choose USDA organic when possible), and the personal care and cleaning products you use (use EWG.org to search the products you're using, vet ingredients, and find better alternatives). "Start with the changes that feel easiest to implement, and go from there," says Dr. Cohen. "Remember, this is a journey. Do one thing at a time, don't let perfection be the enemy of the good, and know that these changes you make over time really can make a positive impact on your health."

Allergies: Why They Happen and What to Do About Them

If you've ever dealt with the telltale signs of an allergic reaction—the sneezing, runny nose, itchy eyes, skin rash, or myriad other symptoms—you know the kind of immediate and often intense reaction your body can have when you're exposed to something your immune system doesn't like. But how and why can your body produce such a violent reaction to something (say, cat dander or tree pollen) that doesn't affect other people at all? And is there anything you can do to change your immune system's response?

Here, allergist and immunologist Zahida Maskatia, MD, walks us through what we need to know about what, exactly, allergies are, why they happen, and what you can do to ease the symptoms.

An allergic response happens when the immune system overreacts to a harmless substance in your environment, known as an allergen. While the immune system works more or less the same in all of us, there are differences in how our immune cells react to different exposures from person to person. For example, your immune system may see cat dander as "danger" and respond to it the way it does all enemies. Your bestie's immune system may see that same cat dander as no big deal—but have an allergic reaction when it comes in contact with tree pollen or peanuts.

Why? Experts don't have definitive answers but point to genetic differences (allergies tend to run in families), early life exposures (the thinking being that early exposure to certain allergens may help the immune system develop tolerance and possibly reduce allergy risk), and even the composition of the bacteria in your gut that make up your microbiome (the more diverse, the more likely you are to avoid allergies).

Anatomy of an Allergic Reaction

What follows is a basic look at what happens before the sneezing, itching, runny nose, rash, or other allergy symptoms set in.

- You're exposed to an allergen—such as pollen, dust mites, pet dander, or certain food proteins—and your immune system overreacts instead of treating it like the harmless substance it is.

- Memory T cells, which are formed during the initial phase of an allergic response, later help your immune system recall the allergen when you're exposed to it again, amplifying your reaction to it.

- Your immune system produces antibodies called Immunoglobulin E (IgE) that sit on the surface of your mast cells and basophils (a type of white blood cell). The next time you come in contact with that same allergen, your IgE antibodies trigger a signaling cascade that leads to the release of inflammatory chemicals, which initiates the inflammatory response you call an allergic reaction.

- Histamine is one of those inflammatory chemicals, and it causes your blood vessels to dilate (leading to redness and swelling), makes your veins more permeable (leading to fluid leakage and swelling), and stimulates your nerve endings (leading to itching and pain). Other inflammatory mediators, including leukotrienes and cytokines, recruit and activate other immune cells, amplifying your body's inflammatory response—and potentially making your symptoms even worse.

- In most cases, an allergic response resolves once an allergen is removed or eliminated from the environment. If you're continually exposed to the allergen (say, pollen when everything starts to bloom in the springtime), regulatory T cells (aka Tregs) help suppress allergic inflammation by releasing anti-inflammatory cytokines.

- If you have severe allergies or repeated exposures to allergens, your allergic response can persist and even become chronic.

What to Do If You Suspect You Have Allergies

While the tactic you choose will depend on the severity and the type of allergy you have, here are some of the most common approaches:

- **Identify and avoid the allergen.** If you suspect you're dealing with allergies, keep notes about your symptoms, including when they happen, how long they last, and how severe they are. There's a good chance some triggers or patterns will emerge that'll help point you to potential allergens.

- **Consider allergy testing to help identify specific allergens.** Skin prick testing and blood tests are the most common methods, but these are recommended only if you have specific symptoms that you and/or your healthcare provider believe are tied to a specific allergen. That's because most of us will test positive for IgE antibodies for allergens that we're not actually allergic to. "It's common for the immune system to get a little overzealous and create IgE antibodies for many harmless substances—and as a result, your IgE may be positive for a substance you *aren't* allergic to," says Dr. Maskatia, who adds that this is why up to 50 percent of positive allergy tests can actually be false positives. If allergy testing is indicated, an allergist or immunologist can assess your test results alongside your thorough health history (including reactions you've had to certain foods or allergens in the past) to give you the best chance of an accurate diagnosis.

- **Know your medication options.** There are a number of both over-the-counter and prescription medications that can help relieve allergy symptoms, including:

  - **Antihistamines**, which block cells from receiving histamine (the key inflammatory chemical released during an allergic reaction).

  - **Corticosteroids**, which reduce inflammation to reduce symptoms.

  - **Decongestants**, which provide temporary relief of nasal and sinus congestion.

  - **Bronchodilators**, which help to improve breathing by opening up airways in those with allergic asthma or exercise-induced airway constriction.

  - **Immunotherapy** (in the form of allergy shots or sublingual immunotherapy, SLIT), which involves exposing you to small, gradually increasing doses of allergens. The theory is that this will desensitize your immune system to the allergen and reduce your reactions to it over time.

- **Be prepared if you have severe allergic reactions.** If exposure to an allergen prompts swelling of the face or throat, difficulty breathing, rapid heartbeat, or loss of consciousness, seek medical help immediately and work with a clinician to establish an emergency action plan for treating your symptoms if they happen again. You might need to carry an epinephrine auto-injector (aka EpiPen), for example, that you can administer yourself in the event you're exposed to the allergen again.

Ask an Expert

I've heard it's important to introduce foods like peanuts into my baby's diet, but I'm scared! Can I put it off until she's older?

As a mom of three, I understand the fear. But the truth is that early exposure to allergenic foods like peanut and egg—which means giving your baby these foods around six months of age and even sooner in some cases—is an incredibly important step you can take to prevent your child from developing food allergies later.

The thinking is that this exposure via the digestive tract teaches a baby's immune system that these foods are harmless. If exposure to allergenic foods happens via the skin—microscopic particles of food allergens in the environment can enter a baby's body via their skin barrier, which isn't as robust as an adult's—the immune system is more likely to see the food as an "invader" and launch an allergic response.

If your baby has severe eczema, they will likely see even greater benefit from early food introduction, but it is also more likely that a food allergy has already developed. To be safe, talk to your child's doctor about the right plan of action for you.

—Zahida Maskatia, MD, allergist, immunologist, and medical director of Latitude Food Allergy Care

Autoimmune Disease: When the Body Attacks Itself

As we've learned so far, a crucial aspect of the immune system is its ability to tell the difference between good and bad. It has to be able to suss out external pathogens (like the novel coronavirus that causes COVID-19) while leaving what's harmless (like tree pollen) alone. It also has to be able to tell when your body's own good cells have turned bad, like if they start multiplying and dividing out of control (read: they've become cancerous) and launch an attack if necessary.

Given this complexity, you can see how the immune system might get things wrong at times and attack *healthy* tissue. When this happens, the result is an autoimmune disease.

There are more than one hundred autoimmune diseases. Depending on where your immune system is attacking, different autoimmune diseases may develop. For example, if your immune system starts mistakenly attacking the cells in your pancreas that make insulin, type 1 diabetes is the result; when it sees healthy skin cells as harmful, you might be diagnosed with psoriasis. (For more on some of the most common autoimmune diseases in women, flip to page 317.)

What Causes Your Immune System to Attack Healthy Tissue—and Why Are Women More Susceptible?

If scientists had definitive answers, they'd be able to spare the 80 percent of the population (78 percent of whom are women!) who suffer from autoimmune conditions from that fate.[4] But there are a few theories for why our immune system can turn on itself, some of which may help explain why women are at greater risk.

» GENETICS

Our genes play a significant role in our susceptibility to autoimmune conditions, and certain autoimmune diseases tend to run in families. There isn't a single gene for autoimmune disease but rather a number of genetic variants found in genes that regulate the immune system. A growing body of research also points to gene-environment interactions, which is when genetic predisposition interacts with environmental triggers, such as infections, pollutants, dietary factors, or stress, to initiate an autoimmune response.[5]

It's also important to note that the X chromosome contains numerous genes involved in immune regulation. Given that women have two X chromosomes (whereas men have only one), scientists hypothesize that this may lead to differences that help explain why we are more susceptible to autoimmune diseases and suffer from them in vastly greater numbers than our male counterparts.

» INTESTINAL PERMEABILITY (AKA LEAKY GUT)

This is a condition that occurs when the tight junctions lining your intestine become more porous, which allows undigested food particles, bacteria, and toxins to leak into your bloodstream. Immune cells recognize these foreign substances as threats and initiate an inflammatory response to neutralize them. The resulting chronic inflammation can lead to immune dysregulation—and increase your risk of autoimmune diseases.[6] Leaky gut can also disrupt the balance of bugs in your microbiome, and the resulting dysbiosis may promote more inflammation, immune dysregulation, and autoimmune responses.

» HORMONAL TRANSITIONS

Puberty, pregnancy, and the menopause transition are all times of hormonal flux that are thought to increase a woman's chances of having autoimmunity triggered.[7] (For more on how each of these transitions impacts the female immune system, flip back to page 302.)

» TRAUMA

Emerging evidence suggests that traumatic experiences may influence immune function and contribute to the development or exacerbation of autoimmune conditions. Traumatic experiences can result in elevated stress hormones for prolonged periods of time, which can cause a dysregulation in the immune system. In fact, up to 80 percent of patients report uncommon emotional stress before the onset of autoimmune disease.[8]

Trauma-induced stress responses (such as inflammation) can also lead to epigenetic modifications, "turning on" genes that may have predisposed you to an autoimmune disease. What's more, the mental health impact of trauma—depression, anxiety, post-traumatic stress disorder (PTSD), and the dysfunctional coping strategies many use to manage these conditions—can further mess with immune function and increase your risk of developing an autoimmune disease.

» AGING

After many years of fighting off countless bacteria and viruses, your immune system has built up an incredible immune memory. However, some experts believe those immune cells responsible for this impressive immune memory may also cause a low level of inflammation, which can lower your threshold for overall immunity—at which point an autoimmune condition may be more likely to develop.[9]

Common Autoimmune Diseases in Women

Despite the fact that autoimmune diseases are so common among women, getting a diagnosis can be a feat. One survey by the Autoimmune Association found that on average, autoimmune patients saw four different doctors over a four-year period before getting an accurate diagnosis—and a whopping 45 percent of those patients had been labeled "chronic complainers" or were told they were "overly concerned" with their health.[10]

Considering the long, often challenging journey it can take to get an accurate diagnosis, it's important to be familiar with some of the most common autoimmune diseases that affect women and their symptoms so you can track what you're experiencing and know which specialists to see to help you figure out what's happening.

» RHEUMATOID ARTHRITIS (RA)

Happens when . . . The immune system mistakenly attacks the tissue lining the joints on both sides of your body.

Common symptoms: Joint pain, swelling, stiffness, and/or tenderness; stiffness in the morning or after sitting for long stretches; extreme tiredness;

weakness. A "flare" refers to symptoms that feel significant after a period of time when you felt better.

» HASHIMOTO'S DISEASE

Happens when . . . The immune system mistakenly attacks the thyroid gland, leading to inflammation and even destruction of the thyroid gland that often results in hypothyroidism, a condition in which the thyroid gland doesn't produce enough thyroid hormone.

  Common symptoms: Fatigue, mild weight gain, sensitivity to cold, constipation, dry skin, brittle nails, hair loss (or slow hair growth), decreased libido, difficulty concentrating or remembering things, and more.

» GRAVES' DISEASE

Happens when . . . The immune system mistakenly produces antibodies that stimulate the thyroid gland to produce too much thyroid hormone (hyperthyroidism).

  Common symptoms: Rapid heartbeat, heart palpitations, weight loss despite increased appetite, nervousness, menstrual cycle irregularities, muscle weakness, and more. Eye disease (bulging eyes, eye irritation, double vision, light sensitivity, or other vision changes) can also be a sign.

» CELIAC DISEASE

Happens when . . . The immune system mistakenly attacks the lining of the small intestine in response to ingesting gluten (a protein found in wheat, barley, and rye), leading to inflammation and damage to the intestinal villi—fingerlike projections that line the intestine walls and help your body absorb nutrients.

  Common symptoms: Gastrointestinal symptoms (abdominal pain, bloating, diarrhea, constipation, gas), fatigue, unintended weight loss, abnormal periods, mood changes (most commonly depression in adults), and more.

» LUPUS

Happens when . . . The immune system mistakenly attacks healthy tissue in various organs and body systems, including the skin, joints, kidneys, heart, lungs, blood vessels, and brain.

Common symptoms: Fatigue, joint or muscle pain, chest pain (particularly when taking a deep breath), headaches, skin rashes (particularly a "butterfly" rash on the face), fever, hair loss, sensitivity to sunlight, mouth sores, and more.

» MULTIPLE SCLEROSIS (MS)

Happens when . . . The immune system mistakenly attacks the myelin sheath, a fatty substance that surrounds and insulates nerve fibers in the central nervous system (which includes the brain and the spinal cord). The resulting damage leads to the formation of scar tissue (sclerosis) along the nerves, which can interfere with the transmission of electrical impulses and cause a wide range of symptoms—which can vary widely and depend on the location and extent of nerve damage within the central nervous system.

Common symptoms: Muscle weakness, numbness or tingling sensations, blurred or double vision, bladder and bowel dysfunction, mood changes, muscle stiffness, muscle tremors, and more.

» SJÖGREN'S SYNDROME

Happens when . . . The immune system mistakenly attacks the body's moisture-producing glands, primarily the salivary and lacrimal (tear) glands, which results in decreased production of saliva and tears. In some cases, it can affect other organs and systems, such as the lungs, kidneys, or liver.

Common symptoms: Dry mouth, dry or itchy eyes, vaginal dryness, dry skin, frequent nosebleeds (which could signal dry nasal tissue), dry throat (which can manifest as coughing frequently), joint or muscle pain, fatigue, loss of sense of taste, light sensitivity, and more.

» PSORIASIS

Happens when . . . The immune system mistakenly attacks healthy skin cells, causing inflammation and abnormal cell turnover, and this rapid overproduction of skin cells leads to thick, red, scaly patches on the skin (most commonly on the elbows, knees, face, nails, genitals, low back, palms, and feet).

Common symptoms: Thick, red patches of skin covered with silvery scales (known as plaques); itchy, cracked, dry skin; skin pain; joint pain; pitted, cracked, or "crumbly" nails.

» SCLERODERMA

Happens when . . . There's an abnormal growth of connective tissue, leading to thickening and hardening of the skin and other organs.

Common symptoms: Thickening and hardening of the skin, joint pain, stiffness (especially in the mornings after waking), fatigue, unexplained weight loss, and more.

» POLYMYALGIA RHEUMATICA (PMR)

Happens when . . . Scientists don't fully understand the cause, but they do know this chronic inflammatory disorder primarily affects the shoulders and hips, and they consider it an autoimmune disease.

Common symptoms: Pain and stiffness in the muscles around the shoulders and hips, which can be particularly severe in the mornings or after periods of inactivity; fatigue; weakness; low-grade fever; loss of appetite; unintended weight loss; and a general feeling of malaise.

» INFLAMMATORY BOWEL DISEASE (INCLUDING CROHN'S DISEASE AND ULCERATIVE COLITIS)

Happens when . . . The immune system mistakenly attacks healthy tissues in the digestive tract. Crohn's disease most commonly affects the end of the small intestine (ileum) and the beginning of the large intestine (colon); ulcerative colitis is characterized by inflammation and ulcers (sores) in the lining of the colon and rectum.

Common symptoms: Abdominal pain and cramping, blood in your stool, diarrhea (which may be bloody), fatigue, unintended weight loss, and more.

Understanding Vaccines: How They Work and Top Questions About Safety, Answered

Among the many health topics for which misinformation is rampant, vaccine safety is at the top of the list—and it's causing record numbers of people to opt out of vaccines for both themselves and their kids. In fact, the World Health Organization considers vaccine hesitancy one of the top global health threats of our time.[11]

While the chasm between pro- and anti-vaxxers grows wider and increasingly politically charged, many people—especially parents faced with decisions about vaccinating their kids—are left with questions. What they need are evidence-based answers. Sadly, when we try to find those answers, most of us are met with behind-the-screen keyboard warriors with an agenda.

To help you navigate this tricky territory, here are some of the questions that frequently come up about vaccines, how they work, and how safe they are—and the science-based answers from Boghuma K. Titanji, MD, PhD.

Q: How do vaccines work?

Vaccines prime the immune system to recognize and respond to specific bacteria, viruses, or other pathogens that can cause disease. If you're exposed to that pathogen in the future, your immune system is able to mount a rapid and robust response that keeps you from developing the disease or reduces its severity if you do get it.

Dr. Titanji describes vaccines as a way to give your body a "cheat code" against something it hasn't seen before. "When you get a vaccine, you're showing your body a piece of something that can cause disease, which prompts your immune system to make antibodies and develop a memory of that virus or bacteria," she explains. "This way, if you encounter that bacteria or virus in real life, your body already has the cheat code and can say, 'I've seen this before and have a library of antibodies for this pathogen, so let's ramp up production of those antibodies to fight the virus.'" The result: You don't get as sick as you would have if your body were seeing the pathogen for the first time.

Q: What's the difference between "natural immunity" and the immunity I get from a vaccine, and is one better than the other?

"Natural immunity" simply means you're not doing anything preemptively to show your body bits of a pathogen before you see it in the real world. The immune response your body develops against any pathogen—whether via an infection or a vaccine—is essentially the same. The advantage a vaccine gives you is that it allows your body to prepare for the pathogen *before* it encounters it. "When someone tells me, 'I'd rather get natural immunity than a vaccine,' I remind them that to get that natural immunity, you will get sick," says Dr. Titanji. "And if it's an infection like meningitis, well, that can kill you within twenty-four to forty-eight hours. Your body may not have enough time to get your immune cells to make the antibodies to fight that bacteria in time for you to be able to successfully recover from that illness.

"On the other hand, if you had a meningitis vaccine before you come in contact with meningitis, your immune system says, 'Oh, piece of cake! We know this bacteria, we have the antibodies that have seen it via the vaccine, so let's quickly ramp up those antibodies and tamp down this infection.'"

It's also important to know that with certain infections, it's better for the immune system to be introduced to the infection through a vaccine than through natural immunity, because the impact of the actual infection on the immune system can be profound. Take the varicella virus, for example—

which manifests as chicken pox and shingles. Once you get this virus, you have it for life, and it hides out in your nerve roots and can get reactivated later in life. Kids who get the chicken-pox vaccine are protected against the varicella virus—meaning they won't get chicken pox as kids *or* shingles later in life.

Q: How are vaccines tested?

Vaccines that are administered today have been through multiple stages of testing, including double-blind, placebo-controlled trials—the gold standard for all drug-safety testing. "Going through all of the stages of these trials usually takes anywhere from ten to twenty years," says Dr. Titanji. "So by the time you're getting that vaccine in your arm, you can rest assured knowing years of work and lots of really good science has gone into it."

Once a vaccine is proven to be effective and safe, it's released to the public. When updates are proposed for existing vaccines, the updated vaccine is tested against the existing one—not a placebo. That's because it would be unethical to withhold from study participants a vaccine that we've already tested and know is safe and effective.

It's also important to note that vaccine safety studies are ongoing and have led to changes in both the components of vaccines and the recommended childhood vaccine schedule. The Vaccine Safety Datalink (VSD) is a tool researchers use to continually look at vaccine safety, determine rates of adverse reactions, and test hypotheses about tweaks to specific vaccines and schedule recommendations. The VSD is a collaborative effort among the Centers for Disease Control and Prevention, multiple managed care organizations, and academic researchers—and includes vaccination and medical records from approximately nine million children and adults.

In a time when vaccines have become such a charged topic, one thing all of us can do is aim to have more productive conversations with our healthcare providers and with one another. "It's important to remember that most of the questions people have about vaccines for themselves and their kids come from a place of wanting to do what's best and safe—not necessarily from an 'antivaccine' stance," says Dr. Titanji. "The more we're able to have open conversations where healthcare professionals educate patients about the vaccines and then give them space to take in that information and leave the door open for them to come back and ask more questions if needed, the better."

Your Game Plan: Science-Backed Tactics to Optimize Your Immune System

Most of us think the goal is to build a "strong" immune system, one we can "boost" with vitamin C and a small army of supplements. But the more accurate aim is for a *finely tuned* immune system, one that works efficiently and effectively to attack what has the potential to cause us harm and make us sick—but doesn't become so overzealous that it starts attacking healthy tissue. The best way to strike this balance and keep your body's defense system working optimally is to get back to the basics, says allergist and immunologist Heather Moday, MD. Here are her go-to strategies for doing just that.

Get at least seven hours of sleep a night. In fact, this might be the most important thing you can do to help your immune system work optimally. That's because the immune system is really active when we're asleep. "At night, the naive T cells in your lymph nodes are presented with new antigens that your innate immune cells have picked up during the day, your NK cells are busy killing viruses and trolling for cancer cells, and your B cells pump out antibodies," says Dr. Moday. "This inflammatory frenzy is your immune system hard at work to keep you healthy." Melatonin (the hormone you've probably heard of as the body's main regulator of sleep and wakefulness) also regulates certain pro-inflammatory cytokines that direct your immune cells to attack and destroy anything that's found its way into your body during the day.

One reason your immune system is so active at night is because cortisol (which has strong anti-inflammatory effects) is at its lowest during the night, so it doesn't interfere. What's more, all this immune system activation requires a lot of energy—which we have more of when we're sleeping and our brain and muscles aren't using as much glucose as they do when we're active during the day. (For expert advice on how to improve your sleep and snag more of it if needed, flip to page 517.)

Hit your stress sweet spot. Too often, women are told to "stress less." But here's something that may surprise you: Cortisol (commonly referred to as the stress hormone) actually has anti-inflammatory properties. When you initially experience a fight-or-flight stress response, your immune system kicks into gear in case you get wounded. White blood cells make their way to your skin, lungs, and GI tract so they're prepared to take on an attack from the outside world. When the threat is over, your immune soldiers retreat.

When stress is acute (and you're not in actual danger), you can think of it as "good" stress that benefits the immune system, honing its function and improving its surveillance capabilities over time. Exercise is a great example of this, says Dr. Moday (more on this next!), as are cold plunges, saunas, and even cognitive challenges. However, when stress becomes chronic, cortisol loses its feedback mechanism and your immune system soldiers don't retreat from their battle stations. The result is chronic inflammation, which tires out your immune system and makes it less effective.

The goal is to be the Goldilocks of stress, says Dr. Moday: You want to get just the right amount to keep your immune system in fighting form, and stay alert to the signs that stress is becoming overwhelming—think things like muscle tension, jaw clenching, anxiety, irritability, or withdrawing from social events—so you're more likely to catch yourself before it becomes chronic.

If you start to feel that unhelpful type of stress, Dr. Moday recommends taking a breathwork break. Her go-to practice is box breathing: Breathe in for a count of four, hold your breath at the top of the inhalation for a count of four, breathe out for a count of four, and then hold your breath for four counts after your exhale. "This pumps the brakes on the stress response," she says.

Move your body. Dr. Moday calls exercise "the best kind of good stress for the immune system." That's because, while your workout prompts some breakdown of muscle tissue and resulting inflammation, your body transitions quickly into restful repair of that damage—which is very beneficial to your immune system. Research backs this up. Those who exercise regularly develop more T cells (those "killer" white blood cells that destroy pathogen intruders) than their sedentary peers.[12]

Here's the good news: All types of exercise are helpful, so choose whatever makes you feel good, says Dr. Moday. "Jog, walk, dance, go on a bike ride, take a yoga class—all of these activities can improve your immune health."

Make your gut microbiome happy. Most of your immune cells can be found in what Dr. Moday calls the immune system central intelligence center: your gut-associated lymphoid tissue (GALT). GALT is a cluster of lymph tissue lining the small and large intestines that contains the highest concentration of immune cells in the body. Why do they live there? Because we interact with most foreign substances in our gut via all the things we eat, drink, swallow, and even breathe in (yes, some of the stuff you inhale makes its way through your esophagus and into your gut). The immune cells in our lymph tissue are in constant communication with the microbes in our gastrointestinal tract to help us decipher what is friend and what is foe. We want to be able to tolerate food, for example, but mount a robust immune response against a pathogen on food that can be dangerous.

"When the gut microbiome is depleted, this important cross talk between our immune cells and gut microbes becomes less robust," says Dr. Moday. "By taking steps to support your microbiome, you're doing what you can to make sure your immune system is as healthy as it can be."

The same things that keep your gut microbiome working optimally also help your GALT, including eating plenty of fiber-rich foods; avoiding processed foods, sugar, and artificial sweeteners; and limiting the use of antibiotics unless necessary. (For a more detailed look at your gut health and the steps you can take to improve yours, see chapter 15.)

• • • • •

We're often sold a bunch of myths about the importance of "boosting" our immune system. But what we really want is a *balanced* immune system—

one that's able to put up a good fight if we encounter a harmful virus, bacterium, or other invader and then return to surveillance mode once the battle has been won. The good news is that following the science-backed steps you've read in this chapter can help you strike this balance and keep your immune system working optimally now and for years to come.

Chapter 12

Pain

*How Women Feel Pain Differently, Why We're Still Told
It's All in Our Heads, and What to Do About It*

> *In medicine, as in the culture at large, women's pain is often treated
> like the drone of a nearby mosquito: constant and annoying, but an
> inevitable part of nature.*
>
> —Jess McAllen, "Endo Days" in *The Baffler*

At least 50 million adults in the U.S. deal with chronic pain—and women make up a higher percentage of that number.[1] Yet when we go to the emergency room with symptoms of heart disease (like chest pain), we can wait ten to fifteen minutes longer than men to be evaluated for possible heart attack.[2] When we seek help for abdominal pain, we're up to 25 percent less likely to be treated with powerful painkillers than men are.[3] And we feel the sting of this gender gap: Multiple surveys have found that nearly half of female respondents say their pain has been dismissed or not taken seriously by a healthcare provider.[4]

Put simply, women's pain is often not taken seriously. This is even more shocking when you consider that research in both animals and humans suggests that females have a greater sensitivity to pain than men and that some painkillers are less effective for us as well.[5]

So why is our pain often ignored and downplayed even by medical professionals, and what can we do to get the relief we need and deserve? We'll tackle these questions and more here.

In this chapter, we'll learn . . .

- **The ins and outs of the body's pain response**, including what's happening in the brain to make us feel pain, the difference between acute and chronic pain, and why chronic pain affects more women than men around the world.

- **The most common chronic pain conditions in women**, why they happen, and the newest thinking on treating each.

- **Specific advice on how to talk about your pain** to clinicians so they can help you find relief faster.

- **How the most common prescription pain medications work**, so you can have a more informed conversation with your healthcare provider about what's best for you.

- **The important role pharmacists can play in helping you treat pain.** When you know what questions to ask, pharmacists can be a great resource for information on how you might treat your pain.

- **How to advocate for yourself when you're in pain** and find a clinician who can help you.

Meet the Experts

Antje M. Barreveld, MD, chief of pain medicine, Newton-Wellesley Hospital, Mass General Brigham, and associate professor of anesthesiology at Tufts University School of Medicine

Esther H. Chen, MD, professor of emergency medicine at the University of California, San Francisco, who has studied gender disparities in pain management

Tina Sacks, PhD, associate professor and doctoral program chair at the School of Social Welfare at the University of California at Berkeley

Maureen Moriarty, ANP-BC, FAHS, FAANP, MS, DNP, headache specialist and associate professor at the Malek School of Nursing Professions at Marymount University

Laura Payne, PhD, director of the Clinical and Translational Pain Research Laboratory at McLean Hospital and assistant professor at Harvard Medical School

Vonda Wright, MD, orthopedic surgeon, sports medicine specialist, and author of *Unbreakable: A Woman's Guide to Aging with Power*

Anita Gupta, DO, PharmD, clinical professor at the University of California School of Medicine, Riverside, and adjunct assistant professor of anesthesiology and critical care medicine and pain medicine at the Johns Hopkins University School of Medicine

Understanding Pain:
What It Is, Why We Feel It, and
Why Women's Pain Is Often Dismissed

For something that can be so straightforward in how terrible it feels, pain is a quite complicated process encompassing several stages and systems of the body. It involves the nervous system and the mind. It impacts our senses and emotions. It can also motivate us to avoid what prompts it and encourage us to rest.

"Pain has widespread implications, not only in day-to-day suffering but also in our ability to care for our families, to be able to work, to feel whole," says Antje M. Barreveld, MD. "Pain is everywhere. We should care about it. And knowing how pain works helps people understand and access the treatment they deserve." Here, Dr. Barreveld walks us through the basics to help us better understand pain.

Most of us understand pain as acute or chronic.

Acute pain is short-term pain that usually comes on suddenly and is often the result of injury, illness, or surgery. It typically dissipates once the underlying cause of the pain is treated.

Chronic pain is long-term pain that can persist beyond an expected recovery period or occurs along with a chronic health condition and can be consistent or come and go.

Pain specialists tend to think about pain in the following categories, explains Dr. Barreveld:

Somatic pain, which is pain related to muscle tissue.

Neuropathic pain, which is pain related to nerves.

Visceral pain, which is pain related to our organs, whether it's the gut or uterus or lungs.

Nociplastic pain (aka centrally mediated pain), which includes brain mechanisms of pain. Pain often starts somewhere specific—say, you cut your finger while chopping onions, pull a muscle playing pickleball, or you're recovering from surgery. Yet no matter where your pain is located or how it started, it gets processed through our spinal cord and our brain. Here's a very basic version of what happens:

- Pain receptors detect potentially harmful stimuli like heat, pressure, vibration, or inflammation, and send electrical signals through nerve fibers.

- Those electrical signals are transmitted to your brain, specifically the dorsal root ganglion, which you can think of like the mothership of pain transmission that communicates with the spinal cord.

- In the spinal cord, there are both ascending and descending pathways to and from the brain, and pain signals can be either amplified or inhibited by various hormones and neurotransmitters. This creates a feedback processing loop.

- Once those electrical signals reach your brain, they travel to various regions responsible for interpreting pain, including the thalamus (which acts as a central hub for receiving and processing pain signals), the cortex (which processes the sensory aspects of pain, like its location, intensity, and quality), and the limbic system (which generates our emotional response to pain, initiating feelings of fear, distress, and anxiety, and helps us form memories of painful experiences to help us better avoid them in the future).

- Your brain then sends signals to your muscles to react to your pain. For example, if you touch something hot, those signals will prompt you to pull your hand away from the heat quickly.

If your pain is acute, you feel pain, and then it goes away. However, if you're dealing with intense, untreated pain or chronic pain that persists over a long period of time, those pain receptors in your spine get repeatedly stimulated. As a result, they become more sensitive and responsive to subsequent stimuli—even if those stimuli are harmless and shouldn't actually cause pain.

Over time, this extra excitability of pain receptors in the spine makes them more efficient at transmitting a barrage of pain signals, which heightens your body's ability to perceive pain even more. This is often referred to as central sensitization (sometimes called the "wind-up" theory of pain), and it's why someone with untreated or chronic pain may become more sensitive to pain than the average person.

"You can think of central sensitization almost like a volume knob," says Dr. Barreveld. "When patients with chronic pain get a pain signal, they hear it at a super loud level, whereas someone who doesn't have chronic pain won't hear pain signals at the same volume, even if it's the same type of pain."

We also know that in addition to chronic pain, anxiety and depression can make people more likely to be hyperexcitable to pain; negative appraisal (which used to be referred to as catastrophizing, or when you expect the worst-case scenario) can also potentially contribute to an increased risk of having higher levels of pain.

But here's the good news: While your brain literally changes when you're in pain in ways that can make you more sensitive to it, treating your pain can reverse those brain changes. Dr. Barreveld references a study of hip replacement patients who had terrible arthritis and discomfort before surgery, where scientists could actually see decreased gray matter density in their brains. Post-op, as the patients' pain dissipated, gray matter density increased.

"This points to the plasticity of the brain, and that chronic pain isn't necessarily a doom and gloom, inevitable consequence," says Dr. Barreveld. "It really is something malleable and changeable."

Women's Pain Is Often Underestimated and Disbelieved. Here's What to Do About It

In an ideal world, all clinicians would investigate women's pain properly and not assume it's exaggerated. Until that happens, Esther H. Chen, MD, who has studied gender disparities in pain management in an emergency setting, explains what we can do to have the best shot at our pain being taken seriously.

- **Be as specific as you can when you talk about your symptoms.** If possible, try to use the most descriptive terms you can when it comes to explaining what you're feeling. For example, you might say, "I have pain in my upper abdomen that gets worse when I eat and feels like a cramping, squeezing type of pain" instead of "My stomach hurts and I just don't feel well." This specificity can help clinicians think of a set of conditions in which the symptoms might fit, says Dr. Chen. "It can be more challenging for providers to deal with vague pain," she adds.

- **Put your pain in context when you're talking about it.** Pain is subjective, which means talking about it in the context of something that's universally understandable can be helpful. You might say something like "The worst pain I've ever had was labor contractions, and what I'm feeling is close to that level of pain."

- **Google your symptoms—and ask your clinician specific questions, especially if you don't feel understood.** Reading a few trustworthy articles about what your pain might mean can help you craft some specific questions that can help your provider better understand what you're experiencing. You might say something like "I've been doing some reading, and I think I have eight out of these twelve symptoms that are listed for this condition; can we talk about this?"

- **Ask someone you trust to join you when you talk to a clinician about your pain.** Not only can this person help you express what you're feeling—something that can feel like a tall task when you're actively in pain—but they can also help your provider understand the context of what you're experiencing.

- **Advocate for yourself.** If you're in pain but haven't been treated, specifically ask for something to relieve your pain—whether it's a pain-relieving medication, a warm blanket, a few pillows to prop up your sore knee, or an ice pack for your head. If you feel like you're not being helped or your pain isn't being taken seriously, ask for a nurse to come in and see you—or even for a different provider. "You don't have to put up with poor care, assuming it's all you're going to get," says Dr. Chen. "There are clinicians who are genuine advocates for women's health." It just may take a bit of time to find one.

How to Talk About Pain: Explaining What You're Feeling

If you're seeing a clinician about pain, Dr. Barreveld says it can help to be prepared to answer the following "OPQRST" questions, which should be part of most pain assessments.

- **Onset:** When did your pain start? What was happening at that time?

- **Palliative and Proactive Factors:** What makes the pain better? Worse? (Include specific activities, positions, or treatments.)

- **Quality:** Describe the pain. Is it burning, sharp, shooting, aching, throbbing, etc.?

- **Region and Radiation:** Where is the pain? Does it spread to other areas?

- **Severity:** How bad is the pain? Does it impact your quality of life?

- **Timing:** When does the pain occur? Has it changed since onset? If so, how?

Racial Inequities in How Pain Is Perceived and Managed

Hidden biases drive many of the differences in how women's pain is viewed and treated compared with men's. Yet for people of color—and especially Black women—the situation is often worse, says Tina Sacks, PhD, who studies racial inequities in health, social determinants of health, and poverty and inequality. "The way pain is perceived and treated among people of color is one of the most persistent health inequities," says Dr. Sacks, "and much of it has to do with the false idea that there is a biological difference between races in how pain is felt and perceived."

Consider a 2016 study of medical students and residents that found that more than half believed at least one false claim about biological differences between Black and white people, including that Black people's skin is thicker, that their blood coagulates more quickly, and that their nerve endings are less sensitive than white people's.[6] "There is no biological basis for this, and yet even some of those educated enough to go to medical school and become physicians have received the message somewhere along the line that Black people are fundamentally different biological entities," says Dr. Sacks. Adding to these biases is the time pressure many clinicians feel—and the stereotyping that can happen when providers have limited time with patients, adds Dr. Sacks. "The American capitalism that shapes our healthcare system impacts everyone, but some of us are more disadvantaged in this system."

For women of color, these truths can feel like an immense burden—and sadly, there isn't always a lot you can do when faced with inequities in treatment. If you find yourself in this position, here's what Dr. Sacks wants you to remember:

- **Playing a game of "what if" is understandable**. Have a sneaking suspicion that if you were living in a different body, you'd be treated differently? That's a normal thought—albeit a heavy burden to carry, says Dr. Sacks. "For so many women of color, going to the doctor involves a lack of certainty because it entails questions like 'Am I being treated badly because I'm a woman? Or because I'm Black? Or because I'm fat? And if I say something, will I get even worse care?' That uncertainty creates a sense of vulnerability and a lack of control over one's health." While acknowledging this won't necessarily change anything, it can help normalize the experience for you.

- **Trust yourself**. Women are often told our pain is all in our heads. There can be a dismissal of our concerns. "Yet while white women may be viewed as crazy, hormonal, or anxious, women of color occupy a different space—we're made to feel that we're disposable and that our pain doesn't matter," says Dr. Sacks. If you're feeling this, try to remind yourself when you're sitting in front of a healthcare provider: *I am living in this body. I am the one who knows what's going on.* "Hold tight to your lived, embodied experience," says Dr. Sacks, who adds that when you're in pain and scared and vulnerable, it can be easy to get talked out of what you know because of a clinician's perceived authority and expertise. "Yes, the provider you interact with has expertise, but you do, too," says Dr. Sacks. "You know what it feels to be in your body. Hold tight to that."

- **Bring someone with you to your appointment if possible**. Having a healthcare advocate is go-to advice for good reason, and it can be especially helpful for people of color who are dealing with acute or chronic pain. "It's incredibly difficult to be in a situation where you're trying to manage anxiety about how you'll be treated, interpret everything your provider is telling you, and deal with the asymmetry of power between you and the person charged with taking care of you," says Dr. Sacks. Having a trusted person in your life by your side as you face all of this can help you navigate these often-tricky waters.

Finally, Dr. Sacks says that, considering the research-proven inequities, it's important to recognize that if you're a person of color, it's likely you'll be treated in a way that is unfair. And while this is disheartening, it can also reinforce that it is not your fault—and embolden you to continue to seek out the care you deserve.

Chronic Pain in Women: The Most Common Pain Conditions, Why They Disproportionately Impact Us, and Symptoms to Keep on Your Radar

Let's take a look at some of the conditions that are more common in women and why.

Headaches

Headaches are one of the most common causes of pain.[7] This is especially true for women, who are roughly one and a half times more likely than men to experience tension-type headaches[8] and two to three times as likely to experience migraine headaches.[9]

Why? "It can be partly explained by hormonal influences," says headache specialist Maureen Moriarty, MS, DNP. Before puberty, migraine incidence is about the same in boys and girls. After that big hormonal transition, about three out of four migraine sufferers are women.[10] While much more research is needed to understand all the factors that contribute to this discrepancy, experts point to estrogen and the role it appears to play in making your blood vessels constrict and dilate.

"If you get migraine headaches, you already have an underlying instability in the blood vessels in the brain, which makes them more reactive when they constrict and dilate," says Dr. Moriarty. "We think that fluctuations in estrogen layered on top of someone who's already predisposed to having this blood vessel instability is part of the story of why women suffer from headaches so much more frequently than men."

For example, one study found that women who get migraines around the time of their period (commonly referred to as menstrual migraines) tend to experience a greater rate of decline in estrogen than women who don't.[11] Migraines also tend to worsen during perimenopause, when estrogen fluctuates, and they often go down in frequency and severity during pregnancy, when estrogen is high and more stable.

» WHY DO WE FEEL HEADACHE PAIN?

Here's what's happening to prompt you to feel the pain of a headache:

- A trigger (for example, stress, muscle tension, certain foods or medications, or enlarged blood vessels) activates pain receptors (aka nociceptors).

- Nociceptors send signals to the trigeminal nerve, which is the nerve that gives us sensation in the face and controls the pain-sensitive structures in the brain. "The brain doesn't feel pain, but there are structures around the brain—like the meninges, which cover the brain, and the cerebral vessels—that do have pain receptors," says Dr. Moriarty.

- The trigeminal nerve continues to shuttle those pain signals to the thalamus, which is like the brain's relay station for pain sensation.

- The thalamus relays pain signals to the cortex, which is when we feel headache pain.

- This process prompts the release of calcitonin gene-related peptide (CGRP), which causes an inflammatory response: Your blood vessels dilate, and your mast cells (the watchdogs of your immune system) get activated and spew out inflammatory chemicals. CGRP also causes pain impulses to be sent from one nerve to another and back again, which keeps you in a continuous feedback loop of pain.

- Headache medications typically work by easing this inflammatory response (thereby reducing pain), narrowing blood vessels (which reduces blood flow and can ease pressure around nerves), or closing off pain pathways. Removing any known triggers of the headache can also help relieve pain over time.

Experts think the same biochemical mechanism is happening whether you have a tension-type headache or a migraine. "While tension-type headache is a distinct form of headache, many people who diagnose themselves with a tension-type headache actually meet the criteria for migraine," says Dr. Moriarty.

» TALK TO YOUR CLINICIAN

When talking to your doctor about your headache pain, Dr. Moriarty recommends describing it as mild, moderate, severe, or incapacitating.

Mild: You know your headache is there, but you'd put it in the "no big deal" category and don't take an over-the-counter (OTC) medication to ease your pain.

Moderate: You know your headache is there, you take something to ease the pain, and you can make it through your day but often feel distracted by your pain.

Severe: You'd classify your pain as very bad and take something to try to ease your pain. You push yourself to get through your day—you can go to work, drive the kids to school, get dinner on the table—but you'd really rather just get into bed.

Incapacitating: Your pain is so bad, you clear your calendar and stay in bed, getting up only to use the bathroom.

Before you make an appointment with a clinician about your headaches, keep track of your symptoms. There's a good chance you'll start to see trends—like your headaches come on right before your period or after you drink wine or deal with a lot of stress. Once you have some of this data, make an appointment with your primary care physician to talk about your headaches specifically—don't just tack this conversation onto the end of your annual physical.

Most important, don't brush off headache pain as no big deal. "Headaches may be common, but they're not normal," says Dr. Moriarty.

Menstrual Pain

Like so many aspects of women's health, we don't have nearly enough research on menstrual pain, especially given the fact that the majority of all people who menstruate will experience it—often so intensely that it prompts us to cancel plans.[12] Many experts say that menstrual pain (dysmenorrhea) has to do with the production and release of prostaglandins in the uterus, which triggers the muscle contractions and shedding of the uterine lining that we call our period. Studies have found that those with menstrual pain tend to have higher levels of prostaglandins than those who don't. Yet this finding isn't entirely consistent—and some scientists aren't convinced higher concentrations of prostaglandins are the whole story.

Laura Payne, PhD, assistant professor at Harvard Medical School, is one of those scientists. She points to the fact that the first line of treatment for menstrual pain is usually nonsteroidal anti-inflammatory drugs, which work by inhibiting the release of uterine prostaglandins, but they don't work for everybody, which means factors other than prostaglandins are likely at play.

What we *do* know is that treating pain rather than powering through it not only can help relieve discomfort in the moment but also may prevent chronic pain from developing later on. "Repeated experiences of pain change how the brain processes pain signals," says Dr. Payne. "When you experience any kind of recurring pain, including menstrual pain, it can lead to changes in your central nervous system that make you more sensitive to pain."

Dr. Payne is studying adolescents who suffer from menstrual cramps and why the condition puts some at greater risk for other pain conditions as they get older. Until we have clearer answers, she urges anyone suffering from the cramping, aching, and debilitating pain around their period to talk to a clinician and do something to ease the discomfort. She also says it's important to talk about this still-too-taboo topic with one another as well: "When we talk about it, we're more likely to realize that this type of pain is valid and that we don't have to hide it."

Menopause

Complaining about aches and pains in midlife and beyond is common for all of us, but for women, there's often a very real explanation for it: the menopause transition.

There are estrogen receptors throughout your entire body, including on your bones as well as on every single muscle, tendon, and ligament in your body. Before menopause, estrogen circulates freely and does multiple *great* things for your musculoskeletal system. It helps:

- Stimulate the cells responsible for bone formation (osteoblasts), which helps maintain bone density and strength. It also inhibits the cells responsible for the breakdown of bone tissue (osteoclasts), which reduces bone loss.

- Promote the production of collagen, which is one of the primary structural proteins in bones and contributes to bone strength and flexibility.

- Contribute to protein synthesis in muscle cells, which helps muscles grow and repair and regenerate, particularly after exercise. It also promotes a balance between fast-twitch and slow-twitch muscle fibers, which are essential for strength and overall muscle function.

- Make your muscle cells sensitive to insulin, which ensures your muscles have enough energy to contract and perform well.

- Reduce muscle inflammation and damage, thanks to its anti-inflammatory properties. It is especially important when it comes to preventing chronic inflammation that can lead to pain.

During perimenopause, estrogen production becomes unreliable. After menopause, "estrogen essentially walks out the door," says orthopedic surgeon Vonda Wright, MD. "And when it does, we lose all of its amazing benefits to our musculoskeletal system." Our osteoblasts don't work as well and our bones get weaker, making us more prone to painful fractures. The cartilage surrounding our joints—that spongy tissue that absorbs shock when we move our body—doesn't get the estrogen it needs and breaks down, prompting us to feel joint pain. When estrogen isn't around to work its anti-inflammatory magic, we also start to get more chronic inflammation—and this often leads to all-over aches, pains, and stiffness (aka arthralgia). This group of pain-related symptoms is increasingly being referred to as the musculoskeletal syndrome of menopause—a phrase Dr. Wright coined to help raise awareness about the many painful symptoms that can surface for women during the menopause transition.

So what can we do about these painful symptoms? Here's Dr. Wright's advice.

Make an educated decision about menopause hormone therapy. "Supplementing with estrogen is often like a salve that soothes all of these symptoms," says Dr. Wright. Educate yourself with science-backed information about hormone therapy and then work with a menopause specialist to get a prescription if it's a good fit for you.

Eat an anti-inflammatory diet. Load up on fiber-rich produce (especially green leafy veggies) and protein (ideally one gram of protein per pound of ideal body weight a day) and cut out all added sugar (which includes alcohol). "You can eat carbohydrates on an anti-inflammatory diet—you just have to make sure they're filled with fiber, not sugar," says Dr. Wright.

Move your body. When you're in pain, it can be tempting to stay sedentary. But this makes pain worse. "Movement flushes out those inflammatory molecules from our joints and we start to feel better," says Dr. Wright.

Lift weights. If you really want to prevent the painful musculoskeletal symptoms that often come along with menopause—or even reverse them if they've set in—strength training is key, says Dr. Wright. But this doesn't mean doing a dozen or more reps with those one-pound dumbbells. The goal is to work up to lifting weights so heavy, you can only do about four reps with good form. "This is the type of weightlifting that actually stimulates muscle growth," says Dr. Wright. "Endless reps with those little pink dumbbells is a waste of your time."

OTHER CHRONIC PAIN CONDITIONS MORE COMMON IN WOMEN

THE CONDITION	WHAT IT IS	SIGNS + SYMPTOMS
Fibromyalgia	A complex condition that causes pain and tenderness in muscles and joints throughout the body.	• Widespread pain, often described as a dull ache, that's lasted for three months or longer • Fatigue that won't go away, even after sleeping well • Brain fog (aka fibro fog) that makes it hard to focus or concentrate
Irritable bowel syndrome (IBS)	A chronic condition that affects the large intestine, leading to changes in bowel movements and/or painful abdominal symptoms.	• Abdominal pain and cramping that's often relieved (or lessened) after a bowel movement • Bloating and gas • Diarrhea or constipation • Changes in the frequency and/or consistency of bowel movements • White mucus in stool
Rheumatoid arthritis (RA)	An autoimmune disease that primarily affects the joints, causing inflammation, pain, and eventually joint damage if uncontrolled.	• Joint pain and swelling on both sides of the body • Joint stiffness lasting more than thirty minutes, particularly in the morning or after periods of inactivity • Persistent fatigue • Low-grade fever (a sign of the inflammatory process) • Unintentional weight loss • Firm lumps of tissue (called rheumatoid nodules) under the skin, especially over bony areas exposed to pressure

THE CONDITION	WHAT IT IS	SIGNS + SYMPTOMS
Osteoarthritis (OA)	The most common form of arthritis, resulting from the degeneration of joint cartilage and underlying bone. It's often referred to as the "wear and tear" arthritis because it's associated with injury or overuse of certain joints, as well as the aging process. Women are more likely to develop OA, particularly after menopause.	• Joint pain during or after movement • Joint stiffness, especially in the hands, knees, hips, and spine • Decreased range of motion, and feeling like a joint isn't as stable or strong as it used to be • A joint that looks noticeably different than usual
Temporomandibular joint disorder (TMJ or TMD)	A group of conditions that affects the jaw joints and surrounding muscles and ligaments.	• Pain or tenderness in the jaw, face, shoulders, and/or neck • Difficulty or pain while chewing • Clicking or popping sounds when opening or closing your mouth • Chronic headaches, migraines, earaches, and/or toothaches • Ringing in your ears (tinnitus)
Chronic pelvic pain (CPP)	Typically defined as pain in the pelvic region that lasts six months or longer. It can impact multiple organs and systems (including the reproductive organs, urinary tract, and gastrointestinal and musculoskeletal systems). CPP can have multiple causes, including: • Endometriosis • Pelvic inflammatory disease (PID) • Interstitial cystitis (a chronic bladder condition causing bladder pressure and pain) • Irritable bowel syndrome • Pelvic floor muscle tension • Uterine fibroids	• Persistent or intermittent pain, ranging from a dull ache to sharp or severe pain in the lower abdomen or pelvis, which can worsen when sitting for long periods • Pain during penetrative sex (dyspareunia) • Severe and prolonged menstrual cramps (dysmenorrhea) that can happen before, during, or after menstruation • Pain with bowel movements or urination • Lower back pain that radiates to the hips • A feeling of pressure or heaviness within the pelvis

Finding Relief: Your Options for Treating Pain, and What to Know About Each One

Pain is one of the most common reasons people seek medical care, and it affects more people than diabetes, heart disease, and cancer *combined*.[13]

Thankfully, we have more pain management treatments available than ever before, and they often include "multi-modal" (using a combination of different therapies to address various aspects of pain rather than relying on a single method) and "team-based" (a collaborative approach where clinicians from various disciplines work together to address the multifaceted nature of pain) strategies.

"Managing pain involves so much more than taking a pill, and many people don't realize this," says Dr. Barreveld. Your game plan could include a combination of the following, listed in no particular order:

- Medications (oral, topical analgesics, suppositories)
- Medical interventions (injection therapies, nerve blocks, surgery)
- Cognitive and mind-body strategies for pain (mindfulness, meditation, cognitive behavioral therapy, group support)
- Physical therapy, occupational therapy, and rehabilitation services
- Exercise
- Dietary strategies
- Sleep strategies
- Alternative therapies (acupuncture, chiropractic care)
- Team-based collaboration and interdisciplinary consultations
- Preventative and integrative medicine approaches

With so many choices, it can be tough to determine the right one for you. Enter this overview, which outlines the new thinking on some of the most common treatment options available.

Pain Medications, Explained Simply

When it comes to taking something to ease your discomfort, you likely turn to over-the-counter pain medications first. Yet when your pain is too intense to be treated by an OTC option, a clinician may prescribe you pain medication. Here are some of the most common ones, as well as some information on how each works and what it's most commonly used to treat.

MEDICATION (AND COMMON BRAND NAMES)	HOW IT WORKS	COMMONLY USED FOR	KEEP IN MIND
Opioids • Morphine • Fentanyl • Hydrocodone + acetaminophen (Vicodin) • Oxycodone (OxyContin) • Codeine • Tramadol	These medications bind to opioid receptors, which are part of the pain messenger system in the body.	The relief of short-term, intense pain due to a medical condition (such as cancer) or a surgical procedure.	These drugs carry a high risk of tolerance and dependence.
Corticosteroids • Oral (prednisone, dexamethasone) • Topical (hydrocortisone and betamethasone ointments, creams, lotions, gels, and more) • Injectable (cortisone shots administered by a healthcare provider)	These medications mimic the effects of hormones produced by the adrenal glands to reduce inflammation and suppress the immune system.	Inflammatory conditions like arthritis, asthma, and autoimmune diseases; some are used for severe inflammation and immune suppression; topical ointments may be used for skin irritation and itchiness.	Short-term side effects can include increased appetite, weight gain, fluid retention, mood swings, and increased blood pressure; prolonged use can lead to more serious side effects, such as diabetes (due to raised blood sugar levels), osteoporosis, and an increased risk of infections, eye conditions (like cataracts and glaucoma), and heart disease.
Antidepressants • Tricyclic antidepressants such as amitriptyline and nortriptyline • SSRIs such as fluoxetine (Prozac) and paroxetine (Paxil) • SNRIs such as duloxetine (Cymbalta) and venlafaxine (Effexor)	Antidepressants may increase levels of neurotransmitters in the spinal cord that reduce pain signals.	Tricyclic antidepressants are commonly used for nerve damage and fibromyalgia; SNRIs are used to treat chronic pain conditions (for example, duloxetine is used for conditions like diabetic neuropathy and fibromyalgia); and SSRIs may help relieve certain types of non-nerve pain.	These medications come with side effects and typically don't work immediately. You may have to take an antidepressant for several weeks before experiencing pain relief.
Antiseizure medications (aka anticonvulsants) • Gabapentin (Neurontin, Horizant, Gralise) • Pregabalin (Lyrica)	These medications originally designed to treat epilepsy can also help manage nerve pain by stabilizing nerve activity and reducing abnormal (and often painful) electrical charges in the nervous system.	Nerve damage (aka neuropathy) caused by diabetes; shingles; chemotherapy; a herniated disc in your spine.	These drugs are usually well tolerated, but side effects may include drowsiness, dizziness, confusion, or swelling in the feet and legs; they are associated with a slightly increased risk of suicidal thoughts or actions.

Ask an Expert

I'm terrified of taking any pain medication because I'm afraid I'll get addicted. Are there things I can do when taking painkillers or opioids to avoid this?

It's understandable that you may have concerns around substance use disorders, and opioid use disorder specifically. Data on the rates of overdose of both prescription and synthetic opioids have been concerning, especially in young adults, raising concerns about how best to treat pain.

However, it's crucial to not let your fear of pain medication keep you from getting any treatment—especially in the early stages of pain, such as right after an injury or surgery. This is because of the "wind-up" phenomenon of pain: When pain receptors in your nervous system are subjected to repeated or high-intensity impulses, your brain becomes increasingly sensitive to pain—which means you'll be more likely to feel pain even when your pain should be dissipating.

If you don't treat pain early and effectively and you experience this nervous system wind-up, it can be difficult to wind *down*. This is why many clinicians will talk about how important it is to treat pain right at the time of injury or surgery; it's very difficult for medications or other pain management treatments to work well as time passes.

While we need more research to understand why some people become tolerant of or dependent on opioids and others don't, we do know that you can lessen the chance of dependence on these medications by following your clinician's orders carefully and making sure you take the medication only as prescribed.

If you're concerned, have a conversation with your clinician before you start taking the medication about their strategy for pain control and whether there are options other than opioids to help control your pain.

The bottom line: Talk through your concerns about opioids with your clinician, who can explain your options—including non-opioid pain medications as well as drug-free strategies—to help you find safe and effective solutions that work for you.

—Anita Gupta, DO, PharmD, clinical professor at the University of California School of Medicine, Riverside, and adjunct assistant professor of anesthesiology and critical care medicine and pain medicine at the Johns Hopkins University School of Medicine

Your Pharmacist Is an Amazing Resource You're Probably Not Using

When you go to the pharmacy to pick up any prescription medication, you should be asked if you'd like any counseling from a pharmacist, who can explain the medication and how to take it, talk through possible side effects, and answer any questions you might have. And if you're like most people, you probably decline by clicking "no" on the screen you sign as you're checking out. However, pharmacists are an incredible source of information—and often they'll have better and more complete answers to our questions about both prescription and OTC medications than our clinicians.

"Pharmacists are highly knowledgeable and have a deep understanding of how drugs work in the body," says Dr. Gupta. "Pharmacist counseling is a free service that too many people don't realize is available and skip over when they pick up their medications."

Here, Dr. Gupta shares five questions you might ask a pharmacist when picking up a prescription or OTC pain medicine:

1. How does this medication work? Knowing the mechanism behind how a drug works can help you make sure you're taking the correct medication and dose for your specific condition.

2. What are the potential side effects? When you know what they are, you'll be quicker to call your clinician if you start experiencing any of them.

3. How should I take this medication? Some drugs work best when taken at specific times of the day or with meals. Certain foods can also interact with medications and reduce their effect.

4. Can this medication interfere with other drugs or supplements I'm taking? Show the pharmacist a list of everything you take—yes, including common dietary supplements, vitamins, and even herbal products—so you can be sure there are no interactions.

5. Why is this medication not working? If you're dealing with pain and your medication stops working, you need to find out why, says Dr. Gupta. "Your pharmacist can call your doctor and work on adjusting your medication or add a nonpharmacologic treatment option to your plan," she says.

Beyond OTC and Prescription Pain Meds: Drug-Free Ways to Ease Pain

These science-backed approaches can help you ease your discomfort without taking medication, and they can also be used in conjunction with medication or other medical treatments to make them even more effective.

- **Sleep.** Getting good-quality sleep is one of the most important things you can do when you're in pain. It helps you regulate your emotions, which can reduce pain-related depression and anxiety. And when you're sleeping well, your body does a better job of repairing inflamed tissue, which can reduce the intensity of your pain and help you heal faster. The kicker is that good-quality sleep can be especially tough to get when you're in pain: Feeling uncomfortable can keep you up at night, and then the poor sleep you get can exacerbate your pain, keeping you in a tricky cycle. If this is you, talk to a clinician who can help you come up with a plan to address your sleep struggles.

- **Exercise.** While your pain may prompt you to want to stay in bed, movement is one of the most powerful pain relievers. When you exercise, blood flows to the muscles and joints and delivers oxygen and nutrients that can help repair tissues and remove waste products, both of which can reduce pain. Exercise also stimulates the release of endorphins, which have been shown to reduce the perception of pain and improve mood. And it prompts your immune system to produce acute inflammation, a temporary increase in inflammation to repair tissues, muscles, and cells—a repair process that'll help you feel less pain over time. Start slow, stick to low-impact movements, and listen to your body. Pushing through severe pain isn't helpful and could make your pain worse.

- **Physical therapy.** This modality often involves using a range of techniques designed to relieve pain and improve movement and strength, including manual therapy techniques (like massage, joint manipulation, and a specific type of therapy called myofascial release that targets the connective tissue around the muscles, called fascia); exercise therapy (targeted strengthening and stretching exercises to improve range of motion, prevent injuries that could exacerbate pain, and build up weak muscles to improve stability and decrease pain); and instruction on self-management strategies (such as proper posture, ergonomics, and activity modification to decrease pain). Physical therapists also use electrical stimulation to interrupt pain signals, as well as ultrasound therapy that uses sound waves to generate heat deep within the body's tissues to promote healing.

- **Cognitive behavioral therapy (CBT).** This is a specific type of talk therapy that can help you change how you think about your pain, learn new ways of dealing with it, and even challenge core beliefs you have about your pain to help you find relief. This style of talk therapy can also include various relaxation techniques to help you manage pain.

Your Game Plan:
How to Advocate for Yourself When You're in Pain

Dr. Vonda Wright sees a lot of female patients in a lot of pain—many of whom have conditions like arthritis and bone fractures or need joint replacement surgery. And she sees a distinct trend among these female patients who are in agony when they come to her: They all brag about how high their pain tolerance is.

"They wear this identity like a badge of honor—as if the only reason they feel like they can finally come to see me to get some relief from their pain is because they've suffered a very long time," says Dr. Wright. "But women deserve to express what they're experiencing and be listened to without judgment." Here, Dr. Wright shares some of the most important things you can do to get the attention your pain deserves.

Track your symptoms. Keep a diary of your symptoms with as many specifics as possible—even if your symptoms seem insignificant. Being able to answer questions in a highly detailed way rather than saying "I don't know—I'm just achier than usual" gives your clinician the best shot at figuring out exactly what's going on. Make notes about what makes the pain worse and what eases it. A pain diary can also help show *you* just how bad your pain is, giving you a clear sense of how much you're suffering and inspiring you to seek help when you need it.

Understand that your chronic pain may be related to your hormones. For 70 to 80 percent of women in perimenopause, chronic pain is due to *arthralgia*, which is total body pain that can be due to the drop in estrogen that happens around menopause and the inflammation that can result, says Dr. Wright. Unfortunately, when many women go to the doctor due to total body pain, they're sent home without a diagnosis and oftentimes with prescriptions for pain medications that aren't likely to work, she adds. If you suspect your pain may be due to the musculoskeletal syndrome of menopause (MSM), which you can read more about on pages 342–343, consider seeing a menopause specialist. A clinician who has been trained in this important life stage is more likely to talk to you about science-backed solutions to treating MSM, which include hormone therapy, anti-inflammatory nutrition, exercise (including strength training), and sleep.

Don't power through your pain. Dr. Wright says she's seen countless patients—mostly women—who've dealt with months of pain without seeking help. When she asks them why, they say, "I don't like to complain." But the problem with this is that waiting to get help often makes the underlying cause of your pain worse. Take frozen shoulder, a condition that can surface during the menopause transition that causes stiffness, pain, and limited movement in the shoulder joint. "If a patient comes in to see me within a week or two of symptoms, we treat it right away with physical therapy, anti-inflammatory medication, and a conversation about menopause hormone therapy and nutrition in an effort to prevent it from progressing," says Dr. Wright. Wait too long to seek treatment and there's a higher chance the condition—and your pain—will progress, which makes both harder to treat.

Talk about your pain to family and friends. Part of what makes pain so hard to deal with is that it's invisible, which means some people aren't going to understand or believe the pain you're in. And the frustration and stress you'll likely feel as a result of not being understood can make your pain worse. Rather than powering through your discomfort silently, talk to a handful of supportive people in your life and be honest about what you're feeling. Sharing the truth about what you're going through is an important step toward feeling fully seen in your pain, and it can also help you shake off that "I have a high pain tolerance" identity—and inspire the other women in your life to do the same.

· · · · ·

Even though women tend to report feeling pain more intensely than men, we often power our way through it and pride ourselves on our "high pain tolerance." However, it's important to remember that pain is your body's way of sending information—and the more you understand those signals, the better a position you'll be in to communicate what you're experiencing to your clinicians and get the pain relief you need.

Chapter 13

Brain Health

What You Need to Know to Fire on All Cylinders and Prevent Cognitive Disease

> *Your brain is your biggest asset. Care for it well so it may last a lifetime. I promise it will be the best investment you can make in your future health.*
>
> —Maria Shriver, from the foreword of *The Menopause Brain: New Science Empowers Women to Navigate the Pivotal Transition with Knowledge and Confidence*

Take a minute to think about your brain right now. For an organ in your body that's arguably one of the most important—enabling you to move, think, and talk, essentially making you *you*—it's remarkable how few of us even consider our brain health until something is wrong. It's time to change that, especially given the cognitive issues that disproportionately affect women.

Consider this: Women are nearly twice as likely as men to be diagnosed with depression, more than twice as likely to develop the most common type of brain tumor (meningioma), and, as we learned in the previous chapter, two to three times more likely to get migraine headaches.[1] And when it comes to Alzheimer's disease, approximately two-thirds of Americans living with the condition are women.[2] Yet despite the many science-backed signs pointing toward brain health issues affecting more women than men, the science is still trying to catch up on finding answers.

The good news is that a number of trailblazing physicians and researchers have discovered sex-specific differences in the female brain that are pointing the way toward those answers. And along the way, they've been uncovering incredible new insights into how the brain works and what we can do to protect our brain health for life.

In this chapter, we'll cover . . .

- **Everything you likely never learned about how your brain works.** Knowing the basics will leave you in awe of your amazing mind and help you understand what steps you can take to optimize your cognitive health.

- **How our hormones—specifically estrogen and cortisol—literally change the female brain.** For example, estrogen has powerful protective effects on the brain, and the precipitous drop in this hormone during the menopause transition helps to explain why women are especially vulnerable to dementia.

- **The brain disorders that disproportionately impact women *and* are often overlooked or misdiagnosed in us.** Understanding what these conditions are and the symptoms of each can help you stay on the lookout for the signs and get the help you need.

- **What you should know about dementia and Alzheimer's disease**, what puts women at risk, and the science-backed steps you can take to put a dent in your risk of developing these conditions.

Meet the Experts

Lisa Mosconi, PhD, neuroscientist, director of the Weill Cornell Women's Brain Initiative and author of *The Menopause Brain: New Science Empowers Women to Navigate the Pivotal Transition with Knowledge and Confidence*

Jessica Caldwell, PhD, director of the Women's Alzheimer's Movement Prevention and Research Center at the Cleveland Clinic

Mimi Winsberg, MD, board-certified psychiatrist and cofounder and chief medical officer of Brightside, a mental health telemedicine service

Shehroo Pudumjee, PhD, clinical neuropsychologist and director of neuropsychology at the Cleveland Clinic Lou Ruvo Center for Brain Health

A Look Inside the Brain: Knowing How Our Brains Are Wired Can Help Us Optimize Our Cognitive Health

The human brain is an incredibly complex organ that's made up of multiple structures and regions, each of which has a specific function. Let's go over the parts of the brain that you'll hear about the most when it comes to **cognition**, which is the technical word for your brain's ability to process all of the information it takes in so you can think, learn, speak, remember, pay attention, and make decisions and judgments.

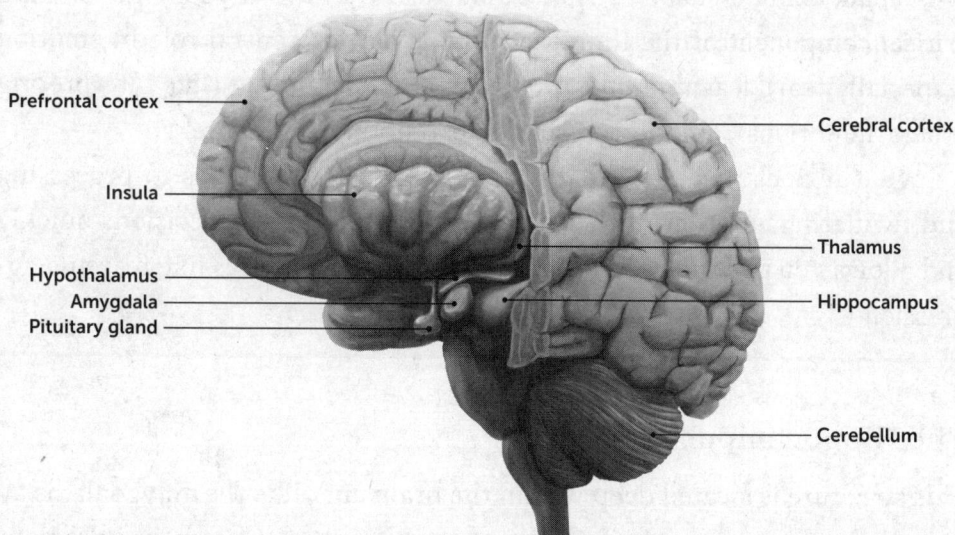

Prefrontal cortex — Insula — Hypothalamus — Amygdala — Pituitary gland — Cerebral cortex — Thalamus — Hippocampus — Cerebellum

The Cerebral Cortex

This is the outermost layer of your brain and makes up about half of your brain's total mass. It's often referred to as gray matter because it is literally gray: It doesn't have a fatty material called myelin covering it, which is what gives other parts of the brain their whitish color.

What it does: It's responsible for things like language, memory, reasoning, learning, decision-making, emotions, intelligence, and personality.

The Prefrontal Cortex

This is located in the frontal lobe of the cerebral cortex (behind the forehead and above the eyes) and receives inputs from other regions of the brain.

What it does: It handles decision-making, planning, problem-solving, memory, emotional regulation, and social behavior. You'll hear the term *executive function* used in relation to the prefrontal cortex because this region is responsible for the type of thinking that controls our behavior and helps us anticipate the consequences of our actions.

The Amygdala

This small, almond-shaped structure sits near the base of your skull and is a critical component of the limbic system. It plays a central role in emotion (especially fear), learning, memory, social understanding (like interpreting others' intentions), emotions related to caregiving, and more.

What it does: It's particularly important when it comes to processing and regulating emotions. It helps you make life-or-death decisions quickly and allows you to form and recognize emotional responses like fear and aggression.

The Hippocampus

This structure is located deep within the brain and, like the amygdala, is an essential component of the limbic system. It's one of the few brain regions where new neurons continue to be generated throughout your lifetime and is larger and works differently in women than in men.

What it does: It works with your amygdala to connect memories to emotions and is also responsible for learning and short- and long-term memory. The hippocampus is densely populated with both estrogen and cortisol receptors, which makes it especially sensitive to fluctuations in these hormones.

The Thalamus

This is an egg-shaped structure located in the middle of your brain, at the top of the brain stem.

What it does: It serves as a relay station for sensory information that travels from movements and senses (except smell) to the appropriate regions in the cerebral cortex. For example, the words you're reading right now are sent to the thalamus, which then sends that information to the specific area in your brain that makes sense of all visual inputs. It's also involved in helping you decide what to focus on out of the vast number of inputs it receives. The thalamus also helps your brain wake up from sleep and maintain wakefulness throughout the day, which is why it's sometimes described as the "gateway to consciousness."

The Hypothalamus

This small structure is located just below the thalamus, deep within the brain.

What it does: Often called the body's thermostat due to its crucial role in regulating many of the body's most vital functions—including body temperature, blood pressure, heart rate, hunger and thirst, sex drive, sleep, and mood—the hypothalamus controls the autonomic nervous system (which is responsible for functions like heart and breathing rate, as well as digestion) and helps regulate the body's response to stress. It also serves as a link between the nervous system and the endocrine system and helps keep the body in the stable state known as homeostasis.

The Pituitary Gland

Located at the base of the brain, just below the hypothalamus, this pea-sized gland is often referred to as the master gland of the endocrine system. It's divided into two main parts: anterior and posterior.

What it does: The anterior (or front portion) of the pituitary gland produces and releases hormones that regulate a wide range of processes, including growth, reproduction, metabolism, and stress response. The posterior (or back part) stores and releases two hormones produced by the hypothalamus: oxytocin and vasopressin (aka antidiuretic hormone, or ADH, which regulates sodium levels and water balance in your body).

The Insula

Also known as the insular cortex or the insular lobe, this region of the brain is situated deep within the cerebral cortex.

What it does: It's important when it comes to regulating emotions, making us feel empathy, and helping us perceive bodily sensations (like temperature and pain). It's also tied to self-awareness and risk-reward behavior.

The Cerebellum

This part of your brain is located at the back of your head, right around where your spinal cord attaches to your brain. It's a small structure (the name *cerebellum* comes from Latin and means "little brain") but has a large number of neurons.

What it does: It's responsible for fine-tuning and coordinating movement, balance, and posture, continuously monitoring movement and helping to detect and correct errors in real time by regulating your gait (walking) and eye movements, keeping you coordinated. It also plays a role in cognitive functions, including attention, language, and memory.

Neurons and Neuroplasticity: Your Brain's Ability to Change

For years, neuroscientists thought the brain was a static lump of cells that declined over time. Researchers now realize that understanding was wrong. The brain is actually quite moldable and ever-changing, able to continually grow new cells, make new connections, and ditch old connections we no longer need. This ability to form and reorganize synaptic connections is called neuroplasticity.

How exactly does the human brain have this capacity to shape-shift? The answer requires a basic understanding of neurons (aka brain cells) and how they work.

Your brain is made up of approximately one hundred billion neurons, and each of them is designed to "talk" to other nerve cells, gland cells, or muscles. They do this communicating via electric signals that travel across synapses, which are tiny gaps between two neurons that transmit and process information. Neurons communicate with one another to regulate all the body processes that keep us alive—from automatic processes like breathing and digesting food to ones that require some thought or intention, like raising an eyebrow when you want to express skepticism or scratching an itch on your leg.

Each neuron looks a little like a tree: It has a cell body (the trunk), axons (the roots), and dendrites (the branches and leaves). Messages come in (as "inputs") via the dendrites and leave (as "outputs") via the axons. The outer layer of your brain tissue (cerebral cortex, aka gray matter) contains the neurons and their dendrites. Deeper in your brain is your white matter, which is where the axons pack together to help the brain exchange information and connect different regions of gray matter.

When a message hits the end of an axon, it triggers the release of chemical messengers called neurotransmitters, which transmit the message via those synapses to other neurons or target cells. Every single neuron can have up to ten thousand connections with other cells—each one sending different messages that allow you to function in the world. The path a neurotransmitter takes from one neuron to another is called a neural pathway, which you can think of as little highways that transmit messages from one brain region to another to help you process information, initiate and control how you move your body, and regulate all your body's physiological functions.

Every time you see something, learn something, make a connection about what's good versus bad or safe versus dangerous, you build a new neural pathway. As a baby, you build countless neural connections—many more than you will need, considering that anytime you learn or experience something for the first time (such as a new toy, color, or movement) a neural connection is made. As you get older, your brain starts to refine its communication network, eliminating neural connections you no longer need (a process called synaptic pruning) so that the ones you *do* need work faster and more efficiently. The years leading up to puberty involve a major remodeling of the brain; a similar burst of synaptic pruning also happens after pregnancy, when the female brain discards neurons and synapses it no longer needs to make room for all the demands of new parenthood.

Everything you do requires information to travel throughout your brain's highly complex network of neural pathways, and oftentimes multiple networks in different parts of the brain are working at once. Thankfully, your brain consolidates information pretty quickly, priming you to think, read, learn, and move through the world without feeling utterly exhausted.

How Hormones Impact the Female Brain: Understanding the Estrogen Factor

As you can imagine, the constant work your brain does to help you function takes energy, and your brain's preferred source for that energy is glucose. In fact, brain cells require a continuous delivery of glucose from the blood. If they don't get enough, the brain slows down production of its chemical messengers (neurotransmitters), which can lead to a communication breakdown between neurons—something you might experience as difficulty paying attention or feeling like you aren't firing on all cylinders.

Now, because the brain is such a crucial organ—and because glucose can be scarce during times of starvation—the human body has a built-in backup system to get the brain the energy it needs when glucose isn't available: ketone bodies. (Yep, the same ketones the "keto diet" is named after.) When you're low on glucose, your body starts to break down stored fat into fatty acids, which are then transported to the liver and converted into ketone bodies, or water-soluble molecules that can cross the blood-brain barrier. However, it's important to remember this isn't your brain's preferred source of fuel.

"When the brain has to switch from using glucose for energy to ketone bodies, it's an extreme change of plans that's not supposed to last for long—at least under normal circumstances," says neuroscientist Lisa Mosconi, PhD.

So what do hormones have to do with our brain getting the glucose it needs? Well, estrogen optimizes how the brain uses glucose, essentially "charging up" brain function, says Dr. Mosconi. Her research has shown that the menopause transition messes with the brain's glucose metabolism, possibly because of the drop in estrogen. That's right: Even if you don't change your diet at all during perimenopause and beyond, your brain burns glucose slower than it once did. Over time, this can affect how brain cells carry information (hello, brain fog!). The menopause transition has also been associated with a decrease in gray matter volume, which may be a sign of an increased risk of future cognitive decline.

Given estrogen's incredibly important functions in our brains, it won't come as a shock that other times in our lives when this hormone is in flux—namely puberty, our monthly periods, pregnancy, and postpartum—can also impact the female brain. Next, let's take a look at how these times of hormonal fluctuation in our lives can impact our brains.

The Major Hormonal Transitions That Impact the Female Brain

» PUBERTY

This big transition in a child's life is often described as a time when sex hormones are "coming online." In girls, a surge of estrogen prompts our reproductive system to mature—and it also prompts changes in the brain's connections, especially the ones related to how we interact with others, our emotional processing, and how we self-regulate.

What also happens during puberty is a neuron pruning that's so intense, there's actually a *decrease* in gray matter. But this isn't as ominous as it sounds! Remember, throughout the first decade or so of life, your brain makes many more connections than it needs. Scientists believe that the release of sex hormones during puberty prompts a pruning of the brain connections that aren't needed anymore, so that the ones that are useful can work more efficiently. Essentially, this brain rewiring that happens during puberty transforms our brains into their adult form.

» THE MENSTRUAL CYCLE

The rise and fall of sex hormones throughout this roughly twenty-eight-day period may actually gently reshape the brain, particularly regions that are in charge of emotions and memory. Just before ovulation, when estrogen and luteinizing hormone rise, brain cells sprout new connections and their connections get stronger, which has been linked to feeling more focused, socially responsive, and verbally fluent. What's more, estrogen can also increase levels of the neurotransmitters serotonin and dopamine, which are linked to happiness and pleasure. After ovulation, estrogen drops and progesterone rises—a combination that's been linked to headaches, irritability, fatigue, sleepiness, and moodiness.

» PREGNANCY AND POSTPARTUM

In many ways, the changes in the female brain that happen during pregnancy and even more so during the postpartum period resemble what you went through during puberty. When you get pregnant, you experience a surge in hormones that prompts a loss of gray matter, as neural connections are pruned away to make your brain more efficient at what it most needs to do: prepare you for being able to tune in to your child's needs. Research has shown that the brain undergoes changes on an almost weekly basis during pregnancy, which supports the hypothesis that pregnancy rewires the brain, reorganizing networks of neurons so you're better able to adapt to your new role as caregiver.

After you give birth, you'll experience another set of hormonal challenges—this time, a drastic drop so severe, many call it a preview of perimenopause.

Even though you may feel like your body and brain have been hijacked and you're sleepier, hungrier, moodier, and more forgetful than ever before, the changes happening in your brain during pregnancy and in the years after having a baby are like an upgrade to your brain's operating system, says Dr. Mosconi—albeit one that may take some getting used to.

» THE MENOPAUSE TRANSITION

When most of us hear the term *menopause* we think about a woman's reproductive system. Yet it's important to know that this big hormonal transition also impacts the brain. In fact, menopause symptoms such as hot flashes, night sweats, anxiety, and insomnia are all *neurological* symptoms that result from the ways that menopause changes the brain, says Dr. Mosconi.

The female brain continuously makes estrogen receptors, which the estrogen binds to so it can travel inside brain cells to communicate information. Yet while scientists previously believed the brain stopped making estrogen receptors shortly after menopause (the thought was that the brain was saying *I don't need estrogen anymore*), Dr. Mosconi's research found that the female brain actually makes more estrogen receptors for years after menopause.

"During the menopause transition, your brain essentially says, 'I need more estrogen, how do I get it?'" says Dr. Mosconi. "Our research found that the brain answers that question by making estrogen receptors, possibly so that the brain can capture every available bit of estrogen when estrogen concentrations are low."

Once you're officially in menopause, your ovaries start to make very small amounts of estrone, a less powerful type of estrogen than the estradiol you made during your reproductive years. (For a refresher on the three different types of estrogen, flip back to page 208.) Yet while estrone does have some benefits, it doesn't do what estradiol did for the brain. Neural connections can start to slow down, brain cells may begin to experience the effects of aging and aren't as likely to get repaired, and the brain becomes less resilient overall. The result? You may become more vulnerable to inflammation, memory lapses, brain fog, and cognitive decline. And while most women's brains experience a rebound once we adjust to our new, low-estradiol state, some don't, which can help explain why Alzheimer's disease disproportionately impacts women.

That said, Dr. Mosconi and a growing number of other experts studying the female brain believe that the menopause transition is actually a renovation project on the brain that often leads to benefits.

"For example, after menopause, all of those neurons and connections between neurons that were needed to support ovulation and enable a pregnancy are no longer needed and can be discarded," says Dr. Mosconi. "It's the brain's chance to get leaner and meaner." What's more, fewer hormonal fluctuations can mean an overall improvement in our emotional well-being and can even lead to a deeper sense of connection with our bodies and our minds, she adds.

"While menopause can be a challenging transition, the idea that this life event puts women at a disadvantage is one rooted in culture rather than biology," says Dr. Mosconi. "By understanding how menopause affects the brain, women can better navigate this phase of life with confidence and resilience."

The Stress Connection: Why Cortisol May Be Just as Important as Estrogen When It Comes to Brain Health

When brain researchers talk about Alzheimer's disease affecting women in greater numbers than men, many point to estrogen. And while we have definitive evidence of estrogen's protective powers in the female brain, it isn't the only hormone at work. Cortisol—aka the stress hormone—plays an important role, too.

How Cortisol Works in Your Brain

The human body is remarkably capable of adapting to stress. When we sense danger, the brain releases neurochemicals and hormones—cortisol being the biggest player—to help us get out of harm's way. But here's the thing about that surge of brain chemicals that put us in fight-or-flight mode and help us stay safe: They're only meant to course through the body for a limited amount of time. When they stick around longer than they should, they exhaust the brain.

That's why there's a feedback loop built into the system, explains Jessica Caldwell, PhD: Your brain gets a message from your body after an acute threat has passed that says, "Let's turn this stress hormone release down!" The part of the brain that gets this shut-it-down signal is the hippocampus, which, as you might recall, is the region of the brain responsible for learning and converting short-term memories into long-term ones.

When stress becomes chronic, the brain stays in protection mode and doesn't stop that cascade of stress hormones. The result? Over time, cells in that brain region start to die and the hippocampus starts to literally shrink, which can lead to memory loss.

The XX Stress Response

When you look at the differences in this stress response between women and men, the results are striking. When women experience chronic stress, we tend to produce more stress hormones than our male counterparts, explains Dr. Caldwell. This can be a great thing when women need to act quickly. However, it's less helpful when stress becomes chronic, because we're less able to tamp down the stress response than men.

Unfortunately, chronic stress becomes incredibly common for many women—especially at midlife. From caregiving (including parenting and taking care of aging parents) and work demands to the menopause transition and all the stress-inducing symptoms it can cause (like sleep deprivation and anxiety), there's a long list of things life throws our way that have the potential to keep us in a heightened stress response. This is particularly risky for women's brain health.

"The off switch for those stress response chemicals is in the hippocampus, which is the part of the brain that's important for taking new memories and shuttling them into long-term storage, and is the first place in the brain that changes in Alzheimer's disease," says Dr. Caldwell. "So when we have chronic stress on the brain, we're essentially putting a burden on top of a system that's already vulnerable to Alzheimer's disease."

Why is a woman's stress response slower to shut off than a man's? While we don't have all the answers to that question, Dr. Caldwell says the hormone estrogen, which helps regulate the stress response, is likely involved.

"My hypothesis is that across midlife, because women lose estrogen at the same time that many of us are undergoing high, chronic stress, there is an interaction there," says Dr. Caldwell. "But stay tuned for more research."

Brain Conditions That May Be More Likely to Be Misdiagnosed or Overlooked in Women, and Why This Is

From migraine headaches to Alzheimer's disease, not only are women more likely to develop certain brain disorders, but we're also at greater risk of misdiagnosis and/or delayed treatment. As a result, many of us endure years of pain, lower quality of life, and even disease progression that might've been prevented. Here are some of the brain conditions most likely to fly under the radar in women and why.

Attention Deficit Hyperactivity Disorder (ADHD)

This neurodevelopmental disorder is marked by an ongoing pattern of challenges that include difficulty paying attention or staying on task, hyperactivity, and/or impulsivity. While most cases of ADHD are diagnosed in childhood, the condition may become apparent for some—especially women—later in life. In fact, while there's a three-to-one ratio of boys to girls diagnosed with ADHD in childhood, diagnoses even out to a one-to-one ratio in adulthood.[3] One reason for this is the different ways ADHD can manifest in boys and girls, says psychiatrist Mimi Winsberg, MD.

"Girls with ADHD are more likely to display inattentive aspects of the condition, such as looking a little spacey or seeming forgetful," says Dr. Winsberg. "Boys are more likely to display the hyperactive aspects of ADHD, such as fidgeting and an inability to sit still—behaviors that are more disruptive and as a result, more likely to be flagged by a teacher or parent for an evaluation."

Given a lack of research on ADHD in females and a persistent stereotype that the ADHD patient is most often male, girls and women are less likely to be assessed, diagnosed, and treated. This can have big consequences, says Dr. Winsberg: Girls who don't get diagnosed are more likely to be subject to trauma, and because they may not perform well in school, they're more likely to suffer from anxiety, depression, and sometimes even eating disorders or self-injurious behavior.

"Unfortunately, another psychiatric disorder can manifest because the primary one—ADHD—isn't getting addressed," says Dr. Winsberg.

Thankfully, we're starting to recognize ADHD in women and the diagnosis gap is narrowing. Between 2020 and 2022, the percentage of women between ages twenty-three and forty-nine newly diagnosed with ADHD nearly doubled.[4]

Autism Spectrum Disorder (ASD)

This neurodevelopmental disorder is caused by differences in the brain that can impact behavior, social interaction, and communication. While it's commonly diagnosed in childhood, like ADHD, the condition can go undiagnosed until adulthood, especially in women. In fact, while boys are nearly four times as likely as girls to receive an autism diagnosis, research suggests that as many as 80 percent of autistic females are undiagnosed as of age eighteen[5]—a delay that comes along with some potentially serious consequences to their physical and mental health, as well as their education and overall well-being.

For many years, it was assumed that autism was a "male" condition—which led to most research being done on male participants and autism assessments and measures (known as ASD traits) being established using a male baseline. What's more, females tend to have different autism traits. They may be better at smiling or making eye contact and more interested in making friends than boys with autism. And because language skills are one way ASD is diagnosed in children—and girls tend to have more advanced language skills than boys—it's possible that girls can better mask some of the symptoms of autism in childhood and go undiagnosed as a result, adds Dr. Winsberg.

Certain Brain Tumors

The most common type of brain tumor is called a meningioma, and it originates in the membranes that surround the brain and spinal cord called the meninges. These brain tumors are more common in women, largely due to the fact that they often contain receptors for estrogen and progesterone, which makes them more likely to grow during big hormonal transitions like pregnancy and perimenopause, and even when taking exogenous hormones (such as fertility medications). Another type of tumor more likely to develop in women is a pituitary adenoma, which is a benign tumor of the pituitary gland and can also be influenced by hormones, particularly prolactin, a hormone that's higher in women, especially during pregnancy and lactation.

Brain Aneurysms

A brain aneurysm is a thin or weak spot in the wall of an artery within the brain (most commonly at the base of the brain, in areas where the arteries branch out), which can bulge out and gradually get bigger over time and can rupture. Most brain aneurysms that haven't ruptured are small and asymptomatic; larger or ruptured aneurysms can cause serious complications, such as bleeding in the brain and surrounding areas, which can be life-threatening.

Research shows brain aneurysms are more common in women by about 60 percent, and after menopause, our risk is double compared with men's. One theory about the reason for this is that the decline in estrogen during the menopause transition may change the brain artery structure and function, increasing the odds of the formation and/or rupture of a brain aneurysm.

Signs and symptoms to be aware of include a sudden, severe headache with nausea or vomiting; confusion; drowsiness; eye pain, blurred or double vision, dilated pupils or sensitivity to light; loss of balance or muscle weakness; stiff neck; speech impairment; seizures; and/or loss of consciousness or other cognitive changes. If you're experiencing any of these symptoms, seek medical care right away.

Concussion

This is a type of traumatic brain injury (TBI) caused by an impact to the head or body that's associated with a change in how your brain functions. When you suffer a blow to your head, the impact can stretch your brain's axons so quickly that they break, which in turn can prompt an electrical "brownout" that causes you to feel dazed and confused and possibly even lose consciousness. Because women tend to have smaller, thinner necks than our male counterparts—and the axons within our brains tend to be smaller and respond worse after a head injury than those in male brains—we are more vulnerable to concussion than men and more susceptible to persistent symptoms. This makes it especially important to do what you can to protect your head from impacts (wear a helmet when biking, skiing, or participating in another sport with a high risk of falls). You'll also want to seek medical attention immediately after a blow to your head, which can help prevent or mitigate any lasting effects of the injury.

Alzheimer's Disease and Dementia: What We Know About What Puts Women at Increased Risk

Alzheimer's disease and *dementia*. These terms are often used interchangeably, but they are distinct conditions, and understanding the difference between them can help you clue in to both your risk factors and symptoms that signal it's time to talk to your healthcare provider. Here, clinical neuropsychologist Shehroo Pudumjee, PhD, walks us through each.

Dementia is an umbrella term used to describe a group of symptoms associated with a decline in memory and/or cognitive function that often (but not always) happens later in life and interferes with everyday activities. It's not a specific disease; it's a syndrome that can be caused by various underlying diseases that affect the brain and cause different types of dementia, including:

- Alzheimer's disease, which is the most common cause of dementia, accounting for 60 to 80 percent of all dementia cases.[6]

- Vascular dementia, which occurs when there is damage to the brain's blood vessels, leading to impaired blood flow to brain cells that can result in cognitive decline.

- Dementia with Lewy bodies, which happens when tiny clumps of protein (called Lewy bodies) build up in the brain, leading to physical changes such as tremors or balance problems and a decline in thinking, reasoning, and function.

- Frontotemporal dementia, which is caused by progressive nerve cell loss in the brain's frontal or temporal lobes, which can cause changes in behavior, personality, and/or language.

- Mixed dementia, which is a condition in which someone has two or more different underlying diseases contributing to the dementia. The most common combination is Alzheimer's disease and vascular dementia, though other types (such as Alzheimer's disease and dementia with Lewy bodies) may also be present. "It's important to note that different types of dementias present with different symptoms," says Dr. Pudumjee. "For example, in one type of dementia we may see memory impairment as the first sign, and in another form of dementia that first sign might be executive functioning degradation. In Alzheimer's disease, impairments in learning, memory, and language tend to be the first symptoms."

Alzheimer's disease is a progressive disease, meaning symptoms gradually get worse over time. Hallmarks of Alzheimer's are the formation of beta-amyloid plaques and tau tangles inside the brain, which accumulate and set off a cascade effect that leads to cognitive decline.

These changes usually start in the part of the brain that affects learning and memory, and as Alzheimer's advances, it leads to increasingly severe symptoms. Some of the most common early signs and symptoms of Alzheimer's include:

- Forgetting recently learned information
- Challenges in planning or problem-solving
- Misplacing things and not having the ability to retrace steps to find them
- Changes in judgment or decision-making, such as errors in judgment when dealing with money
- Difficulty navigating or finding your way in a relatively familiar area

Ask an Expert

What are some of the early symptoms of dementia and Alzheimer's disease that I should see as a sign to get an evaluation?

Is there a significant change from what you or someone you love was able to do in the past? And when I say "the past," I don't mean ten or fifteen years ago but rather, is there a substantial change in the last year or two that feels out of line for what one might expect for one's age?

To put this in context, let's say someone is in their late seventies and they've been living independently and managing their affairs with ease. Then suddenly you start to notice that person is making errors in paying their bills, or maybe they're forgetting to show up for doctor's appointments or family events—and this is out of character for them. That part is important to emphasize because for some people, errors like these have happened all their lives. What you're looking for is a *change* in someone's typical way of being.

Brain Health

It's also important to consider the severity of what's happening. Let's say you go to a new mall, and you have a tough time finding your car when you're done shopping because multiple entrances look similar. This isn't super concerning to me; it's understandable why you might be confused. On the other hand, if you can't remember where you parked your car in a shopping mall you go to all the time, where you know the exits and specific landmarks well, it may be more reason for concern.

Frequency also matters when it comes to any symptoms that feel new and different from someone's prior functioning. One odd error here and there? I wouldn't make too much of it. But if it's happening more frequently, I'd recommend getting evaluated.

Given women's disproportionate risk of Alzheimer's disease, female patients often ask if it's beneficial to get a baseline neuropsychological evaluation even if there are no changes in cognitive function. That baseline can be helpful if two or three years down the line, you notice changes in cognitive function. It gives us a good comparison. However, that baseline testing is less useful if your next evaluation is eight or ten years later. That's because there are natural cognitive changes that happen over time. Are those changes normal or not? That can sometimes be tough to parse out when many years pass between your first and your follow-up neuropsychological exam.

—Shehroo Pudumjee, PhD, clinical neuropsychologist and director of neuropsychology at the Cleveland Clinic Lou Ruvo Center for Brain Health

What You Can Do to Reduce Your Risk of Alzheimer's Disease

Just as heart disease and cancer don't surface overnight, Alzheimer's is also thought to happen after genetic, medical, and lifestyle factors have been adding up throughout your life. Which means there's a lot you can do, no matter how old you are, to bolster your brain health.

Research commissioned by *The Lancet* identified fourteen potentially modifiable factors that account for 45 percent of cases of dementia:[7]

- Less education
- Hearing loss
- High LDL cholesterol (the "bad" kind)
- Depression
- Traumatic brain injury
- Physical inactivity
- Diabetes
- Smoking
- Hypertension
- Obesity
- Excessive alcohol consumption
- Social isolation
- Air pollution
- Vision loss

The good news is that the same study also found that addressing these areas in midlife (between ages eighteen and sixty-five) had the greatest impact in delaying and even preventing the onset of dementia. Translation: Things like treating high cholesterol and depression, exercising regularly, quitting smoking, and prioritizing community really can make a difference when it comes to your brain health.

Why Are Women of Color Even More Vulnerable to Alzheimer's Disease?

The statistics are unsettling: Research suggests that Black Americans are two to three times more likely than non-Hispanic whites to develop a cognitive impairment or Alzheimer's disease.[8] Hispanic Americans are 1.5 times more likely than whites to have dementia.[9] Evidence also suggests that Indigenous people may have disproportionately high rates of Alzheimer's disease and related dementia, too.[10] (Research indicates that Asian Americans have a lower likelihood of developing Alzheimer's and other forms of dementia than other racial groups.)[11]

Why is this? The unsatisfying answer is that scientists don't know. One theory is these populations' higher rates of diabetes, stroke, high cholesterol, and heart disease, which are factors known to correlate with an increased risk of dementia. Another is that exposure to stressful life events, such as repeated exposure to racism, may cause chronic inflammation that accelerates brain aging and makes the brain more susceptible to dementia.

In addition to making lifestyle changes that have been shown to really move the needle when it comes to staving off cognitive issues later in life, one of the best things you can do as a person of color is to consider signing up to be part of medical research—even if you're young and don't have a family history of Alzheimer's. That's because most of the current research on Alzheimer's comes from studies of white people. You might also consider talking to your relatives about our current lack of understanding of cognitive issues in people of color and the importance of changing this through research. If loved ones are hesitant, acknowledge the abuses that happened to people of color in medical research in the past, and talk about the protections that have since been put in place to avoid research discrimination.[12]

Ask an Expert

Should I get genetic testing to help gauge my risk of Alzheimer's?

These days, we hear so much about Alzheimer's disease that the minute you start to feel a little fuzzy or like your memory isn't totally on point, fear can set in, and you might start wondering if you should get genetic testing. But it's important to remember this: Fewer than 1 percent of Alzheimer's cases are caused by genes that cause the disease. There are many other factors that play into whether you'll get a dementia-related illness—and the sum of those factors is greater than any genetic risk you might have.

For example, we know that about 45 percent of current cases of dementia and Alzheimer's disease could potentially have been prevented if we'd known decades ago how lifestyle contributes to risk. Now we have the science that proves that things like getting enough exercise and sleep greatly influence how our brains age—and can even counteract any genetic risk factor you might have. In fact, these lifestyle factors are so important that if you take a genetic test and it shows that you *do* have the APOE-e4 genotype—the strongest genetic risk factor for Alzheimer's—it doesn't mean Alzheimer's or dementia is your destiny.

When it comes to genetic testing, there are essentially two types. One is testing for cause genes, which are known to cause Alzheimer's disease and are quite rare. The other is testing for risk genes, such as APOE e4, which don't cause Alzheimer's disease but do increase your risk of developing the condition.

There are some people for whom knowing that genetic piece helps them stay motivated to eat well, exercise regularly, and do all the other lifestyle habits that are proven to reduce the risk of Alzheimer's disease. Another reason I see women get genetic risk testing is because they have a family history that's not clear. Years ago, dementia wasn't always diagnosed—or it was called senility. For a woman with this type of family history, genetic testing can be clarifying.

On the other hand, there is not a specific set of lifestyle risk changes that we can recommend to you right now if you have a copy of the APOE-e4 gene. If you feel like knowing your genetic risk wouldn't be helpful and would instead just make you anxious, I'd say genetic testing isn't necessary. If there comes a time when the research can support interventions based on genetic status, which is a very real possibility down the line, that recommendation could change.

—Jessica Caldwell, PhD, director of the Women's Alzheimer's Movement Prevention and Research Center at the Cleveland Clinic

Your Game Plan:
Protect Your Brain and Stave Off Disease

Neuroscientists and doctors are starting to change how they think about cognitive decline. Rather than treating symptoms when we're older, experts are urging us to take protective steps *now*.

"The most important thing I want women to understand about their disproportionate risk of Alzheimer's disease is that it can be a wake-up call to take care of yourself," says Dr. Caldwell. So what are the steps you can take, starting immediately, to stay sharp and prevent cognitive decline?

Exercise. This is the first piece of advice Dr. Caldwell shares with people because it is one of the most beneficial things you can do when it comes to reducing your risk of Alzheimer's and dementia and boosting your cognitive function. Aim for 150 minutes of moderate intensity exercise each week as a minimum. Regular strength training is also key for women's bone health as we age.

Follow an anti-inflammatory diet. If you're looking for a science-backed way to eat for your brain health, load up on veggies, herbs, fish, fruits, nuts, beans, and whole grains, and reduce inflammatory foods such as red meat, processed foods, and simple sugars. It's also important to watch your alcohol intake.

"A lot of women don't realize that one drink a day is considered moderate drinking and more than that is heavy drinking," says Dr. Caldwell. "You don't have to have an alcohol-related problem to be having enough alcohol to impact your brain aging."

Get enough sleep. Research shows that women have a harder time falling asleep and staying asleep than men—which is a shame, because not getting enough sleep can essentially put a bigger burden on your brain. Sleep is when the brain clears debris—some of which may be beta-amyloid, the protein that builds up in unhelpful ways in Alzheimer's disease. (Skip ahead to chapter 18 for evidence-based advice on how to get better sleep.)

Prioritize learning at every stage of your life. A growing number of neuroscientists are studying a phenomenon called cognitive reserve, which is the idea that the more you learn and use your brain throughout your life, the more neurons and neural pathways you'll have. This gives you extra capacity to stay sharp as you get older, even if something like cognitive decline or dementia sets in. You might enroll in an online or in-person course that interests you, pick up a musical instrument, or start a hobby that requires you to learn a new skill. Engaging in intellectual conversations that stimulate your memory and critical thinking (hello, book club!) also counts. And combining movement with learning—say, by listening to a podcast on your daily walk or taking a pickleball class where you're learning new skills—is a double-whammy brain booster.

"If you're already getting a daily intellectual challenge from the work you do or other pursuits, you don't need brain games right now," adds Dr. Caldwell. "If that's the case, go ahead and focus on a different step toward protecting your brain health."

Put down some of your "mental load." It turns out doing most of the planning work in the household—remembering to make doctors' appointments, signing up kids for summer camps, thinking about next year's family vacation, the list goes on—can mean cognitive problems later in life, says Dr. Caldwell.

"While having some mental load keeps us learning and making new, beneficial neural connections, it becomes problematic when you're continuously stressed because of all you have to handle," she says. To strike a balance, it's important to really think about what's on your plate and take a few things off your to-do list if you need to. Enlist help if you can and try to accept that not everything you need to do may get the attention (or perfection) you want to give it. This "good enough" attitude can take some time to embrace. But think of it as a step in the right direction for your brain now and for years to come.

• • • • •

We've made a lot of progress when it comes to what we know about women's brain health and some of the factors that make us more vulnerable than men to various brain conditions and neurodegenerative disease. Yes, there's much more research that must be done. But with a greater understanding and awareness of our distinct challenges and the steps we can take to make our brains more resilient, we can strengthen our cognitive reserve, meet the challenges of aging, and do what we can to help shape our cognitive health now and in the future.

Chapter 14

Heart Health

Why Cardiovascular Disease Is a Woman's Issue,
Too—and How to Gauge Your Risk

> *The medical community is misogynistic, and too many of us—*
> *cardiologists included—still think heart disease is a man's disease.*
> *Nobody is talking to women about the female-specific risk factors of*
> *heart disease, so we need to empower women to bring them up with*
> *their doctors when they don't.*
>
> —Martha Gulati, MD, director of preventive cardiology and associate
> director of the Barbra Streisand Women's Heart Center in the
> Smidt Heart Institute at Cedars-Sinai Medical Center and former
> president of the American Society for Preventive Cardiology

Many of us are prone to think of heart disease as something that's more likely to happen to men. Or we assume it's something that'll happen to older women. Or women who don't exercise as much as we do. Or who don't regularly go to the doctor. That is, we find ways to distance ourselves from the very real fact that heart health is something that all women—every one of us—should be concerned about.

Some important statistics:

- Heart disease kills more women than *all forms of cancer combined*.[1]
- One woman dies of heart disease every minute.[2]
- Nearly 45 percent of women twenty and older are living with some form of heart disease—and many don't realize it.[3]
- What's worse, our physicians aren't always helping us correct course and get the care we need. In fact, women are less likely to receive preventive cardiac care[4]—and if we're hospitalized for a heart attack, we're less likely to receive treatment and more likely to die than men.[5]

These facts aren't meant to scare you but rather to help you see that, as women, we are uniquely susceptible to heart issues throughout our lives. When we understand this, we can take steps to keep our hearts healthy and reduce our risk of cardiovascular disease.

In this chapter, we'll learn . . .

- **The anatomy of the heart**, zeroing in on recent research that shows some fascinating differences between the female heart and its male equivalent.
- **What, exactly, heart disease is, the mechanism behind how it develops, and the female-specific risks**. For example, did you know that pregnancy is considered a woman's first stress test for her heart, and that complications such as a history of miscarriages, preeclampsia (high blood pressure during pregnancy), and gestational diabetes significantly increase a woman's risk of cardiovascular disease?
- **The heart attack symptoms that far too many women ignore** because they're often more subtle than the shortness of breath and crushing chest pain most men experience.
- **The alarming rise of heart attacks in young people, especially younger women**, and why the outcomes tend to be worse for us than they are for our male counterparts.
- **All about cholesterol**, including what it is, why LDL (the "bad" kind of cholesterol) causes so much harm, and the truth about cholesterol-lowering medications (like statins).

- **The specific things you can do to take charge of your heart health,** no matter how old you are or your current risk of cardiovascular disease.

Meet the Experts

Martha Gulati, MD, director of preventive cardiology and associate director of the Barbra Streisand Women's Heart Center in the Smidt Heart Institute at Cedars-Sinai Medical Center and former president of the American Society for Preventive Cardiology

Skyler St. Pierre, MS, mechanical engineer and PhD candidate at Stanford University's Living Matter Lab

Jennifer Mieres, MD, associate dean and professor of cardiology at the Donald and Barbara Zucker School of Medicine at Hofstra/Northwell Health

Stacey E. Rosen, MD, cardiologist, senior vice president of women's health and executive director of the Katz Institute for Women's Health, and president of the American Heart Association

Jayne Morgan, MD, cardiologist, vice president of medical affairs at Hello Heart, and former executive director of the largest healthcare system in Georgia

Suzanne Steinbaum, DO, cardiologist specializing in preventive care, author of *Dr. Suzanne Steinbaum's Heart Book: Every Woman's Guide to a Heart-Healthy Life*, and founder and CEO of Adesso by Heart-Tech Health, a med-tech innovation for women's cardiovascular prevention, health, and wellness

A Look Inside Your Heart: A Brief Anatomy Lesson

You know your heart pumps blood throughout your body—a function that's crucial to keeping you alive. However, it's helpful to have a slightly more in-depth understanding of the heart's anatomy and how it works. Here's what you need to know.

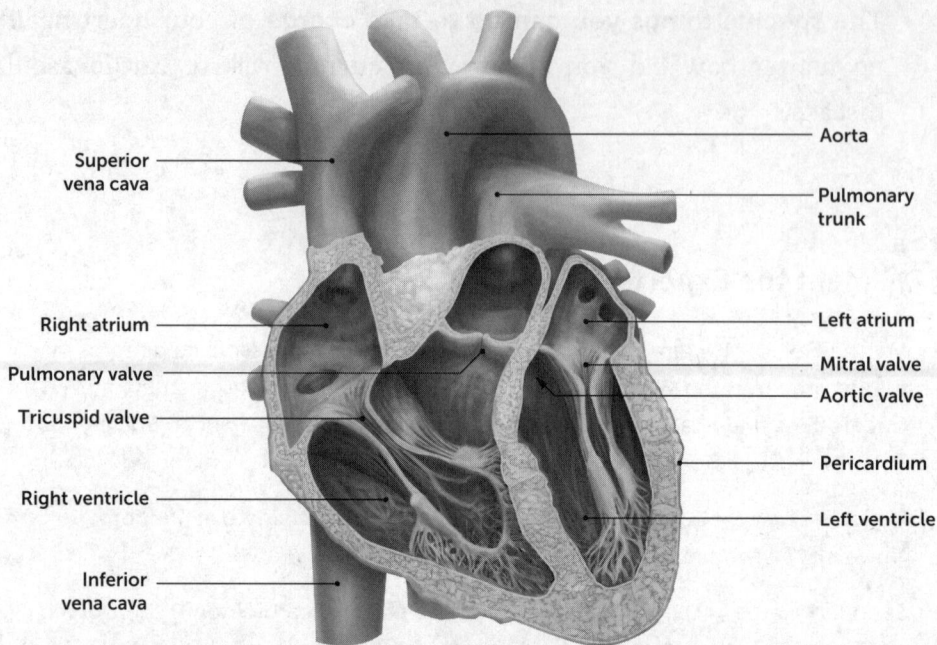

Superior vena cava — Aorta — Pulmonary trunk — Right atrium — Left atrium — Pulmonary valve — Mitral valve — Tricuspid valve — Aortic valve — Right ventricle — Pericardium — Left ventricle — Inferior vena cava

Chambers: The heart has four chambers. The two upper chambers are called atria (the right atrium and left atrium) and the two lower chambers are called ventricles (right and left). Blood flows from the body to the atria and from the atria to the ventricles. The ventricles then pump blood out of the heart to the rest of the body.

Valves: There are four heart valves that open and close to keep blood flowing in one direction. The heart valves include the tricuspid valve (between the right atrium and the right ventricle); the pulmonary valve (leading from the right ventricle to the pulmonary arteries); the mitral valve (between the left atrium and the left ventricle); and the aortic valve (leading from the left ventricle to the aorta).

Aorta: The largest blood vessel in the human body, the aorta's primary function is to carry oxygen-rich blood from the heart to the rest of the body.

Inferior vena cava: This is your body's largest vein, and it carries oxygen-depleted blood back to your heart from the lower part of your body.

Superior vena cava: This is your body's second-biggest vein, and it brings oxygen-depleted blood from your upper body to your heart.

Pericardium: This is a protective sac that wraps around your heart and produces fluid that allows for smooth, frictionless movement of the heart.

The heart has a "plumbing" system and an "electrical" system, each with distinct functions that work together to ensure effective blood flow throughout your body. The "plumbing" system is your heart's blood vessels, or the pathways through which blood flows. The heart's "electrical" system controls the rate and rhythm of the heartbeat, ensuring the heart chambers contract in a coordinated way to effectively pump blood.

The XX Heart: How the Female Heart Is Different—and Why That Matters

For many years, experts didn't think there were any noteworthy differences between the male and the female heart. Sure, they assumed ours was smaller, given our smaller-than-male body size. Yet they didn't study what anatomists call microstructural architecture—the smaller blood vessels and arteries that bring blood to and from the heart.

At Stanford University's Living Matter Lab, mechanical engineer Skyler St. Pierre is on a mission to change this. After all, cardiovascular disease in women is still underdiagnosed and undertreated, and research suggests that one reason for this is that our criteria for diagnosing heart disease (things like cutoffs for high blood pressure and cholesterol, and other tests for heart disease) are based on what we know about the male heart.

"The female heart is *not* just a small version of the male heart," says St. Pierre. "The more we understand how a woman's heart is different, the more likely it is that our diagnostic criteria will change—and that cardiac disease will be diagnosed in women as early and reliably as it is in men." Here, St. Pierre shares some of the key differences in the female heart.

Smaller Arteries and Thinner Artery Walls

The female heart is about 25 percent smaller than the male heart, with arteries smaller in diameter than men's, even after accounting for body size.

Why it matters: Smaller coronary arteries in the female heart can be more difficult to visualize clearly during certain diagnostic procedures. Similarly, they can be more challenging to work with during therapeutic procedures like coronary angioplasty, where a surgeon stretches or widens a narrowed portion of a blood vessel. Plaque buildup in the microvascular system is also harder to detect in women's smaller blood vessels, which makes it more likely to go unnoticed. This leads to women going to the doctor with more diseased hearts than men, because men are diagnosed with and treated for heart disease at earlier stages.

Faster Resting Heart Rate (RHR)

Women tend to have a lower stroke volume (the amount of blood that gets pushed out every time the heart contracts), so the thinking is that the heart rate increases to help push more blood per minute.

Why it matters: A higher RHR can be a risk factor for cardiovascular disease, according to research. For women with known heart disease or who are at high risk for heart disease, it can indicate increased strain on the heart or poor cardiac function. Some research also suggests that RHR may increase during the menopause transition.

Lower Blood Pressure

Women may have a lower "normal" blood pressure than their male counterparts.

Why it matters: For years, the normal upper limit for systolic blood pressure in adults (the first number in a blood pressure reading, which measures the force of the blood against the artery walls as your heart beats) has been 120 mm Hg. Consistently higher than that and it qualifies as hypertension, which puts you at risk for cardiovascular disease (CVD). Yet new thinking is that this normal upper limit for systolic blood pressure may be slightly lower in women. This could mean women spend more time with high blood pressure before being treated, which can lead to a higher risk of CVD.

Heart Disease:
What It Is and How to Gauge Your Risk

The term *heart disease* is tossed around a lot, and many of us don't know exactly what it means. Plaque buildup in the heart's arteries that causes heart attack? Heart failure? Arrythmia? Yes, yes, and yes—and more, says Martha Gulati, MD, a cardiologist who specializes in women's heart disease prevention. *Heart disease* (aka cardiovascular disease) is an umbrella term for several conditions. These are some of the most common in women:

- **Coronary artery disease (CAD, aka ischemic heart disease):** This is the most common type of heart disease in the U.S. and a leading cause of heart attacks. It happens when plaque builds up in the arteries in the heart over time, causing them to narrow and partially or totally blocking the flow of blood.

- **Arrhythmia:** This is a heart rhythm that can be too fast, too slow, or erratic. Common types include:
  - Atrial fibrillation (AFib)
  - Atrial flutter
  - Ventricular tachycardia (VT)
  - Ventricular fibrillation (VFib)
  - Bradycardia (resting heart rate slower than sixty beats per minute)
  - Tachycardia (resting heart rate faster than one hundred beats per minute)

- **Heart valve diseases:** These are conditions that affect any of the heart's four valves. They can happen with age, or you can be born with abnormalities in your heart valves. Common types include bicuspid aortic valve (a congenital heart defect); regurgitation (which can happen when a valve doesn't seal tightly and allows blood to leak backward); or stenosis (a valve opening that is too small).

- **Cardiomyopathies**: Diseases of the heart muscle, including:
  - Peripartum cardiomyopathy (which happens to women only during or immediately after pregnancy)
  - Dilated cardiomyopathy
  - Hypertrophic cardiomyopathy
  - Restrictive cardiomyopathy
  - Arrhythmogenic right ventricular dysplasia

- **Heart failure**: When the heart can't pump blood efficiently to meet the body's needs. There are two types of heart failure you'll hear about based on ejection fraction, which is essentially how efficiently your heart pumps blood.

  - **Heart failure with reduced ejection fraction (HFrEF, pronounced "hef-ref")**: Often referred to as systolic heart failure, this type is more common in men and occurs when the heart muscle does not contract effectively and thus a lower percentage of the blood in the left ventricle is pumped out with each beat.

  - **Heart failure with preserved ejection fraction (HFpEF, pronounced "hef-pef")**: Often referred to as diastolic heart failure, this type is more common in women and occurs when the heart muscle contracts normally but the ventricles do not relax as they should and cannot fill properly with blood.

- **Broken heart syndrome (aka stress cardiomyopathy or takotsubo cardiomyopathy)**: This can occur after an extremely stressful situation and/or emotions, serious physical illness, or surgery. While it causes symptoms similar to those of a heart attack (shortness of breath, chest pain), there are typically no blockages in the coronary arteries and the condition is usually temporary.

How Heart Disease Develops

What happens to a healthy heart over time to cause problems? The answer is an unsatisfying "It depends." Heart disease is typically the result of multiple processes, influenced by a combination of genetic, lifestyle, and environmental factors. Yet while it's often thought of as a disease of age and something we don't have to really worry about until we're older, it can begin as early as your teens and twenties and progress over decades. Here are some of the contributing factors:

- **Atherosclerosis:** This is a hardening of your arteries due to a buildup of plaque over time. The lining of the arteries in your heart (called the endothelium) is made up of a single layer of cells that provides a smooth surface for blood to flow. Over time, factors like high blood pressure, smoking, or high levels of cholesterol in the blood damage the endothelium—and you can think of that damage to the artery like a little cut, says cardiologist Jennifer Mieres, MD. LDL cholesterol (aka the "bad" kind) can then enter the arterial wall through those little cuts, which triggers an immune response.

  "Just like your skin heals a cut by creating a scab, your body tries to heal damage in the lining of your artery," says Dr. Mieres. The only problem? That "scab" is plaque, which can lead to problems in the heart over time.

- **Hypertension:** This is chronic high blood pressure, which is when the force of blood pushing against the walls of your arteries is consistently too high. Over time this damages your arteries and can put you at greater risk for heart attack, stroke, and other problems.

- **Diabetes:** Over time, high blood sugar levels can damage blood vessels, leading to atherosclerosis. This condition is also likely to coexist with other risk factors for heart disease, such as hypertension and too much "bad" LDL cholesterol.

- **Lifestyle choices:** While you can't do anything about your age, gender, family history, and genes—all nonmodifiable risk factors for developing heart disease—you can make changes when it comes to some known contributors, including your diet (eating too much saturated fat and sodium can contribute to CVD), lack of physical activity (which contributes to obesity, hypertension, and poor cardiovascular health), smoking (which can raise triglycerides, lower your "good" HDL cholesterol, damage cells that line your blood vessels, and increase your risk of atherosclerosis), and drinking alcohol (which raises blood pressure, increases the risk for heart rhythm problems, and makes you more likely to develop heart disease).

Understanding Your Risk Factors

When it comes to assessing your personal risk of developing heart disease, it's crucial to know about *all* the factors that play a role so you can have more informed, personalized discussions with your healthcare providers. Unfortunately, the risk calculators you'll find online—the same ones many clinicians use—are still based on male markers for heart disease and don't take into account female-specific risk factors, like having experienced complications during pregnancy, radiation to the left chest during chemotherapy, or hot flashes during the menopause transition. So while they're a good starting point—after all, some modifiable and nonmodifiable risk factors are the same in both women and men—there are many other factors that must be considered when looking at a woman's individual risk.

Here, Stacey E. Rosen, MD, walks us through what all women should be talking to their healthcare providers about to gauge their risk of heart disease. If your clinician doesn't ask you specifically about these things, bring them up yourself.

"I want all women to feel empowered to know the relevant information about their risks for heart disease and come to their doctor visits ready to talk about it," says Dr. Rosen. "In some cases, you'll have to be the one to take the initiative to bring up these points, but it's so important you do." Here's what needs to be on your radar:

- **Blood pressure.** This is a major risk factor for heart disease and is often called a "silent killer" because you may not experience symptoms. Keep in mind that emerging research indicates that women might be more vulnerable to heart attack and stroke at a lower blood pressure than men. One study analyzed about twenty-eight thousand people over an average of nearly thirty years and found that women with "healthy" blood pressure (100 to 109 mm Hg) had the same cardiovascular disease risk as men with hypertension (130 to 139 mm Hg).[6]

- **Cholesterol.** This waxy, fatlike substance is made by the liver and also found in certain foods. When we take in more cholesterol than our bodies can use, it can build up in the walls of the arteries and, over time, lead to a narrowing that can decrease blood flow to the heart, the brain, and other parts of the body. (For more info on cholesterol, flip to page 399.)

- **Type 2 diabetes.** This condition prompts sugar to build up in the blood, which can, over time, damage your blood vessels as well as the nerves that control your heart.

- **Obesity.** Carrying excess body fat is linked to a number of factors that contribute to heart disease, including diabetes, high "bad" LDL cholesterol and triglyceride levels, low "good" HDL cholesterol, and high blood pressure.

- **Ethnicity.** Black Americans have a disproportionately higher risk of hypertension, stroke, and heart disease.[7] Indigenous Americans are 1.5 times as likely to be diagnosed with coronary heart disease compared with their white peers, and heart disease is also more common among those of Latin and South Asian descent.[8]

A Surprising Connection to Heart Disease: Your Gynecologic Health History

While most of us think our reproductive health history is a topic for our gynecology visits, it can also give your cardiologist a better picture of your risk of heart disease, says cardiologist Jayne Morgan, MD. If your healthcare provider doesn't bring up these topics when they start asking you about your heart health, be proactive and bring them up yourself.

- **Your menstrual cycle and menopause status.** Women who have a cycle that's shorter than twenty-two days or longer than thirty-four may have an increased risk of certain cardiovascular conditions, such as coronary heart disease, heart attacks, and atrial fibrillation.[9] You'll also want to talk about how old you were when you started and stopped menstruating: Both early and late menarche (the first occurrence of menstruation) pose risks for heart disease later on. While going through menopause doesn't cause cardiovascular disease, it does mark a point when women's cardiovascular risk factors can accelerate. And if you went through menopause early (before age forty), either naturally or surgically (if your ovaries were removed), your risk for a number of heart issues may be elevated.[10]

- **PCOS status.** Has a clinician ever suspected you have PCOS or diagnosed you with the condition? (For more on what this is, flip back to page 118.) A significant proportion of people with PCOS have insulin resistance, and elevated insulin levels over time impact blood vessels and can contribute to the development of atherosclerosis. Chronic inflammation, hypertension, and obesity—all risk factors for cardiovascular disease—are also common in those with PCOS.

- **History of miscarriages.** Some research has shown a link between recurrent miscarriages and a higher risk of developing cardiovascular diseases later in life.[11] While the mechanism isn't fully understood, theories propose that certain factors—such as endothelial dysfunction, hormonal imbalances (like PCOS), autoimmune conditions, and inflammation—might increase the risk of both miscarriage and cardiovascular issues. Mental health considerations are also a factor, as miscarriage can lead to stress, depression, and anxiety—all conditions that can impact heart health.

- **Pregnancy complications.** Nearly every major system of a woman's body has to work harder to take on the massive feat of growing a fetus, and the cardiovascular system is no exception. To nourish the baby, blood volume increases by 30 to 50 percent, which means the heart has to pump more per minute—essentially working faster and harder throughout your pregnancy. It's important to realize that pregnancy-related issues such as gestational diabetes, gestational hypertension, and preeclampsia or eclampsia put you at greater risk for cardiovascular conditions later on. No matter how long ago you were pregnant or how healthy you are now, it's important to contact your healthcare provider and ask for a cardiac workup if you experienced any of these pregnancy complications, says Dr. Morgan.

- **Having a low-birthweight baby.** Delivering a full-term baby who is considered small for gestational age (SGA) may put a woman at an increased risk for heart disease later on. While the reasons for this association aren't entirely understood, experts believe certain conditions that increase the risk of having an SGA baby (think hypertension, preeclampsia, certain autoimmune diseases, insulin resistance, and lifestyle factors like poor nutrition or smoking) also contribute to a higher risk of heart disease.

- **History of hot flashes.** Think this annoying symptom of the menopause transition is benign? Think again. Vasomotor symptoms are associated with higher blood pressure, higher blood sugar levels, and higher LDL ("bad") cholesterol. Research also shows that women who have more frequent hot flashes have an increased risk for heart attacks, stroke, and other cardiovascular disease as they get older.[12]

- **History of cancer treatment.** When radiation is administered to tumors in the chest area (as it is in some cases of breast cancer), there's potential for radiation exposure to the heart. Certain chemotherapy drugs may also damage the heart muscle, potentially causing heart issues years after cancer treatment. While the risk is very low and depends on the dose, duration, and type of treatment you have, it's important to make sure your clinician knows if this is part of your medical history.

Heart Attacks and Strokes: Why They Happen and What Puts Women at Risk

Symptoms of Heart Attack in Women—and How They're Often Different from What Men Experience

When you picture a heart attack, you might think of crushing chest pain, shortness of breath, or pain shooting down your arm. While these are classic symptoms, there are several more subtle signs that can easily go unnoticed—especially in women, says Dr. Morgan.

"Unfortunately, the symptoms of heart attack in women are still considered atypical, which is a sad reflection of our sexism in medicine," she says. "Who's to say women aren't having the typical symptoms?"

Given the subtlety and variability of symptoms, women often underestimate the seriousness of their situation, writing off what they're feeling as "normal" attributes of the aging process or chalking it up to simply having a lot on their plate, adds Dr. Morgan. Make sure these lesser-known symptoms are on your radar:

- **Chest pain (aka angina) that feels like pressure, squeezing, or tightness**—not necessarily the shooting or stabbing pain many of us associate with heart attack. It's also important to know that while angina tends to get worse with physical activity and go away with rest in men, women can be more likely to have angina while at rest.

- **Pain in the upper neck, jaw, back, or stomach (including pain similar to indigestion or acid reflux)** that seems to come out of nowhere.

- **Shortness of breath**, especially if it's sudden and unexplained.

- **Cold sweat, nausea, dizziness, or lightheadedness,** which may feel like the flu is coming on and can occur without any chest discomfort.

- **Unexplained fatigue,** which can sometimes last for days.

- **Unexplained changes in sleep patterns,** including waking up due to difficulty breathing.

- **Anxiety,** or a sense of impending doom that you can't pinpoint to anything in particular.

You may read this list of symptoms and wonder how you'll be able to tell if what you're experiencing is a heart issue or just run-of-the-mill fatigue, anxiety, indigestion, or illness. Here's the truth: These symptoms may be nothing to worry about or they could be the subtle early-warning signs that you're having a heart attack. That's why experts recommend calling your provider if you're experiencing any of these symptoms and asking specifically about diagnostic tests for heart disease.

Heart Attacks Are on the Rise in Younger People (and the Outcomes Are Worse for Women)

While heart attacks in young people are rare, rates are rising—particularly among women ages thirty-five to fifty-four.[13] Experts don't yet understand exactly why, but they do point to research showing that healthcare providers are more likely to dismiss heart attack symptoms in women and underdiagnose risk factors like high blood pressure, high cholesterol, diabetes, and obesity.

What do we do with this information? For starters, more of us need to recognize we *are* at risk for heart disease, and this is especially true if we have one or more known risk factors. We also need to talk to our healthcare providers about our risk—something that shouldn't be on us to do but is, given many clinicians' misunderstandings that younger patients are at low risk of heart disease. And we must realize that our twenties, thirties, and forties are a prime time to focus on the lifestyle habits known to prevent heart disease, says cardiologist Jayne Morgan, MD.

"Yes, it comes back to the basics here: A healthy diet, regular exercise, no smoking, and making sure you're getting enough sleep really can make a difference," she says.

SCAD: What It Is, and Why It Happens to Mostly Women

Spontaneous coronary artery dissection (SCAD) happens when a tear develops inside an artery in the heart, creating a split in the wall of the artery that often results in a loose flap of tissue that can slow or block blood flow to the heart. The result? Heart rhythm problems, a heart attack, or even sudden death. Up to 90 percent of SCAD patients are women, and they are typically otherwise healthy and have few risk factors for heart disease.[14] For some patients, a stent or surgery may be necessary to fix the tear in the wall of the heart's artery; other times, SCAD can heal without treatment.

While researchers don't have definitive answers as to why SCAD develops, they do point to factors such as genetics, hormonal influences, abnormalities in the arteries, or inflammatory issues—all of which can be made worse by physical or emotional stressors, which are also commonly reported by patients with SCAD.[15]

Given that most SCAD patients are healthy young women (their average age is forty-two years old) who don't have conventional risk factors for heart disease, it's important to keep these symptoms in mind:

- Chest pain (including pressure, tightness, or heaviness)
- A rapid heartbeat (sometimes experienced as a fluttery feeling in the chest)
- Pain in the arms, shoulders, back, neck, stomach, or jaw
- Excessive sweating
- Extreme tiredness
- Nausea and/or vomiting

- Dizziness and/or lightheadedness
- Fainting or loss of consciousness
- Headache

What Is a Stroke, and Why Is It Closely Tied to Heart Health?

Heart attack and stroke are often referred to as a pair when you're talking about cardiovascular disease risk. That's because the most common type of stroke—called an ischemic stroke—occurs when the blood supply to a part of the brain is reduced or cut off completely, often due to fatty deposits that have built up in the blood vessels or a blood clot that travels through the bloodstream, most often from the heart. Like an ischemic stroke, a transient ischemic attack (TIA) is caused by a temporary decrease in blood supply to part of the brain. The key difference is that with a TIA, the blockage of blood flow to the brain is temporary and symptoms (similar to those of a stroke) are also temporary. It's important to note that even though symptoms of a TIA go away, it is a medical emergency.

The other main type of stroke is a hemorrhagic stroke, which occurs when a blood vessel in the brain leaks or ruptures. This could be due to uncontrolled high blood pressure or an abnormal bulge in the blood vessel wall, called an aneurysm.

» SYMPTOMS OF A STROKE

It's crucial to know the symptoms of a stroke and get emergency help immediately if you or a loved one are experiencing any of them. The American Stroke Association uses the acronym FAST as a helpful tool to remember the key warning signs.

F: Face drooping

A: Arm weakness

S: Speech difficulty

T: Time to call 911

Heart Health

Additional symptoms can include:

- Numbness of the face, arm, or leg, especially if it's happening on only one side of the body
- Confusion
- Trouble seeing, outside normal vision issues you may have
- Difficulty walking
- Severe headache

If you've ever experienced these symptoms but they passed quickly, you might've had a TIA. In these cases, symptoms often fade by the time people get to the emergency room. However, it's still crucial to be evaluated immediately, as nearly one in five people with a possible TIA will have a full-blown stroke within three months.[16] Your healthcare provider can order brain and blood vessel imaging, blood work to screen for diabetes and high cholesterol (known risk factors of stroke), and an electrocardiogram (to check heart rhythm).

» TAKE THESE STEPS TO REDUCE YOUR RISK OF STROKE

Stroke is common: Every forty seconds, someone in the U.S. has one.[17] But about 80 percent of all strokes are preventable, according to the American Heart Association.[18] Want to reduce your risk? Follow these steps:

Step 1: Manage your health conditions. High blood pressure, atrial fibrillation, type 2 diabetes, and high cholesterol all increase your risk of having a stroke, so it's crucial to come up with a plan to get these under control. Stress is also associated with an increased stroke risk and should be considered an important factor to control, not written off as a fact of modern life you can't do anything about.

Step 2: Maintain a healthy weight. Individuals with obesity or a high body mass index have a higher stroke risk, especially those who carry excess fat around their midsection. In fact, research shows even normal-weight women with excess abdominal fat may be at increased risk for both stroke and heart disease compared with those who carry excess weight in their legs.[19]

Step 3: Eat and exercise for your health. You've likely heard this advice so frequently it almost sounds like white noise. Yet while you know that moving your body regularly and fueling it with nutritious foods is a good idea, you might be surprised by the extent to which it can really move the needle when it comes to reducing stroke risk. One study found that people who sit for thirteen hours a day or more increase their risk of stroke by 44 percent.[20] Other research has found that following a Mediterranean diet (which is rich in whole grains, fruits, vegetables, and legumes) is associated with a reduced stroke risk, particularly in women.[21]

Cholesterol 101: What It Is—and What You Need to Know About the Drugs That Help Lower It

When you hear the term *cholesterol*, you likely think one thing: How do I keep my numbers optimally balanced to prevent heart disease? Here's what you need to know to do just that.

First, What Exactly Is Cholesterol?

It's a waxy, fatlike substance that's found in all cells of the body. It's an integral component of cell membranes and is needed to build cells and make vitamins and several important hormones. Your liver makes all the cholesterol your body needs; but certain foods also contain cholesterol, which may increase the amount that circulates in your blood and can cause problems at too-high levels.

The fatlike nature of cholesterol means it's not water-soluble and can't travel in the blood on its own. So it hitches a ride on carriers called lipoproteins that transport it throughout the body. The two main types of lipoproteins are low-density lipoprotein (LDL) and high-density lipoprotein (HDL).

LDL cholesterol is referred to as the "bad" kind because when you have excessive amounts of LDL, it starts to deposit cholesterol on your artery walls, causing plaque buildup. (To geek out on how this happens, keep reading.)

HDL cholesterol is known as the "good" kind because it carries LDL cholesterol away from the arteries to the liver, where it's either reused or excreted, ensuring that excess cholesterol doesn't build up. This is why higher levels of HDL have been associated with a lower risk of cardiovascular disease.

Triglycerides are a type of fat we get from food (mostly from fats, like butter) that gets stored in the body's fat cells to use for energy when needed. And while triglycerides aren't cholesterol, they're an important part of the picture because high levels—especially in combination with high LDL or low HDL—can increase the risk of heart disease.

Lipoprotein(a), also known as Lp(a) and pronounced "Lp little *a*," is a type of lipoprotein that's genetically inherited and can cause plaque buildup and a resulting increased risk of cardiovascular disease.[22]

ApolipoproteinB, also known as apoB, is the main protein found in Lp(a) and LDL. Similar to Lp(a), high apoB numbers are linked to an increased risk of heart disease.[23]

What Determines Cholesterol Levels—and How to Keep Yours in the Optimal Range

There are multiple factors that play a role in determining cholesterol levels in the body, some of which we can control and others we can't.

- **Diet.** While dietary cholesterol is now thought to play a smaller role than previously believed, saturated fats (found in meat and dairy products) and trans fats (found in processed foods) potentially increase triglycerides and LDL levels.

- **Exercise.** Regular physical activity can boost HDL and potentially reduce LDL and triglycerides.

- **Age and gender.** As we get older, cholesterol levels tend to rise—and this is especially true for women after menopause. Before the menopause transition, women often have lower LDL levels than men. Postmenopause, LDL often climbs.

- **Genetics.** *Familial hypercholesterolemia* is a fancy term for high cholesterol that runs in your family. People who have it make too much LDL cholesterol and can't get rid of it—frustratingly, sometimes even with changes to their diet and lifestyle.

Ask an Expert

Why does a woman's risk of heart disease increase so dramatically after menopause?

The lining of the arteries, which is called the endothelium, protects the arteries. When the endothelium becomes stiff, damage can occur.

This stiffness can be due to several factors, such as high blood pressure, elevated blood sugars, smoking, inflammation, and high levels of cholesterol in the blood. During the menopause transition, a decrease in estrogen also causes the endothelium to get stiffer and less pliable—and, as a result, more likely to get damaged. That drop in estrogen also causes increases in cholesterol, blood pressure, risk of insulin resistance, risk of diabetes, and weight (especially in the abdominal area), all of which put you at greater risk for heart disease.

When the endothelium is damaged, lipids, inflammatory cells, and other substances have a greater chance of accumulating in and on the artery walls and forming a plaque. This buildup of plaque and the consequent narrowing of the arteries is called atherosclerosis.

Only in the past twenty years have cardiologists learned that atherosclerosis develops differently in women and men, likely thanks to estrogen. While both female and male hearts have estrogen receptors, the primary estrogen women have in abundance during their reproductive years is believed to have several benefits on the heart, including:

- Promoting vasodilation, or a widening of blood vessels that can lead to reduced blood pressure and improved blood flow

- Increasing HDL cholesterol (the "good" kind that protects the heart)

- Decreasing LDL cholesterol (the "bad" kind that contributes to atherosclerosis) and inhibiting its oxidation, which may help stave off plaque development.

These cardio-protective benefits of estrogen help to explain why after menopause—when estrogen drops significantly—the female heart starts behaving more like the male heart and is at a two to six times increased risk of developing atherosclerosis, ultimately leading to heart disease.

—Suzanne Steinbaum, DO, cardiologist specializing in preventive care, author of *Dr. Suzanne Steinbaum's Heart Book: Every Woman's Guide to a Heart-Healthy Life*, and founder and CEO of Adesso by Heart-Tech Health, a med-tech innovation for women's cardiovascular prevention, health, and wellness

Rx, Explained: Cholesterol-Lowering Medications

While you can try to steer cholesterol toward optimal levels by eating the right foods, exercising, maintaining a healthy weight, and quitting smoking, your doctor might prescribe one of these common cholesterol-lowering medications if your lifestyle changes don't make enough of a positive impact on your levels.

CATEGORY OF DRUGS	HOW THEY WORK
Statins	These block a specific enzyme your liver needs to create cholesterol. This helps decrease LDL ("bad") cholesterol and triglycerides and may increase HDL ("good") cholesterol.
Bile acid sequestrants	These bind to bile acids, preventing their absorption. The liver needs cholesterol to make bile acids, and it pulls that cholesterol from your blood, ultimately lowering your cholesterol level.
Cholesterol absorption inhibitors	These help prevent your body from absorbing and storing cholesterol in your liver. They also improve the way cholesterol is cleared from the bloodstream.
Fibrates	These reduce the amount of very-low-density lipoprotein (VLDL), which in turn lowers your triglyceride levels. (VLDL particles carry triglycerides throughout the body.) Fibrates also increase the amount of HDL ("good") cholesterol you make.
PCSK9 inhibitors	These are newer LDL ("bad") cholesterol–lowering agents, developed for those who can't tolerate statins or for whom statins don't sufficiently lower cholesterol levels. They lower LDL cholesterol by blocking PCSK9, a protein that destroys cholesterol-clearing receptors in the liver, which in turn allows the body to remove more cholesterol from the blood.
Niacin (nicotinic acid)	This B vitamin limits the production of blood fats in the liver, which may help lower triglycerides and LDL ("bad") cholesterol.
Adenosine triphosphate-citrate lyase (ACLY) inhibitors	These block the production of cholesterol in the liver.

The Truth About Statins—and Why Many Women Refuse to Take Them

What is it about cholesterol-lowering medications that inspires so many of us to beg our doctors to postpone prescribing them, promising we'll work to lower our cholesterol on our own by exercising more and eating healthier? Research shows that one in five people who are at high risk of heart attack or stroke refused their doctor's statin prescription—and women are 20 percent more likely than men to reject these cholesterol-lowering meds and 50 percent more likely to never accept the recommendation.[24] (The scientists who conducted this study found that the people who refused statin therapy developed higher LDL or "bad" cholesterol levels, and it took them three times longer to get those levels down than the patients who went on statins right away.) Even among people sixty-six and older who've had a heart attack and have been told they'll need lipid-lowering medications, upward of 40 percent stop taking statins within two years of their cardiovascular event, according to research.[25]

What's behind our collective reluctance to take cholesterol-lowering drugs? Many cardiologists point to the misguided perception that women are less likely than men to be at risk of cardiovascular disease, which makes us think medications that lower cholesterol are unnecessary. Another reason may be an aversion to the potential side effects of these drugs (such as high blood sugar and muscle weakness or pain), which are less common than people think, says Dr. Rosen.

"Cholesterol-lowering medications are one of the greatest discoveries of modern medicine, and a class of drugs most people tolerate very well," she says. "There's this misconception that statins are overprescribed and too difficult to take, but the truth is that the data is quite robust regarding safety, efficacy, and significant risk reduction for heart attack and stroke when used in the appropriate population."

Your Game Plan: How to Take Charge of Your Heart Health, No Matter How Old You Are

In an ideal world, your primary care physician would start asking the kinds of questions that screen for your risk of heart disease starting in your early twenties. In reality, we're far from this optimal scenario. Not only do most women underestimate their risk of heart disease, but many healthcare providers do, too. Just 22 percent of primary care doctors and 42 percent of cardiologists report feeling well prepared to care for their female patients' hearts, according to one study.[26] That same research found that nearly 71 percent of women almost never raised the issue of heart health with their physician, assuming their doctor would bring it up. It's time to change this. Here, Dr. Gulati explains where to start.

Talk to your doctor about your heart health *now*—not after you've lost weight or finally quit smoking. The good habits that lead to optimal heart health have been drilled into most of us, so we know when we have room for improvement when it comes to making diet, exercise, and other lifestyle changes that'll make our doctors proud. However, it's important not to put off a heart health checkup until you've made those changes—and unfortunately, it's something a lot of us do. A whopping 63 percent of women admit to putting off going to the doctor at least sometimes, and 45 percent of women canceled or postponed an appointment because of concern about going on a scale and being weighed.[27]

If your clinician launches right into concerns about your weight, request that you discuss that particular aspect of heart disease risk after going over other factors. (For more on how to talk to your clinicians about weight, skip ahead to page 564.)

Understand your risk of heart disease—and find a clinician who does, too. While science has come a long way in recent years in terms of what we know about the female heart and cardiovascular disease, there's still a lot of ground to cover, including around awareness. One decade-long study by the American Heart Association found that fewer than half of all women recognize that heart disease is their leading killer.[28] And this number is decreasing. Sadly, the greatest declines in awareness were among women under the age of thirty-five, as well as among Black and Hispanic women—groups in which heart disease is on the rise.

Unfortunately, many healthcare professionals also aren't aware of how big a risk heart disease is for women. If you bring up heart disease risk factors that are on your radar and your provider dismisses you, find another healthcare practitioner, says Dr. Gulati.

Take steps that are proven to help your heart. While heart disease can feel scary—and the fact that it's the number one killer of women can feel downright overwhelming—it's important to remember that it is a preventable disease. Even better, making just a few changes that feel doable (like exercising, eating a heart-healthier diet, and prioritizing your sleep) really can move the needle when it comes to staving off cardiovascular issues.

• • • • •

Heart disease is the leading cause of death in American women, and yet heart problems are often underrecognized and undertreated. But here's the good news: There is a lot each of us can do to take matters of our heart into our own hands. The more you know, the better able you'll be to accurately assess your risk, take action, and advocate for the cardiology care you deserve.

Chapter 15

Gut Health

*What to Know About Your Gastrointestinal
Tract and Microbiome to Optimize Your
Health and Prevent Disease*

> *Poop shame is real—and it disproportionately affects women, who
> suffer from higher rates of irritable bowel syndrome and inflamma-
> tory bowel disease. In other words, the patriarchy has seeped into
> women's intestinal tracts. Let's call it the pootriarchy.*
>
> —Jessica Bennett and Amanda McCall, "Women Poop. Sometimes at
> Work. Get Over It." in *The New York Times*

T he term *gut health* gets tossed around to such an extent these days it
can seem, at times, like the gut is some part of our body that is at
once the source of all our health woes and in perpetual and desperate need of fixing. The truth is that a healthy gut *is* important for our overall
health and well-being—but the topic can prompt a lot of confusion, given
that it can mean a number of things.

Our resulting uncertainty can lead to all kinds of missteps, from spending too much money on probiotics to dismissing red-flag gastrointestinal

(GI) symptoms like bloating, constipation, or changes in our bowel movements. Not only that, but the sexist double standards that women have been up against for ages when it comes to talking about (and, heaven forbid, getting caught) burping, farting, and especially *pooping* haven't exactly helped us get comfortable tracking our GI symptoms or talking about them with our healthcare providers.

It's time to collectively change that—and the best way to start is with the information in the pages that follow.

In this chapter, we'll learn . . .

- **The anatomy of your gastrointestinal tract** so you understand how each of the parts of this system works to help you digest your food, and what makes a woman's gut different from a man's.

- **Some of the most common GI disorders in women**, including why they're more likely to happen to us and the best ways to treat each.

- **What "leaky gut" is** and why it puts you at an increased risk for digestive and other health woes.

- **All about the gut microbiome**, what it does, and the science-backed strategies that can help you boost the health of yours.

- **What you need to know about poop**, why it's essentially a diagnostic tool for our gut health that we produce every day, and why more of us need to be looking at (and talking about) ours.

- **Why colon cancer** rates are on the rise among young people, the reasons women are more often dismissed by clinicians when they report symptoms of the disease, and symptoms to stay on the lookout for.

- **The straightforward steps you can take to improve your gut health** and, as a result, optimize many other aspects of your overall health.

What, Exactly, Is Gut Health?
Understanding What This Catchall Phrase Entails

It can be tricky to decipher what the term gut health entails. Is it shorthand for the microbiome or the GI tract? Does it involve digestive issues such as bloating, gas, and constipation?

The truth is that "gut health" encompasses a wide range of conditions that impact multiple organs that run from your mouth to your anus, as well as other organs that supply enzymes and digestive juices to the organs of your GI tract, says gastroenterologist Rabia de Latour, MD. Let's take a look inside the "gut" to get a better sense of what we'll explore in this chapter.

Your gastrointestinal (GI) tract includes your:

- **Mouth:** This is where food and liquid enter your GI tract, and the act of chewing, along with your saliva, starts to break food down for digestion. (Though digestion begins even before you eat, when the thought, sight, and smell of food trigger your salivary glands to produce saliva, which contains enzymes that help break down food.)

- **Esophagus:** Your tongue pushes food into the esophagus, where muscles there automatically move it down toward your stomach.

- **Stomach:** There's an upper muscle in your stomach that relaxes to allow food and liquid you've consumed to enter your stomach; there's also a lower stomach muscle that contracts to mix that food and liquid with digestive juices—namely gastric acid (aka hydrochloric acid, or HCl). This digestive stew (called chyme) slowly empties into your small intestine.

- **Small intestine:** Your small intestine is lined with muscles that continue to mix food and digestive juices and push the mixture farther through your GI tract. It may be called "small," but this organ is about twenty feet long and is where most of the digestive process happens. Fingerlike projections called villi line your small intestine to increase its surface area, helping nutrients pass through the intestinal lining and into your blood so they can travel throughout your body. The waste products of this digestive process (including undigested food, fluid, and even old cells from the lining of your GI tract) then move into your large intestine.

- **Large intestine (aka the colon):** This tubelike organ follows from the small intestine and ends at your anal canal, and while it's much shorter than the small intestine (it's approximately six feet long), it's wider—which is why it's called the large intestine. This is where food waste becomes stool.

- **Rectum and anus:** At the lower end of your large intestine is the rectum, which stores stool until it's pushed out of your anus during a bowel movement.

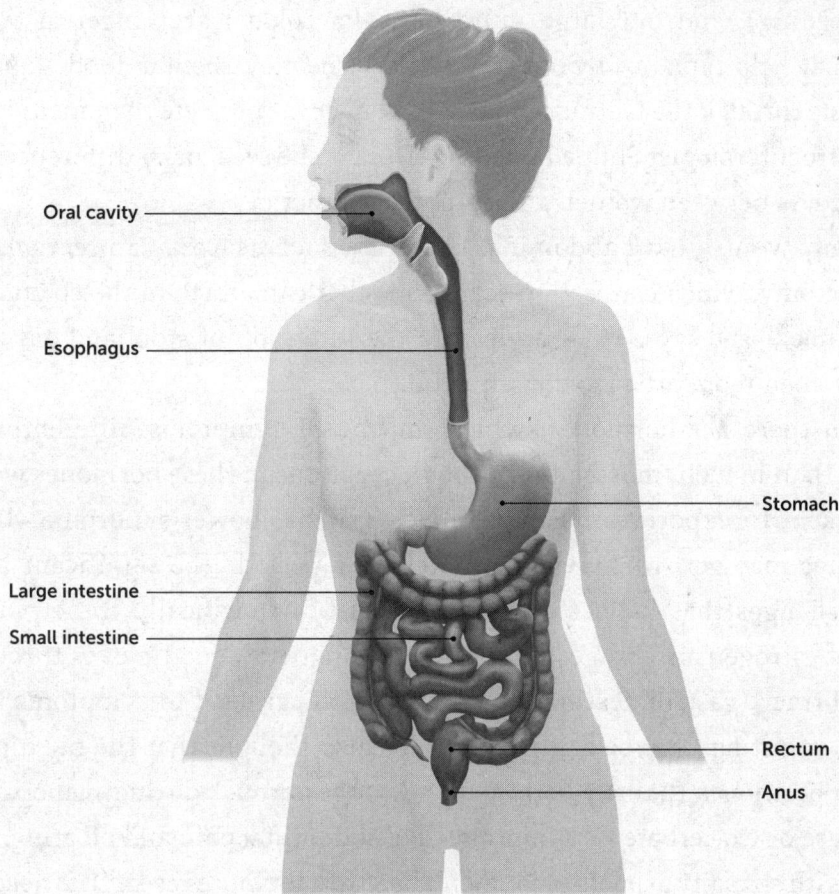

Oral cavity

Esophagus

Stomach

Large intestine

Small intestine

Rectum

Anus

The Female Gut: What's Different About *Our* Gut Health?

Like so many things in the human body, the organs and structures that make up the gastrointestinal tract are similar in females and males—but have enough variation that certain GI symptoms and disorders are more prevalent among women.

One obvious anatomical difference is the presence of additional organs in our abdomen and pelvis—the uterus, uterine tubes, and ovaries. What's more, a handful of small studies on cadavers have found that women's small intestines are up to thirty centimeters longer than men's (likely due to our need to better absorb fat and other nutrients during pregnancy and breastfeeding), and our large intestines (aka colons) are longer as well, which may help explain why our GI "transit" (the movement of food, liquids, and waste through the GI tract) takes a bit longer to complete than men's.[1]

Gastroenterologist Shilpa Ravella, MD, says she sees many differences in GI disorders between women and men in her practice.

"Many women have abdominal surgeries, such as Cesarean sections or hysterectomy, which can lead to scar tissue that can attach to the colon and cause kinks," she says. This can lead to the retention of stool and gas and make women more prone to constipation.

Then there are hormones, which impact GI symptoms differently in women than in men, mostly due to the fluctuations in these hormones we're more likely to experience. For example, irritable bowel syndrome (IBS) symptoms may get worse when you get your period. The significant hormonal changes that happen during pregnancy—specifically the elevated levels of estrogen and progesterone—can change how food moves through your GI tract (gastrointestinal motility), which can lead to symptoms like nausea, vomiting, and/or constipation. It's also thought that the big dip in ovarian hormones (namely estrogen and progesterone) during menopause may cause or exacerbate GI symptoms like abdominal pain and bloating.

As with so many aspects of women's health, a lot more research is needed to more fully understand these sex differences in the GI tract and how they lead to different health conditions. Until those studies are done, having even a basic understanding of the GI tract differences we do know about can help you stay clued in to any symptoms you're experiencing.

What Is Leaky Gut? Zooming In on Your Intestinal Barrier

Your small and large intestines are essentially one long, winding tube that has multiple layers of mucus and epithelial cells that act as a barrier between your gut and the rest of your body. These protective layers that make up your gut barrier work in multiple ways to let the good stuff (like nutrients and beneficial by-products of your gut bugs, such as short-chain fatty acids) pass through and keep the bad stuff (like bacteria, viruses, and other pathogens that hitch a ride into our bodies on the food we eat) out, says functional medicine practitioner Amy Myers, MD.

There are layers of mucus coating your intestines, and these layers secrete special proteins called immunoglobulins (aka antibodies), which your immune system makes to fight infections. These antibodies trap pathogens and physically remove them from your body via your stool. This mucus layer is also rich in carbohydrate-like structures, which your gut bugs like to feed on if they don't get the fiber they're really craving.

Under those mucus layers is a layer of epithelial cells that are held together by tight junctions. You can think of them as a drawbridge that opens and closes to allow small nutrients to be absorbed into the bloodstream. Beneath those tight junctions are immune cells that protect you against foreign invaders that could penetrate your tight junctions.

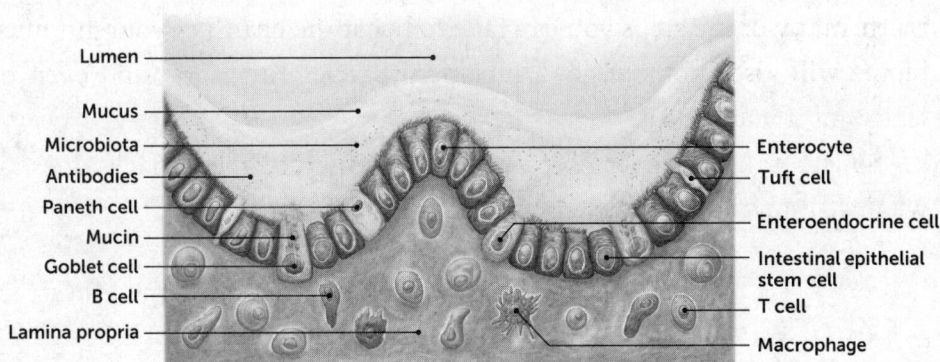

If your intestinal barrier is working optimally, it'll succeed in its role of being a good interface between the external and the internal. However, factors like an unhealthy diet, stress, drinking too much alcohol, and taking antibiotics or other pharmaceuticals can cause the protective gut lining to weaken—and the tight junctions that lie beneath the intestine's lining can open up and stay open. This is sometimes referred to as increased intestinal permeability—or, more commonly, "leaky gut"—and it means that everything from tiny, undigested particles of food to bacteria, viruses, and other pathogens can more readily pass through the protective layer in your intestine walls and get absorbed into your bloodstream.

"When food particles, microbes, and other foreign invaders that should've been passed out of your body make their way into your bloodstream, your immune system responds by attacking them," explains Dr. Myers. Like most immune responses, this creates inflammation—and your body's inflammatory response can cause a range of digestive issues (think gas, bloating, and diarrhea) and even symptoms you may not link to your gut, such as mood issues (like depression and anxiety), skin issues (like acne, eczema, or rosacea), and symptoms of hormonal imbalance (such as irregular periods and premenstrual syndrome). Research links leaky gut to intestinal diseases, such as inflammatory bowel disease and irritable bowel syndrome; it's also associated with autoimmune diseases (such as celiac disease, psoriasis, lupus, Hashimoto's thyroiditis, and rheumatoid arthritis) as well as obesity, type 1 diabetes and even heart disease.[2]

While there are multiple approaches that can help promote a healthy gut barrier and heal one that's been compromised, here's the research-backed truth: Many of the steps you can take to boost the health of your gut microbiome will also promote good intestinal barrier function—and even heal leaky gut if you have it.

So let's take a deeper dive into the gut microbiome, what it does, and what we know about how to boost the health of yours.

Meet Your Gut Microbiome: How the Ecosystem of Bacteria in Your Gut Impacts Your Health

You've undoubtedly heard of your microbiome, the trillions (yes, *trillions*) of microbes, including bacteria, that live in and on your body. These bugs are everywhere—on your skin, in your mouth, on every strand of hair on your head. If you get pregnant, the breast milk you produce even has its own microbiome. And while these bugs that make up what we call the microbiome are everywhere in and on you, the vast majority of them live in your large intestine. This is known as your gut microbiome—and it's also a big part of what many refer to when they talk about "gut health."

What Does the Gut Microbiome Do?

Turns out there's a very good reason most of your microbiome is located in your gut: It's because your gut also houses a significant portion of your body's immune cells. Your gut bugs, which are part of the outside world and take up residence in your gut over time, start to train your immune system at birth so it learns what can stay in the body and what must get "attacked" and go. Those immune cells also help to get rid of the many pathogens that pass through your GI tract every day.

Your gut bacteria play other important roles as well. For example, some of the bugs in your large intestine extract nutrients from the food you eat so they can then produce health-promoting vitamins, enzymes, and other metabolites such as short-chain fatty acids. (Short-chain fatty acids are powerful anti-inflammatory molecules in the body.) Some gut bugs help make neurotransmitters that impact your mood, your cognitive function, and even how energized you feel. And others regulate the gut's secretion of hormones like ghrelin, leptin, and insulin, which play a role in sensations you know as hunger, satiety, and food cravings.

A specific group of bacteria in your gut actually mediates the estrogens circulating throughout your body. This posse of gut bugs even has its own name: *the estrobolome.*

Meet Your Estrobolome

Researchers have defined a group of bacteria in the gut microbiome that are specifically involved in estrogen metabolism. And while both women and men have an estrobolome (because hormones aren't gender-specific, as we've been taught to believe, and men have estrogen floating around their bodies, too!), the monthly swings and menopausal dip in estrogen that women experience may cause significant changes in the female estrobolome, explains women's hormone expert Carrie Jones, ND.

Here's what we know (so far) about how the bugs that make up the estrobolome work: They produce an enzyme called beta-glucuronidase, which can convert inactive estrogen that's been metabolized and "marked" for elimination back into active forms that then get sent back into circulation in your body. (For more detail on estrogen as well as our other hormones, flip back to chapter 8.) An imbalance (or dysbiosis) of the microbes that make up the estrobolome can mean you make either too much or too little beta-glucuronidase—and have either too much or too little estrogen circulating through your body as a result. And this surplus or shortage of estrogen can show up as health conditions ranging from PMS to worsening endometriosis, says Dr. Jones.

So how can you promote a good balance of bacteria in your estrobolome? This is a continually emerging field of study, but what scientists know as of now is that many of the same things that boost the health of your gut microbiome will keep your estrobolome thriving, too.

How to Boost the Health of Your Microbiome

Experts are learning more and more every day about the vast world of bacteria living in and on us, and the many roles it plays in human health. Here's what we know so far about some of the best things you can do to improve the health of your gut bugs. The best part? Your gut bugs are quick to respond to positive changes.

"The composition of the bacteria in your gut can shift within one to three days," says Gail Cresci, PhD, RD, who studies the gut microbiome and probiotics. To help them shift for the better:

- **Eat foods that'll actually reach your gut bugs (e.g., dietary fiber).** The microbes that make up your gut microbiome need to eat in order to survive, just as you do, and each of these bugs has its preferences when it comes to what it likes to feed on. In a healthy microbiome, bugs prefer dietary fiber as their fuel source. Thanks to the different fibers in fruits, vegetables, and other plants and the fact that our bodies cannot digest fiber, the fiber in these foods makes its way through your GI tract and meets up with the bugs in your large intestine. Then various microbes feed on the fiber (as well as unabsorbed proteins and fats) and produce different by-products, or metabolites. For example, certain microbes that prefer eating fermentable soluble fiber (mostly found in beans and legumes) can produce a short-chain fatty acid called butyrate, a substance that fuels colon cells and helps support the immune system, strengthens the gut lining, reduces inflammation, and even modulates how our DNA is expressed to stave off disease. This is one reason why study after study shows a diet rich in plant-based foods promotes a gut microbiome linked to better health.

- **Starve your bad bugs.** Just as feeding your microbiome's health-promoting bugs will help them thrive, depriving your bad bugs of the food they like best can help the overall balance of your microbiome. Top offenders are simple sugars, artificial sweeteners (like sucralose, aspartame, and saccharin), animal meat, and processed foods, says Dr. Cresci. When these sugars, proteins, and fats make it to your large intestine, your "bad" gut bugs feast on them and multiply, crowding out the "good" bacteria, which can lead to negative health outcomes. Need more inspiration to lay off the simple carbohydrates and sugar? These fiber-lacking foods get absorbed quickly and don't typically make it to the bugs in your colon. Because, like you, your gut bugs don't like to go hungry, they start noshing on the protective mucus layers that line your colon. The result? A compromised immune system and a weakening in the gut barrier that keeps your gut lining intact—aka leaky gut.

- **Take antibiotics only when necessary.** The antibiotics we rely on to treat bacterial infections—everything from strep throat to UTIs—are one of the greatest medical advancements of our time. Yet while these drugs are designed to target and kill infection-causing bacteria, they don't distinguish between harmful and beneficial bacteria. Which means when you take antibiotics, they can kill the good microbes with the bad, reducing your gut microbiome's diversity in a way that can take months (or even years) to restore. If your healthcare provider prescribes an antibiotic, be sure you understand what bacterial infection it's treating, which is a good way to make sure it's absolutely necessary.

- **Keep stress in check.** It may sound far-fetched that feeling stressed could lead to changes in your gut microbiome. Yet thanks to the complex network of nerves, hormones, and immune system molecules that connect the gut microbiome to the brain—often referred to as the gut-brain axis—physical and emotional stress can have a significant impact on the balance of bugs in your gut microbiome. Chronic or acute stress has been linked to a reduction in microbial diversity (the opposite of what we're going for when it comes to optimizing health), and it can also make the lining of the gut more permeable, increasing the risk of bacteria passing through the gut barrier and causing inflammation and other problems.[3] What's more, the gut-brain axis is bidirectional, meaning not only does stress affect the microbiome, but the microbiome may also influence the body's response to stress. So all the steps you take to keep the ecosystem of microbes in your gut healthy when life feels fine have a good chance of paying off when the inevitable stress does show up in your life.

- **Move your body.** Exercise has been linked to a boost in beneficial bacteria and a decrease in potentially harmful bacteria.[4] It's also known to have a positive impact on the immune system, and when that's well functioning, your immune cells can help your gut microbiome maintain an optimal balance of bugs.

Ask an Expert

There's a lot of contradictory information about probiotics. Do they improve gut health—or are they a waste of money?

Probiotic supplements are beneficial microbes that are similar to those that are found in your gut. There are situations where a probiotic may be beneficial. For example, it may provide some symptom relief if you're dealing with irritable bowel syndrome (IBS), ulcerative colitis, diarrhea associated with antibiotic use, or a *Clostridioides difficile* (*C. diff*) infection. But given the fact that there are hundreds of different strains of both lactobacillus and bifidobacterium (the two types of bacteria most commonly found in probiotics), and each strain can act differently and have different effects, it's nearly impossible to know if the probiotic supplement you buy will help *your* particular symptoms.

It's also important to know that independent agencies that test probiotic supplements for the "live, active cultures" they claim to have on their labels often find that they aren't as potent as they purport to be. Why? Because our gut bacteria are mostly anaerobic, which means if they're exposed to oxygen, they'll die. This makes it difficult to extract them from the gut and turn them into a supplement. One of the reasons most probiotics contain bifidobacterium and lactobacillus is that both can handle some oxygen, which means they're easy to culture and grow in large amounts. Yet just because these probiotics can *survive* oxygen exposure doesn't mean they *thrive* in oxygen—and they will degrade over time. When you put these probiotics in a capsule that sits on a store shelf for a while, they're going to lose their viability.

Research on probiotics is ongoing, with scientists aiming to figure out which strains of probiotics may be most beneficial in treating certain conditions and also how to make supplements filled with good but oxygen-hating bacteria more viable. For example, we're studying a specific type of probiotic strain called bacillus, which forms spores that remain dormant until they get into the right environment—like the dark, zero-oxygen environment of the colon—where they then become active.

Until we know more, focus on eating a diet rich in foods that contain fiber and/or live active cultures. Fiber-rich fruits and vegetables and fermented foods, such as yogurt, kimchi, and sauerkraut, are likely to give you viable bacteria and come with other health-boosting benefits.

—Gail Cresci, PhD, RD, gut microbiome researcher with Cleveland Clinic's Digestive Disease & Surgery Institute and director of nutrition research with Cleveland Clinic's Center for Human Nutrition

Gut Pain and Problems:
Signs Something Is Wrong and What to Do About It

Given the sex-specific differences in our GI tract, it's no surprise that there are certain GI symptoms and disorders women are more likely to experience than men. Here are some of the most common GI disorders in women, why they're more likely to happen to us, and the treatment options for each.

Gastroesophageal Reflux Disease (GERD)

This is a chronic disorder that typically involves the persistent backflow of stomach acid into the esophagus, causing symptoms ranging from heartburn and regurgitation to chest pain, difficulty swallowing, and a chronic cough. When the lower esophageal sphincter—the ringlike muscle at the bottom of the esophagus that allows food to pass down from the mouth into the stomach—doesn't work properly, it allows stomach contents to flow back into the esophagus (acid reflux). Acid reflux is common; nearly a third of adults in the U.S. get it weekly. When acid reflux becomes more frequent and severe, it becomes GERD. (Note that heartburn is a symptom of acid reflux and GERD and isn't a condition in itself. Heartburn can also be a sign of other problems, such as a peptic ulcer or heart trouble, so it's important to see your clinician if it's persistent rather than popping antacids and thinking your heartburn is no big deal.)

» TREATMENT

Depending on the severity of symptoms and underlying causes of GERD, one or more of the following may be used:

- Lifestyle modifications, such as avoiding "trigger" foods that make your symptoms worse, eating smaller, more frequent meals, and losing excess weight

- Over-the-counter antacids, which neutralize stomach acid

- Prescription H2 blockers (which reduce stomach acid production) and proton pump inhibitors (which provide longer-lasting relief by reducing stomach acid production)

- Procedures—both minimally invasive and surgical options—that tighten or strengthen the lower esophageal sphincter

Irritable Bowel Syndrome (IBS)

This is a condition that impacts the small intestine and colon and can cause recurrent abdominal pain (often described as a cramping sensation that stops only after a bowel movement); changes in bowel habits that may include diarrhea, constipation, or alternating bouts of both; and bloating and gas. While the exact cause of IBS isn't fully understood, it's thought to involve an interplay of multiple factors, including gut motility, changes in the gut microbiome, and communication between the gut and the brain. IBS affects women about twice as often as men for reasons that aren't entirely understood, though hormonal fluctuations (IBS symptoms can worsen predictably based on your menstrual cycle) and psychosocial factors (like stress, anxiety, and depression) may trigger or exacerbate symptoms.

» TREATMENT

This involves managing (and hopefully alleviating) symptoms, as there is no known cure for IBS. Tactics include:

- Diet modifications, such as boosting fiber intake and avoiding foods that exacerbate symptoms

- Medications, such as antidiarrheal drugs, laxatives, and prescription drugs

- Lifestyle changes, such as stress management, regular exercise, and optimizing sleep

- Cognitive behavioral therapy, which can address the psychological aspects of IBS for people whose symptoms are influenced by stress and anxiety

Indigestion (Dyspepsia)

This is characterized by discomfort or pain after eating and while you're still digesting your meal. And while all of us can relate to this feeling—especially after eating the wrong thing or scarfing down a meal too quickly—for some, indigestion happens every day. Some research shows that a type of indigestion called functional dyspepsia (which is diagnosed if there's no obvious cause of the indigestion) occurs more often in women than men, and that it affects quality of life more significantly in women.[5]

» TREATMENT

Most approaches to managing and treating indigestion are similar to the recommendations for GERD:

- Diet tweaks

- Over-the-counter medications and, in some cases, prescription medications

- Managing stress and avoiding smoking (both can exacerbate symptoms)

Gallstones

These are small, hardened pieces of bile that form within the gallbladder (a small organ that sits just beneath the liver). Bile is a fluid produced by the liver and stored in the gallbladder that helps us digest food. Gallstones don't always cause symptoms; but when they get trapped in the ducts that carry bile from the gallbladder to the small intestine, they can lead to nausea and abdominal pain, among other symptoms.

Women are two to three times more likely than men to develop gallstones, particularly through the childbearing years,[6] and hormones are most likely responsible for our increased risk: Estrogen increases cholesterol in the bile and progesterone slows gallbladder emptying, a combination that increases the chances of gallstone formation.

» TREATMENT

If gallstones aren't causing symptoms, a watch-and-wait approach is usually recommended. If symptoms are severe or your gallstones are causing a blockage and leading to other complications, surgery to remove the gallbladder may be needed.

Constipation, Bloating, and Diarrhea

These conditions are often grouped together because they are common symptoms of IBS. Here's a brief explanation of each:

- **Constipation**: This may involve infrequent bowel movements, hard or lumpy stools, and straining during bowel movements.

- **Bloating**: This is a feeling of fullness in the belly, often due to gas, which can cause pain and what looks like swelling (aka distension).

- **Diarrhea**: This is loose or watery stools.

These are all more common in women, though the reason isn't fully understood. More hormonal fluctuation, slower colonic transit and gastric emptying (food and waste tend to move through and out of the female GI system more slowly than they do in males), and a higher likelihood of scar tissue on the colon resulting from prior abdominal surgeries (such as C-sections and hysterectomies) are all thought to be possible contributing factors.[7]

» TREATMENT

The best way to manage each of these GI woes will be different depending on the underlying cause but may include diet tweaks, changes to how much water you're drinking, exercising more, and possibly even an OTC or prescription medication. It's also important to talk to your healthcare provider about the prescription medications you're taking that could be causing GI symptoms.

Small Intestinal Bacterial Overgrowth (SIBO)

This happens when there is excessive growth of bacteria in the small intestine, which normally contains a relatively small amount of bugs compared with the large intestine. These bacteria then feed off the undigested food in your small intestine (they especially love sugar, starches, and alcohol), which causes these carbohydrates to ferment. The result? Gas that you'll experience as burping, farting, and bloating, as well as a range of other potential symptoms, including chronic diarrhea, vitamin and mineral deficiencies due to malabsorption of nutrients, and inflammation that can lead to everything from skin rashes to the development of autoimmune disease over time.

» TREATMENT

Antibiotics are often prescribed to reduce the bacterial overgrowth in the small intestine, in combination with dietary changes that restrict certain types of carbohydrates (like fruits, starchy veggies, dairy products, grains, sugars, and sweeteners) that can promote bacterial growth. It's also important to try to address the underlying cause of SIBO, such as abnormalities in the small intestine that create pockets where bacteria can accumulate or conditions that affect the normal movement of the small intestine, such as an intestinal obstruction or an autoimmune disease like scleroderma, which can slow down intestinal transit and lead to bacterial overgrowth.

Candida Overgrowth (Candidiasis)

This is a fungal infection that's caused by an overgrowth of *Candida albicans*— a form of yeast that lives in your mouth, on your skin, and in your gut microbiome. In your gut, it helps break down food so it can be absorbed. When candida grows out of control, it can damage the mucus layer that protects your gut cell wall, which allows candida and other bugs to permeate the gut lining and get into the bloodstream, where they can invade other tissues and cause everything from skin issues and vaginal infections to brain fog, mood swings, and autoimmune disease if left untreated. A candida overgrowth can also worsen existing digestive diseases.

» TREATMENT

Your healthcare provider will likely recommend an antifungal medication to treat the overgrowth of yeast. You can also eliminate foods candida loves to feed on, which include anything with yeast and foods high in sugar or refined carbohydrates.

Let's Talk About Poop—and Why You Should Look at Yours

Your stool (aka poop) can provide valuable insights into your gut health. Stool tests—yes, when you scoop a tiny sample of your poop and send it to a lab to be analyzed—can test for things like infection, inflammation, and even colon cancer.

Your healthcare practitioner may recommend a stool test along with other diagnostic tools—things like your personal and family medical history and a physical exam—to diagnose gastrointestinal issues. However, there's also a lot you can tell about how well (or not) your GI tract is working by really looking at your stool, says gastroenterologist Rabia de Latour, MD.

"Being able to talk about your poop if your gut health feels off can give your healthcare practitioners helpful insight that can lead to a quicker diagnosis and treatment for your symptoms," says Dr. de Latour.

Because so many of us find it tough—and maybe a little mortifying—to describe our poop, healthcare professionals use the Bristol Stool Chart, which is essentially a scale to show the different kinds of bowel movements.

Types 1 and 2 may point to constipation.

Types 3 and 4 are considered "normal" or "healthy" stools that are ideal.

Types 5 and 6 are considered loose stools, with type 5 considered borderline diarrhea and type 6 considered diarrhea—even though they're not liquid.

Type 7 describes very loose stools or fully liquid diarrhea, which is most often caused by infection (if it's an acute issue), though chronic loose stools are typically not due to infections.

As for how often you should be pooping, there's a wide range of what's considered normal. If you're pooping at least three times a week (fewer than three bowel movements a week is defined as constipation) and you're not having pain or any other symptoms, that's okay. What's most important is any sudden changes in your usual bowel movement habits. For example, going from pooping once a day to pooping just three times a week—or vice versa—is something to bring up with your clinician for evaluation.

TYPE 1
Separate hard lumps, like nuts (hard to pass)

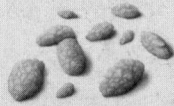

TYPE 2
Sausage-shaped but lumpy

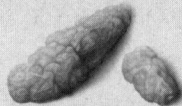

TYPE 3
Like a sausage but with cracks on its surface

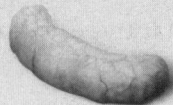

TYPE 4
Like a sausage or snake, smooth and soft

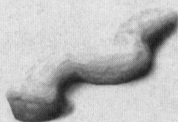

TYPE 5
Soft blobs with clear-cut edges

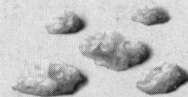

TYPE 6
Fluffy pieces with ragged edges, a mushy stool

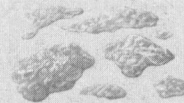

TYPE 7
Watery, no solid pieces, entirely liquid

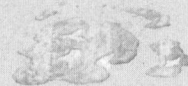

Colon Cancer Is on the Rise—and Symptoms Are More Often Dismissed in Women

You've likely heard the alarming statistics: Colorectal cancer (a term used to describe both colon and rectal cancer, and often used interchangeably with *colon cancer*) is the third most common cancer diagnosed in both women and men around the world.[8] And while cases have declined over time, people under fifty-five make up about 20 percent of all colorectal cancer cases—a significant jump from 11 percent in the mid-1990s.[9] Diagnoses in people under age fifty-five also tend to be more advanced than colorectal cancers detected in older people, which could help explain why this type of cancer is the leading cancer-related death in men under fifty and the second leading cancer-related death, just behind breast cancer, in women under fifty.[10]

The facts are admittedly scary. Yet what's even scarier is that experts have yet to pinpoint *why* more of us are being diagnosed with this disease at younger ages (eating more ultra-processed foods? living more sedentary lives? obesity?), and there's a growing conversation around the fact that women may be more likely than men to be dismissed by their doctors when they report colon cancer symptoms.

For example, a common symptom of colorectal cancer is rectal bleeding, which is often presumed to be hemorrhoids (little clusters of vascular tissue, smooth muscle, and connective tissue that form along the anal canal). Other signs of colorectal cancer, such as abdominal pain, unexplained weight loss, and blood in the stool, may also be brushed off as nothing to be alarmed about when instead they should prompt healthcare practitioners to do further testing. One Colorectal Cancer Alliance survey found that 75 percent of young colorectal cancer patients and survivors saw at least two physicians before getting a correct diagnosis—and 40 percent said their symptoms and concerns were dismissed by their healthcare providers.[11]

What's more, colon cancer can develop without clear early warning signs, which is why routine screening is essential for early detection. That's when precancerous or cancerous growths are highly treatable. (More on screening options next.) However, there are a few symptoms that should raise a red flag and prompt you to get in touch with your healthcare provider.

- **Unexplained change in bowel movements**, such as diarrhea, constipation, or a feeling of incomplete bowel movements. Narrow, pencil-thin stools can also be a sign of colon cancer.

- **Blood in your poop**, which can be bright red or much darker than what you consider blood's "normal" hue.

- **Unintentional weight loss**, especially if it's significant.

- **Persistent and unexplained fatigue, weakness, and anemia**, likely due to iron deficiency.

- **A mass or lump** in your abdomen.

- **Abdominal pain**, such as cramps or even just a feeling of discomfort that won't go away. This is especially concerning if it comes along with one or more of the other symptoms listed here.

It's important to say here that if you're experiencing one or more of the above symptoms, try not to freak out. Yes, these can be signs of colon cancer. But they may also be symptoms of a benign GI condition. Call your healthcare provider, talk about your symptoms, and ask specifically about getting screened for colon cancer if your doctor doesn't bring it up.

Colon Cancer Screening

» WHEN TO START

While the guidelines for who needs a screening and when vary depending on your age and family and personal medical history, the current guidelines for average-risk adults are to get colonoscopies starting at age forty-five.[12] If your screening colonoscopy shows no signs of cancer or precancer, your healthcare provider will likely recommend you get another colonoscopy in ten years. If you had polyps removed, you may need your next colonoscopy in one to seven years. And if you are considered at high risk for colon cancer due to family or personal history—for example, you may be at increased risk due to an autoimmune disease, such as ulcerative colitis—you may need screening starting at a younger age (usually forty, as the risk of colon cancer before this age is still low), and at more frequent intervals than every ten years.

» YOUR SCREENING OPTIONS

The most comprehensive screening test for colon cancer and the one considered the "gold standard" is a colonoscopy, where a gastroenterologist uses a long, flexible tube with a light and a camera at the end of it to examine your rectum and colon. This is an outpatient procedure that involves some preparation (typically involving following specific dietary restrictions and taking laxatives to empty your colon fully in order for your doctor to see your colon lining), anesthesia (to help you relax and prevent discomfort), and possibly one or more biopsies during the colonoscopy if your healthcare provider finds polyps or tumors.

Another option is a fecal immunochemical test (FIT), which involves collecting your own poop (usually at home) and sending it to a lab, where it's tested for signs of blood, which can be a sign of precancerous polyps or colorectal cancer. There's also a stool DNA test (marketed as Cologuard in the U.S.), which looks for both signs of blood and signs of cancer DNA. If either test is positive, which suggests there could be a risk of cancer, you'll likely be told to schedule a colonoscopy. While these stool tests can detect colon cancer, they are more likely to miss polyps, which can be removed during a colonoscopy so they don't grow and possibly develop into cancer over time.

What's a Polyp?

Polyps are growths on the lining of the gastrointestinal tract that can vary in size, shape, and type. While polyps are common and many are harmless, some types have the potential to develop into colon cancer over time. (Thankfully, it takes about ten years for a colorectal polyp to change from benign to cancerous.)

Colonoscopy is the best way to check your colon for polyps, as it allows your clinician to see the entire colon lining and remove any polyps they find. (The same endoscope your clinician uses to look at the lining of your colon during a colonoscopy has a wire snare attached to it, which gets looped around a polyp to detach it from your colon's lining so it can go to the lab for testing.)

Removing polyps during a colonoscopy is common and an important cancer-prevention measure, as early detection and removal of precancerous polyps can significantly reduce your risk of developing colon cancer.

Your Game Plan:
How to Optimize Your Gut Health

Once you know the many ways your gut health impacts so many other aspects of your overall health, you'll likely want to take steps to improve yours. Here, Dr. Rabia de Latour shares her top tips for keeping your GI tract happy and healthy.

Get specific when you're talking to your healthcare practitioners about your "gut health." *Gut health* is a vague term that could mean any number of things, which is why going into the "gory" details about your poop, farting, burping, and more—symptoms many women, in particular, have been taught to be ashamed of—is exactly what's going to help your provider suss out what's going on. For example, rather than saying something like "I think my gut health is off," be specific about what is happening to make you think you've got gut issues, such as "I've had diarrhea for the last two weeks, my farts are stinkier than ever, and I feel bloated and crampy when I wake up in the morning."

Look at your poop before you flush. "You have a free diagnostic tool that you create yourself—hopefully every day—that tells you so much about what's going on in your body," says Dr. de Latour. "Yet if you're like most people, you're flushing it down the toilet before looking at it, and you're missing out on a lot of information about your health as a result."

That's right: Your poop can give you clues about so many things, like how hydrated you are, whether you're getting enough fiber in your diet, and even if something is amiss in your colon (for example, super-thin stools prompt doctors to wonder if there's a growth in the colon that's changing the shape of the stool, which requires screening to find out what's going on). So start clueing in to the color, consistency, shape, and even smell of your poop. Take notes and talk to your doctor about what you see. (Flip back to pages 425–426 for a chart to help you know what to look for and get specific in your descriptions.) This is a great thing to bring up at your annual physical and is especially important to track and talk to your provider about if you're experiencing any GI-related symptoms.

Talk about your poop with your friends and kids. In addition to paying attention to your own stools, it's a great idea to start talking more freely about poop when the timing feels right. There's a lot of social anxiety around pooping in public, and it's causing many of us—especially women and young girls—to avoid pooping when we need to. The result? Constipation and other gut-health issues that can persist for *years*. Together, we can collectively try to normalize pooping and how it's a sign of health to poop regularly, and the best way to start is by making it less taboo to talk about. While you're at it, let's normalize farting, too, which the average human does upward of twenty times a day.

Drink more water and eat more fiber. By and large, many of our gut-health issues can be improved if we're well hydrated and eat a wide variety of fiber-rich fruits and vegetables. Just as your stool can tell you a lot about your health, your urine can, too. Take note of your urine output (how much you're urinating) as well as its color (is it clear, light yellow, or dark yellow?): If you're not peeing much and it's darker in color, increase your water consumption, which helps to both soften stool and add bulk to it, making it easier to pass through your intestines and reducing the risk of constipation.

As for fiber—which promotes regular bowel movements, supports a healthy and diverse gut microbiome, and is linked to a lower risk of colorectal cancer, among many other benefits—aim for at least twenty-five grams of total dietary fiber per day and thirty different plant foods (think fruits, veggies, grains, legumes, nuts, and seeds) each week, a diet plan that's linked to better bowel movements and a significantly more diverse microbiome. On average, American adults eat ten to fifteen grams of total fiber a day and ten or fewer different plant foods each week—so most of us have some room for improvement. Do you experience GI pain, bloating, and gas when you eat more plant-based foods? Increase your fiber intake gradually, and drink plenty of water throughout the day as you do, which can help keep those GI symptoms at bay as your body adjusts to the additional fiber.

Keep stress in check and prioritize exercise and sleep. You already know certain "healthy lifestyle habits" are good for your overall health, but it turns out they're especially helpful when it comes to good gut health. Mindfulness-based practices proven to help you feel less frazzled—things like breathing exercises, meditation, yoga, or whatever works to help you calm down—put you in a parasympathetic state, otherwise known as your rest and digest mode, which is key for optimal digestion. Too much time spent in the opposite ("fight or flight") state can influence the gut in negative ways. Gut motility can be altered (which can lead to symptoms like diarrhea or constipation); stomach acid can increase (which can cause heartburn); and the permeability of the gut lining can increase. Even the composition and diversity of your gut microbiome can be impacted.

Not only does exercise help from a stress perspective (it's a proven way to reduce stress hormones and boost feel-good endorphins, which helps us relax), but the sheer act of moving your body stimulates the muscles in the GI tract, which can help promote regular bowel movements.

Getting the recommended seven to nine hours of sleep a night also plays a significant role in improving gut motility, appetite regulation, and the composition of your gut microbiome. Sleep can also help you better manage stress, which in turn helps gut health and any GI symptoms you may be dealing with.

· · · · ·

With your newfound understanding of gut health, you'll feel armed with the information you need to keep your gastrointestinal tract working well, make sure the ecosystem of bugs that live in your intestines (your gut microbiome) stays happy, and take the science-backed steps proven to move the needle the most when it comes to optimizing your gut health.

Chapter 16

Skin Health

What You Need to Know to Take Care of Your Largest Organ

> *Skin is a strange little miracle.*
>
> —Brooke Jarvis, "Rethinking the Science of Skin" in *The New Yorker*

When you think about your skin, there's a good chance the first thing that comes to mind is how it looks. That's understandable, considering that skin is one of the first things others notice about us—and having clear, glowing skin is baked into the beauty standards that women, in particular, are held to.

However, what so many of us forget in our quest for a "perfect" complexion is the fact that skin is the body's largest organ and one of its main functions is *protection*. Your skin needs to keep out potentially harmful invaders like bacteria and chemicals while letting in enough moisture to keep you hydrated. The superhighway of tiny blood vessels in your skin regulates your body temperature. Sensory receptors in each layer of your skin send messages to your brain, which allows you to sense and respond to the environment around you. Skin even produces a pigment called melanin that forms a protective cap over your skin cells' DNA—kind of like tiny little umbrellas shielding that DNA from damaging ultraviolet light.

What we see on our skin as blemishes can be outward signs of something happening under the skin's surface, which is why it's helpful to understand the basics of what skin is and why different skin conditions can surface.

In this chapter, we'll learn . . .

- **The basic anatomy of your skin**, including what it's made of, how it changes over time, and the mix of bugs that make up your skin microbiome.

- **Some of the most common skin conditions**, including the symptoms, treatments, and underlying causes of each.

- **How sunscreen works**, why it's your best protection against skin cancer and the signs of aging, and how to choose from the different types you'll find on store shelves.

- **What you need to know about skin cancer.** We'll cover how it develops, the different types (and what each type typically looks like), and the skin cancer screening guidelines you should know.

- **Some of the most common cosmetic procedures that can improve the appearance of your skin**, including injectables, laser skin resurfacing, and microneedling.

- **The specific steps you can take to keep your skin healthy and looking great**, including the healthy skin habits top dermatologists follow—and the stuff they steer clear of.

Meet the Experts

Diane S. Berson, MD, associate professor in the department of dermatology at Weill Cornell Medical College of Cornell University

Tamia Harris-Tryon, MD, PhD, associate professor in the department of dermatology at UT Southwestern Medical Center

Ellen Gendler, MD, clinical associate professor of dermatology at Ronald O. Perelman Department of Dermatology at NYU Grossman School of Medicine

Elizabeth Tanzi, MD, associate clinical professor of dermatology at The George Washington University School of Medicine and Health Sciences

Jody A. Levine, MD, director of dermatology at Plastic Surgery & Dermatology of NYC

What Is Skin, Anyway? What You Need to Know About Your Body's Largest Organ and How It Works

We use words like *glowing* to describe our ideal complexion. Yet even though how our skin looks and feels is important, there's so much more to skin health than appearance. Here, Diane S. Berson, MD, shares what we need to know.

Your Skin Is Your Body's Largest Organ

That's right, it's an organ just like your brain or your liver, and plays a critical role in keeping you alive and well, thanks to its ability to perform a number of essential functions, some of which include:

- **Protection:** Your skin is a physical barrier against injury, pathogens, and other harmful substances. It also protects you against ultraviolet (UV) radiation from the sun by producing melanin.

- **Regulation:** Your skin regulates your body temperature by producing sweat as well as dilating blood vessels (a widening that increases the speed of blood flowing to and within the skin and allows more heat to be lost, lowering body temp) and constricting them (a narrowing that helps you conserve heat).

- **Immunity:** There are special cells in the top layer of your skin (the epidermis) called Langerhans cells that detect and fight pathogens. Think of them as your body's first line of defense against infections from the outside world.

- **Sensation:** Your skin contains millions of nerve endings that detect things like touch, pressure, pain, and temperature, providing you with sensory feedback from the environment.

- **Absorption and excretion:** Your skin is able to absorb certain substances, such as medications and toxins, and get rid of some waste products via sweat.

- **Synthesis of vitamin D:** When your skin is exposed to UV radiation from the sun, it makes vitamin D, a hormone that's essential for bone health and immune system function as well as nerve connections to the brain, healthy blood vessels, and more.

Your Skin Has Three Main Layers

» THE EPIDERMIS

This is the outermost (and thinnest) layer of your skin, and what you can see and feel. It's primarily made up of cells called keratinocytes, which produce a protein (keratin) that makes your skin strong. Those keratinocytes have estrogen receptors on them, which helps explain why when estrogen drops in menopause, your epidermis gets thinner, your skin gets dry and itchy, and your skin barrier weakens. The epidermis is also where you'll see tiny openings in your skin (called pores) that are essentially the tops of hair follicles, which release sebum (a waxy, oily substance that the body's sebaceous glands produce to protect and moisturize the skin).

» THE DERMIS

Lying just beneath your epidermis, this is your thickest layer of skin and is made up of connective tissue, blood vessels, nerves, and hair follicles, as well as sweat glands and sebaceous glands. The cells in this layer of skin are called fibroblasts, and they're responsible for making collagen and elastin, which maintain your skin's connective tissue. They also help skin regenerate when it's been injured. The fibroblasts have estrogen receptors on them as well. As you lose estrogen after menopause, the receptors in your fibroblasts fade away. This is why postmenopausal skin isn't as plump and elastic as it was when you were younger: The less estrogen you have, the less productive your fibroblasts—and the less collagen and elastin your skin makes.

» HYPODERMIS (AKA SUBCUTANEOUS TISSUE)

This is the deepest layer of your skin and is made up mostly of fat (adipose tissue). It also contains some collagen, blood vessels, and nerves. This layer helps insulate your body, absorbs shocks, and anchors your skin to its underlying structures (like your muscles and bones).

Meet the Microbiome on Your Skin

Just as there are communities of microorganisms in your gut that you likely think of when you hear the word *microbiome*, your skin is teeming with millions of microscopic bugs.

You have microbes that produce peptides and ceramides, which help keep skin supple and moisturized. (And yes, this is one reason you see skin care products with peptides and ceramides in the ingredients list.) The microbes on your skin also play a key role in teaching your immune system what's okay—and what's a potentially harmful pathogen it needs to respond to.

Think of your skin like soil and your skin's microbes as plants, says Tamia Harris-Tryon, MD, PhD, who studies the skin microbiome: Just as you want the dirt you plant a garden in to have all kinds of nutrients to help the right plants grow, you want the right set of nutrients in your skin to encourage microbes at the skin surface that perform various jobs to keep your skin healthy. Do things that mess with your skin barrier and you're essentially altering the terrain on which these microbes grow and thrive. The result can be an overgrowth of "bad" bacteria and a vast reduction in "good" bacteria, and your skin may become more sensitive and prone to acne, irritation, inflammation, and hyperpigmentation.

While research is ongoing to understand what prompts changes in the skin microbiome, some of the biggest offenders seem to be environmental factors (especially exposure to UV radiation and pollution), irritants (including excess detergents in skin care products), and a poor diet, says Dr. Harris-Tryon.

Common Skin Conditions in Women: Symptoms, Treatments, and What We Know About the Underlying Causes of Each

In a world where beauty standards remain unforgiving, women often feel pressure to have flawless skin—something that can feel unattainable when you're dealing with an unpredictable flare-up of acne or rosacea. Here are some of the most common skin conditions women face and some of the treatment options for each.

Acne

This is the most common skin condition in the U.S., affecting approximately fifty million of us every year.[1] It happens when your skin's hair follicles get clogged by sebum (aka oil), bacteria, or dead skin cells. The result? Pus-filled bumps (pimples), small red bumps (papules), blackheads, whiteheads, and/or painful, large lumps (nodules) or pus-filled lumps (cysts) under your skin. Changing hormones, which can increase your skin's sebum production, are a common culprit.

» TREATMENT

There are three main strategies when it comes to treating acne:

- **Topical treatments**, such as over-the-counter (OTC) medications with benzoyl peroxide, salicylic acid, and sulfur, as well as prescription options like topical retinoids, antibiotics, and azelaic acid.

- **Oral medications,** including a blood pressure drug (spironolactone), oral contraceptives, and oral retinoid. Antibiotics have also been a longtime treatment, but in recent years there's been a push to avoid using them, in an attempt to combat drug resistance.

- **Dermatologic procedures,** such as light therapy, chemical peels, or drainage and extraction of large cysts.

Dermatitis

This is a broad term that refers to conditions that cause inflammation (-itis) of the skin, usually seen as redness, rash, swelling, itching, blisters, cracking (or scaly) skin, and pain. There's atopic dermatitis (eczema), contact dermatitis (which is caused by direct contact with an irritant or allergen), seborrheic dermatitis (dandruff or cradle cap), and many more types.

» TREATMENT

There are a number of treatment options, and which one you choose depends on the type of dermatitis you have and where it is on your body. There are topical treatments (such as corticosteroids to reduce inflammation and itching and moisturizers to keep skin hydrated and prevent irritation and dryness), oral medications (like antihistamines or, in severe cases, systemic corticosteroids), and phototherapy (controlled exposure to UV light, which can help reduce some types of dermatitis). It can also be helpful to switch up your skin care routine if you're dealing with dermatitis: Use mild, fragrance-free personal care products and bathe and wash your face in lukewarm water instead of hot to avoid further irritating your skin.

Hives (aka Urticaria)

These raised, itchy welts can show up anywhere on your skin and vary in size. Acute hives (ones that last six weeks or less) are typically caused by an allergic reaction: Immune cells in your skin called mast cells respond to allergens by releasing histamine, which causes the swelling under your skin that you see as hives. Chronic hives last for longer periods of time and can be caused by viral or bacterial infections or another chronic health condition, such as lupus, which activates those mast cells in your skin. Women are about twice as likely as men to experience chronic hives,[2] and our hormones may be to blame: Mast cells have estrogen and progesterone receptors on them, and fluctuations in these hormones around the menstrual cycle can trigger hives.

» TREATMENT

OTC or prescription antihistamines are a common first line of treatment for hives because they help relieve the itching and swelling. For severe or chronic cases, prescription corticosteroids or immune modulators may be prescribed. Regardless of which treatment option you land on, it's essential to identify and avoid known triggers. Sometimes this will be easy: Let's say you take a new medication and break out in hives a few hours later; you can be pretty confident in the connection and then avoid that drug in the future. Oftentimes, figuring out what's causing your hives—especially if they're chronic—will be trickier. Keep notes on what foods you eat and any medications you take, as well as your menstrual cycle and stress levels. This can help you pinpoint what's causing your hives and help inform your next steps.

Shingles (aka Herpes Zoster)

This incredibly painful skin condition is actually a reactivation of the varicella zoster virus, which is the one that causes chicken pox. About one in three people in the U.S. will develop shingles in their lifetime, and women are slightly more at risk of getting it than men, though the reason is unclear. Your risk also increases as you age, or if you have a weakened immune system.[3]

If you ever had chicken pox (likely as a kid), you were probably told it was a one-and-done illness. And while that's usually true, the virus never leaves your body. It becomes dormant (or inactive) and hangs out in a part of your spinal nerve root. When the chicken pox virus reactivates, it usually travels along a single nerve pathway in your skin and can cause the distinctive, painful shingles rash, which is often on just one side of the body and commonly appears on the chest, belly, back, or face.

One of the most important things you can do to prevent shingles is to get vaccinated, which can boost your immune system's ability to combat the varicella zoster virus if it's reactivated in your body.

» TREATMENT

If you suspect a shingles rash, it's important to seek help right away and get treatment—not only to help with pain management but also to prevent serious complications, including vision problems (which can happen if your rash spreads to one or both eyes) or postherpetic neuralgia (PNH), which can prompt pain that persists in the affected area even after the rash has healed. Treatment options include:

- Antiviral medications, which help stop the replication of the reactivated chicken-pox virus and are most effective at reducing the severity and duration of shingles when started within seventy-two hours of the appearance of a rash

- Pain relievers, ranging from OTC to prescription options depending on the severity of pain

- Anticonvulsants, such as gabapentin (Neurontin) and pregabalin (Lyrica), as well as certain antidepressants may be used to manage nerve pain

It's also crucial to keep shingles rashes clean and dry, which will help avoid secondary bacterial infections. To prevent infection and scarring, avoid scratching your skin and apply cool, wet compresses to soothe skin as needed. Making sure you rest and keep stress in check (admittedly tough to do when you have a painful rash taking over parts of your body) is also important.

Melasma

This common skin condition causes flat, dark, discolored patches, primarily on the face—particularly on the cheeks, nose, forehead, and chin and above the upper lip. One of the reasons melasma is more prevalent in women than in men is its association with hormonal changes: Elevated levels of estrogen and progesterone are thought to stimulate the production of melanin, which in turn can lead to hyperpigmentation when skin is exposed to UV rays and visible light.

This is why melasma is so common during pregnancy (up to 50 percent of pregnant women will get it, leading to its becoming known as the mask of pregnancy[4]), particularly in the third trimester, which is when estrogen and progesterone are very high. Women taking oral contraceptives or menopause hormone therapy are also more susceptible to melasma.

The most important step you can take to prevent melasma and to keep it from getting worse is to protect your skin with a tinted mineral sunscreen or makeup product that includes iron oxides. (For more on what to look for in sunscreen, skip ahead to page 447.)

» TREATMENT

Topical medications can help prevent new pigment formations by inhibiting the production of melanin or increasing cell turnover (to target the symptoms of melasma). Oral tranexamic acid (OTA) has also been shown to inhibit the production of melanin in the skin. There are also a handful of procedures your dermatologist can do, including a chemical peel (which exfoliates the top layers of your skin to reduce pigmentation) and certain laser and light therapies (which work by breaking down pigment in the skin). However, keep in mind that many of these procedures aren't safe during pregnancy, so it's important to talk through treatment options with a highly trained clinician, such as a dermatologist, physician's assistant, or nurse practitioner who specializes in skin health.

Rosacea

This chronic condition most often affects the face, causing redness (including visible blood vessels under the skin's surface) and acne-like bumps on the cheeks, nose, forehead, and chin that typically flare up and then retreat. While the exact cause of it isn't well understood, and experts don't know why rosacea is more common in women than in men, it likely involves a combination of genetics (it runs in families and most often affects those with fair skin) and certain triggers (including sun exposure, extreme temperatures, stress, spicy foods, alcohol, and irritating skin care products).

» TREATMENT

As with many skin conditions, there are multiple treatment options for rosacea, including topical and oral medications as well as laser and light therapies—all of which work to reduce redness and inflammation. Using skin care products with gentle, nonirritating ingredients and avoiding known triggers can also help keep rosacea symptoms in check.

Psoriasis

This is a chronic autoimmune condition that primarily affects the skin and typically presents as areas of thick, discolored, dry skin that are often covered with scaly-looking "plaques." They're commonly found on the elbows, knees, face (including inside the mouth), scalp, fingernails and toenails, palms and feet, lower back, and/or genitals. Some research shows that psoriasis may impact slightly more women than men, and the mental health toll may be greater for us: Women are more likely to experience stress, worry, and shame as a result of psoriasis.[5] And while a lot more research is needed to more clearly understand what causes it, genetics, immune system dysfunction, and certain triggers (such as viral or bacterial infections, skin injuries, stress, smoking, heavy alcohol use, and certain medications) are thought to be risk factors.

» TREATMENT

Both topical and oral medications are often used as a first line of treatment to reduce inflammation and slow skin cell turnover, which can ease symptoms. A new class of medications called biologics target specific parts of the immune system and are used in more severe cases of psoriasis. And lifestyle changes—such as avoiding known triggers and managing stress (which can trigger or worsen symptoms)—may be helpful as well.

Stretch Marks (aka Striae)

These discolored, sunken, scar-like lines in your skin happen when the skin is stretched or shrinks quickly. When this happens, the collagen and elastin fibers in the middle layer of your skin can break, which is what causes these lines. While most of us associate stretch marks with pregnancy (up to 90 percent of all people who are pregnant develop them[6]), they can also happen during puberty as well as during other times of body changes, whether you're building muscle or gaining or losing weight.

» TREATMENT

With time, stretch marks can fade. Yet for stubborn lines that persist, there are a few options that may improve the appearance of stretch marks, including:

- **Topical retinoids**, which promote collagen production. However, these are not recommended during pregnancy.

- **Laser treatments**, which can help stimulate collagen production and reduce the redness of new stretch marks.

- **Microneedling**, which uses tiny needles to create tiny injuries in the skin, which in turn stimulates the production of collagen and elastin.

- **Moisturizers** containing hyaluronic acid and shea butter, which help keep skin hydrated and may improve its texture.

Cellulite

That dimpled, lumpy, cottage cheese–like skin commonly found on the thighs, hips, butt, and belly is the result of little deposits of fat that push through the connective tissue under the skin and create an uneven surface. And while cellulite happens to all of us, it's much more common in women and occurs in 80 to 90 percent of females.[7] This may be due to our higher levels of estrogen, which influences fat distribution and encourages the storage of fat in our hips, thighs, and butt—all areas where cellulite is most common.

» TREATMENT

The unsatisfying truth is that there are very few treatments that successfully reduce the appearance of cellulite. The FDA has approved a handful of treatments for cellulite, including a minimally invasive laser treatment (called Cellulaze) and other procedures that involve breaking up the tough bands beneath the skin that cause us to see cellulite. Topical treatments (such as retinol creams) and lifestyle changes (such as regular exercise) may also help. However, it's important to remember that none of the currently available treatments are permanent—which means that finding some acceptance for this often inevitable aspect of our changing bodies is also key, no matter what cellulite-reduction tactics we try.

Sunscreen 101: How It Protects You, What Ingredients to Look for, and More

To understand sunscreen and how it works, it helps to have a basic understanding of what happens when ultraviolet (UV) light from the sun hits our skin.

There are two main types of UV radiation:

- **UVB radiation** (aka the sunburning rays) causes sunburn and directly damages the DNA in your skin cells, which can eventually contribute to skin cancer.

- **UVA radiation** (aka the tanning rays) penetrates deep into your skin and can contribute to both skin cancer and photoaging, such as wrinkles and age spots.

When UVB rays hit our skin, they interact with a protein in the skin called 7-DHC, which is then converted into vitamin D_3—the active form of vitamin D that helps our health in so many ways. But here's the catch: Those UVB rays also damage your DNA. This damage can trigger an inflammatory response in the skin: Cytokines and prostaglandins are released, which leads to the classic symptoms of sunburn (redness, swelling, pain) and an increase in blood flow to the affected area.

That DNA damage can also prompt cells to start mutating when they replicate, which can disrupt normal cell function and can lead to the development of cancerous cells over time. Repeated UVB exposure and multiple sunburns increase your risk of developing skin cancer due to repeated damage done to the DNA in your skin.

UVA rays penetrate even deeper into your skin than UVB rays and stimulate your melanocytes—the cells responsible for producing melanin. Yes, this is what gives certain skin tones a "tan," but it's also responsible for uneven skin pigmentation and age spots (aka hyperpigmentation)—both of which are hallmarks of "photoaging" as we get older. When UVA rays penetrate deep into your dermis, they also produce free radicals that damage your collagen and elastin fibers. Over time, this breakdown results in wrinkles, fine lines, sagging, age spots, and uneven skin tone.

Slathering on the broad-spectrum sunscreen is one of the best ways to protect your skin against both UVA and UVB rays. Here, dermatologist Ellen Gendler, MD, explains how, exactly, sunscreen works and what you need to know to make sure the sunscreen you use is keeping you optimally protected.

How Sunscreen Works

There are two types of sunscreens, and they work similarly to protect your skin:

- **Chemical sunscreens** work by absorbing both UVA and UVB rays and converting them into heat, which is then released from the skin. This process prevents the UV radiation from penetrating your skin and causing damage. In the U.S., the only chemical sunscreen ingredient currently approved by the FDA that shields well against UVA rays is butyl methoxy dibenzoylmethane (aka avobenzone), says Dr. Gendler.

- **Mineral sunscreens** (aka physical sunscreens) also work by absorbing some UV light and reflecting UV light. They contain ingredients like zinc oxide and titanium dioxide, which protect against UVB rays and, to a lesser extent, UVA rays. Many tinted mineral sunscreens and makeup products contain an ingredient called iron oxides, which help protect against visible light (which is light you can see, such as from the sun and computer screens, and plays a role in the development of melasma).

In recent years, there's been a lot of talk about mineral sunscreens being "safer" because of a pervasive myth that they're not absorbed by the skin but rather sit on its surface and act as a physical barrier—like a "block." However, it's a myth that mineral sunscreens act as a physical barrier to sunlight, says Dr. Gendler.

"The truth is mineral sunscreens work by absorbing light and reflecting some light in the same way that chemical sunscreens do," says Dr. Gendler. "One is not safer than the other."

The bottom line: The best sunscreen is the one you'll use consistently, and any sunscreen is better than not using sunscreen.

What to Look for in a Sunscreen

The Skin Cancer Foundation recommends everyone use a broad-spectrum SPF 15 sunscreen or higher every day, and SPF 30 or higher if you'll be spending time outside.[8] Apply sunscreen to all exposed areas of your skin about twenty minutes before heading into the sun, and reapply every couple hours (or immediately after sweating or swimming, as moisture and/or toweling off can remove the protective SPF layer on your skin). And yes, you need to wear sunscreen even when it's cloudy, as UV rays still reach the Earth's surface (and our skin) on overcast days.

If you're looking to maximize your sun protection, Dr. Gendler recommends buying chemical sunscreen in Europe, Asia, Mexico, or South America, where products often contain ingredients that protect against a broader range of UVA rays than the ingredients in products sold in the U.S.

"If you use a broad-spectrum sunscreen made in the U.S., you can protect yourself from sunburn, but you will likely tan," says Dr. Gendler. "This is because the UVA protection in U.S. sunscreens is more limited, and UVA is the light that leads to tanning. UVA also penetrates the skin deeper than UVB and is believed to contribute in large measure to the development of skin cancers and precancers, as well as pigmented spots that are typical in aging skin."

Look for products that contain the following ingredients, says Dr. Gendler. These are UV-absorbing filters that are not yet approved by the FDA but are available in some other countries:

- Ecamsule (Mexoryl SX)
- Drometrizole trisiloxane (Mexoryl XL)
- Methoxypropylamino cyclohexenylidene ethoxyethylcyanoacetate (MCE or Mexoryl 400)
- Bemotrizinol (Tinosorb S), which appears on ingredient lists as bis-ethylhexyloxyphenol methoxyphenyl triazine
- Bisoctrizole (Tinosorb M or methylene bis-benzotriazolyl tetramethylbutylphenol)
- Diethylamino hydroxybenzoyl hexyl benzoate (Uvinul A Plus)
- Phenylene bis-dephenyltriazine (TriAsorB)
- Bis-(diethyaminohydroxybenzoyl benzoyl) piperazine (BDBP)

Ask an Expert

I keep hearing about the numerous benefits of vitamin D, and how using sunscreen prevents the production of this important hormone. Should I expose my skin to the sun, even just for a few minutes, before putting on my sunscreen?

It's true that vitamin D is very important for overall health. However, the first thing to know is that sun exposure doesn't always guarantee your body will make enough vitamin D. I've seen patients who live in warm climates and are in the sun all the time who are low in vitamin D. Plus, even if you use sunscreen, you're likely still getting enough sun exposure that will impact your body's production of vitamin D. For example, it's possible (and common) to get tan despite slathering on sunscreen when exposed to the sun on a regular basis. That's because sunscreen doesn't block 100 percent of UV rays.

If your vitamin D level is low, there are plenty of safe options outside of UV exposure, including eating certain foods (fatty fish like salmon and tuna are great sources, and foods like milk, yogurt, and breakfast cereals are often fortified with D) and supplementing (the Skin Cancer Foundation recommends the average person between ages one and seventy get 600 international units, or IU, a day).

If you still want to go out in the sun for vitamin D production, here's my advice: Do it first thing in the morning or later in the afternoon, which are times when you're at a lower risk of burning your skin. And never expose your face, neck, or chest to the sun unprotected, as these are areas that are already getting enough sun exposure over the course of your lifetime. Minimizing sun exposure is the most important step to reduce your risk of skin cancer while helping to slow down the signs of skin aging.

—Elizabeth Tanzi, MD, associate clinical professor of dermatology at The George Washington University Medical Center

Skin Health

Skin Cancer: What You Need to Know to Prevent It, Spot It, and Get It Treated

Skin cancer is the most common form of cancer in the U.S., and one in five of us will develop it in our lifetime.[9] Yet here's the good news: It remains one of the most preventable types of cancer and is also highly treatable, especially if detected early. Here, dermatologist and skin cancer survivor Elizabeth Tanzi, MD, fills us in on what we need to know.

First, How Does Skin Cancer Develop?

Most cases of skin cancer are the result of overexposure to UV radiation from the sun or tanning beds, which can lead to mutations in genes that regulate cell growth and division—ultimately causing skin cells to grow uncontrolled. Once cancerous cells have formed, they can develop mechanisms to evade detection and destruction by the immune system, which allows the mutated cells to proliferate and form a mass (aka tumor).

All of us have protective mechanisms within our skin that repair the DNA mutations caused by exposure to UV rays. Dr. Tanzi likens it to a game of whack-a-mole: When we're young, our skin defenses are robust and quick to stamp out damaged skin cells before they can turn into skin cancer. The lower layer of skin sends growth factors to the upper layers and essentially says, "Hey, turn on the processes to find and remove damaged cells!" Yet as we age, the lower layer of skin gets tired and slows down its production of those growth factors. The result: Our skin loses some of its protective mechanisms and skin cancer is more likely to develop.

Your skin type also plays a big role in your risk of developing skin cancer: The lighter your skin, hair, and eyes, the higher your risk of developing skin cancer. That's because you make less melanin, which protects against UV radiation. Other risk factors include immune health (if you're immunosuppressed due to certain medications you're taking or if you've received an organ transplant, your immune system's surveillance isn't as robust and may miss developing cancer cells) and genetics (a family history of skin cancer can increase your risk).

Types of Skin Cancer, What They Look Like, and How to Treat Each

There are three main types of skin cancer. Here's what to know about how each forms, what each typically looks like, and how dermatologists treat each one.

TYPE OF SKIN CANCER	WHAT IT IS	WHAT IT TYPICALLY LOOKS LIKE	TREATMENT
Basal cell carcinoma (BCC)	The most common type of skin cancer, which develops in the basal cells located in the outermost layer of your skin (epidermis).	A round pimple with blood vessels surrounding it; a scar that slowly expands; a pearly or waxy bump that may bleed; an open sore that doesn't heal or that heals and then comes back.	Surgical excision where the tumor and a margin of surrounding tissue are removed; Mohs surgery (a layer-by-layer removal of the cancerous tissue where each layer is examined to ensure no cancer cells remain).
Squamous cell carcinoma (SCC)	The second-most-common type of skin cancer, which develops in the squamous cells in the epidermis.	A red, scaly, or crusty patch of skin or a sore that may bleed; a raised growth that has a lower area in the center; a wartlike growth; an open sore that doesn't heal or that heals and then comes back.	Like BCC, SCC is typically removed via surgical excision or Mohs surgery. Cryosurgery (freezing the cancer cells), photodynamic therapy (where light-sensitive agents and blue light are used), and even some topical medications may also be options.
Melanoma	The most dangerous type of skin cancer due to its potential to spread to other parts of the body, though highly curable if caught early. It develops in melanocytes, the cells in your skin responsible for producing melanin, the pigment that gives skin its color.	A new mole or an existing mole that changes in size, shape, or color. Melanoma can also appear as scaly patches, open sores, or raised bumps.	The first line of treatment involves surgically removing the tumor along with a margin of surrounding tissue. If the melanoma has high-risk features, a sentinel lymph node biopsy may be performed to check if the cancer has spread. Imaging such as a CT, MRI, or PET scan may also be used to see if melanoma has spread.

Pre–Skin Cancers to Keep on Your Radar

Precancerous skin lesions are abnormal growths or changes in skin that have the potential to develop into skin cancer if they're left untreated. Here's what to keep on your radar.

TYPE OF PRE–SKIN CANCER	WHAT IT IS	WHAT IT TYPICALLY LOOKS LIKE	TREATMENT
Actinic keratosis (AK)	The most common type of pre–skin cancer, which can develop into squamous cell carcinoma if not treated. Note: Just 5 to 10 percent of AKs turn into skin cancer but having them is a sign of sun damage—and raises your lifetime risk for skin cancer.	Small, dry, scaly, crusty patches of skin that won't go away and can be red, light or dark tan, white, pink, flesh colored, or a combination of colors. Sometimes they can be easier to feel (like a rough, dry patch of skin) than to see.	Topical medications, cryotherapy (freezing the lesion with liquid nitrogen to destroy abnormal cells), photodynamic therapy, laser therapy, or excision.
Atypical moles (dysplastic nevi)	These unusual-looking moles can resemble melanoma but are typically benign. That said, they have a higher risk of becoming malignant than regular moles. Having multiple atypical moles increases your risk for developing melanoma.	Larger-than-normal moles that have an irregular shape, are varied in color (pink, red, tan, brown, and/or black), and can be flat or slightly raised.	Regular skin exams to check for changes to moles. A biopsy may be necessary, which involves removing part or all of the mole (and oftentimes a margin of surrounding tissue) so it can be examined.

Skin Cancer Screening: What You Need to Know and Do to Catch Skin Cancer as Early as Possible

Here's a stat that might inspire you to start scanning your body for unusual-looking spots: More than half of women's melanomas are detected by women themselves, and we tend to catch them earlier than men do, which often leads to cancer being identified at earlier stages and better outcomes as a result.[10]

It only takes five minutes to do a thorough job: Examine your body in a full-length mirror, doing your best to check everywhere—including tough-to-see areas like your back, scalp, and butt, as well as places you may not think to look, like the soles of your feet and between your toes. You can use a hand mirror to get a glimpse of those spots or ask your partner or a friend to give those areas a once-over.

The most important thing to clue in to is anything that's changed over time, says Dr. Tanzi.

"Look for anything that makes you stop and say, 'Hmmm, that hasn't always been there' or 'That mole looks bigger or stranger than before,'" she says.

When you look at your moles, think ABCDE:[11]

Asymmetry (perfect circles are usually okay; lopsided shapes are not)

Borders (moles with smooth, well-defined borders are typically normal; stay alert to moles with irregular, blurred, or ragged borders)

Color (you want it to be uniform, not varied)

Diameter (bigger than six millimeters is a warning sign)

Evolving (look for moles that have changed in color, size, or shape, or are inflamed, itch, or bleed)

If you have a mole or other type of spot (aka lesion) on your body that has one or more of the ABCDEs, schedule an appointment with a dermatologist to get it checked out. Here are some other signs of precancers and skin cancers to look out for:

- A red patch or a scaly bump or lump
- A shiny, pearly bump that looks translucent or waxy
- A spot that's itchy or painful
- A change in skin texture, like a patch of dry skin that won't go away
- A sore that bleeds, develops a crust, and doesn't seem to heal
- A craterlike sore with blood in the center
- A wartlike growth
- A scar-like growth

If you see any of these signs, schedule an appointment with a dermatologist for an expert assessment.

The Full-Body Exam: How to Make the Most of Your Appointment

Starting around age twenty, it's time to start getting an annual head-to-toe inspection of your skin. This is done at a dermatologist's office and involves a clinician thoroughly examining your skin to detect skin cancer or other skin conditions as early as possible.

While the Skin Cancer Foundation recommends you see a dermatologist once a year starting at age twenty, you may need more frequent checks if you're at higher risk of skin cancer (which includes having a history of indoor tanning, sunburns, and/or unprotected exposure to UV radiation; a lighter skin tone; red hair; a family history of skin cancer; and/or atypical moles).

Here's how to prep for your appointment:

- **Bring a list of concerns or changes you've noticed**. Give yourself a body scan before your appointment so you can point out anything that looks unusual or new.

- **Arrive with clean skin**. Don't wear makeup, nail polish, or heavy moisturizing lotions, which can mask suspicious-looking spots.

- **Wear your hair loose**. Your clinician will take a thorough look at your scalp, which is a common spot for skin cancers.

Common Cosmetic Treatments, Explained

Cosmetic dermatology has become more popular—and accessible—than ever before. From injectables like Botox and fillers to in-office treatments like lasers and microneedling, the options for enhancing your appearance can seem endless. Here, Jody A. Levine, MD, director of dermatology at Plastic Surgery & Dermatology of NYC, walks us through some of the most requested procedures and what you need to know about each.

Injectables

Commonly used to improve the appearance of skin and reduce the signs of aging, there are a few different types of injectable substances that have different effects.

» BOTULINUM TOXIN (AKA BOTOX)

Botulinum toxin is a protein produced by a bacterium (*Clostridium botulinum*). It temporarily stops the nerve cells where it's injected from releasing the neurotransmitter (called acetylcholine) that prompts muscles to contract. When that neurotransmitter isn't released, the muscles don't get the message to move, which in turn relaxes them.

When injected into specific spots on your face, Botox reduces the muscle activity that leads to "dynamic" wrinkles—lines caused by muscle movements, such as forehead and frown lines as well as crow's-feet around the eyes—making them less noticeable. This muscle relaxation typically lasts three to four months, at which point your muscles will start contracting again, prompting your wrinkles to return.

Potential side effects: Complications are rare when experienced clinicians (like board-certified dermatologists or plastic surgeons) are administering the injections. Bruising or swelling at the site of the injection can happen. Drooping eyebrows or eyelids are another potential side effect, which is usually caused by the Botox spreading to (or being injected into) other muscles unintentionally and is temporary.

» DERMAL FILLERS

These are injections that can plump up wrinkles, restore volume, and lift the skin in specific areas of the face, including the lips, cheeks, nasolabial folds (aka smile lines), and under-eye hollows. As we age, we lose muscle, fat, bone, and collagen, and our skin begins to sag. Fillers put back some of that volume that's been lost over time.

There are multiple types of dermal fillers, each of which has unique ingredients and works in a specific way. Here are some of the most common.

TYPE OF FILLER	BRANDS	HOW IT WORKS
Hyaluronic acid (HA)	Juvéderm, Restylane, Belotero Balance	HA attracts and holds water in the injected area, plumping the skin and smoothing out wrinkles.
Calcium hydroxylapatite (CaHA)	Radiesse	CaHA particles are suspended in a gel carrier that's gradually absorbed by the body, while the CaHA stimulates collagen production and provides volume.
Poly-L-lactic acid (PLLA)	Sculptra	PLLA works gradually to stimulate collagen production, with results appearing over several months as new collagen forms.
Polymethyl methacrylate (PMMA)	Bellafill	This filler contains "microspheres" of PMMA suspended in a collagen gel. While the collagen gel provides immediate volume (and smooths wrinkles), the PMMA microspheres stay in place and prompt the body to produce its own collagen.

Potential side effects: The most common include mild pain, redness, swelling, and bruising at the site of the injection. Less common but more serious risks include infection at the injection site, allergic reaction to the ingredients in the filler, and lumps under the skin. One of the most serious risks is filler being accidentally injected into a blood vessel, which can lead to tissue death (aka necrosis) and even blindness if injections are in vessels that feed the eyes.

It's important to note that if you had a hyaluronic acid–based filler injected and hate the results, it can be reversed. Hyaluronic acid is a sugar molecule that's easily broken down by an enzyme called hyaluronidase, which can be injected into the filler to correct results you don't like. If you had one of the other fillers, you'll have to wait it out until your body breaks it down over time.

Laser Skin Resurfacing

Lasers, which direct intense beams of light energy, have been used for many years to improve the appearance of acne scars, fine wrinkles, uneven skin color or texture, and sun-damaged skin. Different types of laser treatments are used depending on the specific skin issue you're treating and the outcome you're looking for. There are ablative laser treatments, which destroy the outer layer of your skin while at the same time stimulating collagen production in the underlying layers, and nonablative laser treatments, which work similarly to ablative lasers but are less aggressive and have a shorter recovery time.

» FRACTIONAL LASERS

Fractional lasers can be ablative or nonablative and work by creating microscopic columns of heat damage in the skin in a grid-like pattern as opposed to damaging skin all over. Leaving some skin untouched by the laser allows the skin to heal and regenerate itself more quickly, which reduces downtime. Emerging research shows that nonablative fractional lasers stimulate certain growth factors that may reduce the risk of squamous cell and basal cell carcinomas.[12]

Potential side effects: Redness and swelling are the most common side effects and are generally temporary. Skin color changes can also occur in some cases, and this side effect is usually temporary. There's also a risk of bacterial, viral (especially herpes simplex), or fungal infections after laser resurfacing treatments, as well as scarring, which is more likely to happen if you don't care for your skin properly during the healing process. (Whatever you do, don't pick at your itchy, dry, peeling old skin as your new skin starts to emerge!)

Microneedling

This minimally invasive cosmetic procedure is growing in popularity and being offered in many nonmedical settings; there are also a growing number of do-it-yourself options in the form of "microneedling pens" and "dermarollers" you can use on your face at home. The promise: Making tiny holes in the top layer of your skin triggers a natural healing response, which increases blood flow to the skin, and helps stimulate the production of collagen and elastin, which improves your skin's texture and tone.

Potential side effects: Redness and swelling are very common and typically last a few hours to a few days after your procedure; mild bruising and skin irritation, as well as dryness and peeling, may also happen as skin heals and regenerates. Less common (but more serious) side effects include infection (which is more likely to happen if skin isn't properly cleaned before the procedure), hyperpigmentation, and scarring.

Your Game Plan:
The Most Important Steps You Can Take to Keep Your Skin Healthy (and Looking Great) at Every Age

As women, we're bombarded with skin care advice. Figuring out what actually works—or even where to start when it comes to sorting through all of the information—can feel overwhelming. But taking steps for healthy, great-looking skin doesn't have to be so complicated, says Dr. Tanzi. While information about the best products and procedures will always change, Dr. Tanzi says these are the timeless steps you can take to protect your skin *and* keep it looking great now and for years to come.

Get to know your skin. Simply becoming aware of your skin—what moles and birthmarks you have, what skin conditions you're prone to, and what's normal (and not) for you—can keep you clued in to changes, which is the key to getting care when skin conditions like cancer are most treatable.

"I had a melanoma on my leg that looked like a tiny black dot, but the warning sign for me was that it was *new*," says Dr. Tanzi. "If you know your skin, you're in a better position to spot anything that's new or changing in size, shape, color, or feel—all signs that you should get it checked out by a dermatologist."

Have a "sun strategy." While you've undoubtedly heard that using sunscreen is important, it shouldn't lull you into thinking that you're totally protected and can lie in the sun safely, says Dr. Tanzi, who recommends thinking of sunscreen as a second line of defense against UV rays.

The first line is having what she calls a good sun strategy, which means avoiding direct sun exposure during the peak sun hours each day (around 10:00 a.m. until 4:00 p.m.). Can you walk on the shady side of the street? Can you sit in the shade at the park or under an umbrella at the beach? If you love golf or tennis, can you play early in the morning or late in the afternoon? If you can't avoid midday sun exposure, can you wear protective clothes and a wide-brimmed hat to protect your skin?

"Living a healthy, active life is going to mean you're exposed to the sun," says Dr. Tanzi. "But having a sun strategy and sticking to it faithfully can go a long way toward preventing the cumulative sun damage that happens over the course of your life."

• • • • •

It's okay to focus on how your skin looks. It can help you stay alert to changes and inspire you to see a dermatologist who can diagnose and treat skin conditions, including skin cancer. Yet it's also important to know that skin health entails so much more than quick complexion fixes and product trends. With an understanding of your body's largest organ, you can treat surface-level concerns while also considering the bigger picture about the ways your skin can be a window into your overall well-being.

Part III

Optimize Your Health

The Road to
Strength and Resilience

Chapter 17

Mental and Emotional Health

Understanding Depression, Anxiety, Trauma, and Addiction—and Proven Ways to Feel Better

> *The most beautiful people we have known are those who have known defeat, known suffering, known struggle, known loss, and have found their way out of the depths. These persons have an appreciation, a sensitivity, and an understanding of life that fills them with compassion, gentleness, and a deep loving concern. Beautiful people do not just happen.*
>
> —Elisabeth Kübler-Ross, *Death: The Final Stage of Growth*

In recent years, there's been a lot of talk about our collective mental health crisis. And while women and men alike are struggling in new and profound ways, there are some sex-specific differences to the challenges we face when it comes to our mental health.

For one, women are about twice as likely as men to be diagnosed with depression.[1] We also experience post-traumatic stress disorder (PTSD) at two to three times the rate of our male counterparts,[2] and we have a two to three times higher lifetime risk of generalized anxiety disorder.[3] Even conditions that were once more prevalent in men, like alcohol abuse and drug addiction, are now on the rise in women.

Thankfully, more of us are talking to professionals and to one another about our mental health struggles, in large part because the stigma around many of these conditions has decreased in recent years. Mental health is a broad topic, so for this chapter we're going to focus on some of the most common conditions that affect women, to give you a starting point to stay alert to symptoms and get help if you find yourself struggling.

In this chapter, we'll learn . . .

- **What depression and anxiety really are**, the sex and gender differences that may contribute to women's higher likelihood of being diagnosed with these conditions, and the information that'll help you distinguish between a case of the blues and clinical depression.

- **How to ease everyday anxiety**, what's physically going on when we feel this common emotion, and science-backed tactics that can help you use anxiety to your advantage.

- **The most common prescription medications for depression and anxiety**, how each one works, and potential side effects to keep on your radar.

- **What you need to know about trauma**—and the many ways traumatic situations can impact our physical, mental, and emotional health.

- **The underacknowledged details of addiction**, and what all of us can do to destigmatize substance use disorders and best support those who are struggling.

- **Some of the most popular types of therapy** to help you manage your mental and emotional health, plus information on what each style entails so you can find the one that feels best for you.

Meet the Experts

Carrie Wilkens, PhD, cofounder of the Center for Motivation & Change and author of *Beyond Addiction: How Science and Kindness Help People Change*

Katherine Morgan Schafler, LMHC, psychotherapist and author of *The Perfectionist's Guide to Losing Control: A Path to Peace and Power*

Tanmeet Sethi, MD, integrative family medicine physician specializing in trauma, complex mental health, and guided psychedelic medicine and author of *Joy Is My Justice: Reclaim What Is Yours*

Wendy Suzuki, PhD, professor of neural science at New York University and author of *Good Anxiety: Harnessing the Power of the Most Misunderstood Emotion*

K. Ashley Garling, PharmD, pharmacist and clinical assistant professor at the University of Texas at Austin College of Pharmacy

Depression, Anxiety, and Trauma: Why Women Are Most Vulnerable—and What We Can Do About It

Women are at a twofold greater risk of experiencing depression and anxiety compared with men, thanks to a combination of biological and sociocultural factors. We're also more likely to be impacted by sexual abuse, domestic violence, and gender-based discrimination, which can contribute to the development of depression and anxiety disorders. Knowing the symptoms of each can help you get the support you need.

Depression

Maybe you can't seem to shake a sense of sadness or are finding that things you used to love doing don't hold the same appeal. Perhaps you feel sluggish all the time or wonder if anything you do matters. But how can you tell if you're dealing with an ordinary case of the *blahs*—or something a clinician would diagnose as depression? That can be a tricky question to answer, even for mental health practitioners. After all, depression can manifest differently from person to person and symptoms can vary greatly in severity and duration. However, knowing the common symptoms of depression is a good place to start.

» ARE YOU DEPRESSED—OR JUST IN A FUNK?

The reality is, it's normal for your mood to fluctuate. Sometimes you'll be able to pinpoint what's making you feel down. Other times you may have no clue as to why you can't shake off sadness, even when everything in your world seems to be going well. But if one or more of these symptoms persist for two weeks or longer, or they significantly interfere with your quality of life, you might be dealing with depression.

Some of the most common symptoms of depression include:

- Persistent sadness, hopelessness, a feeling of "emptiness"
- Loss of interest or pleasure in activities or hobbies you once liked to do
- Significant changes in appetite and/or eating habits, leading to weight loss or gain
- Insomnia (difficulty falling or staying asleep) or sleeping too much (hypersomnia)
- Feeling tired, sluggish, or physically drained more often than not
- Difficulty concentrating, focusing, remembering details, or making decisions
- Experiencing intense feelings of worthlessness
- Being unusually restless, agitated, and fidgety
- Feeling unusually slow, either physically or mentally or both
- Experiencing physical symptoms like headaches and/or digestive issues
- Having thoughts of death or suicide, including making plans for suicide or attempting suicide

There's no shame in experiencing depression. If you suspect you might be depressed, schedule a time to talk to your healthcare provider or mental health specialist.

» THE TYPES OF DEPRESSION

Depression isn't just one condition. Here's how the American Psychiatric Association classifies depressive disorders in the *Diagnostic and Statistical Manual of Mental Disorders*, 5th edition (DSM-5), including some of the symptoms of each.

DEPRESSIVE DISORDER	SYMPTOMS
Disruptive mood dysregulation disorder (DMDD)	Chronic, intense irritability and frequent anger outbursts in kids, with symptoms usually starting before the age of ten.
Major depressive disorder	Depressed mood (feeling sad, low, and/or worthless) that interferes with daily activities most of the time for at least two weeks. Other symptoms may include sleep problems, loss of interest in activities, and a change in appetite.
Persistent depressive disorder (PDD)	Depressed mood that occurs for most of the day, for more days than not, for at least two years (or at least one year for children and adolescents). Major depressive episodes may occur during PDD.
Premenstrual dysphoric disorder (PMDD)	Significant mood disturbances and other symptoms (including irritability, mood swings, depression, anxiety, and fatigue) that occur repeatedly in the days leading up to menstruation and get better around the start of the cycle or shortly after. This is a severe form of premenstrual syndrome (PMS).
Substance/medication-induced depressive disorder	Symptoms of a depressive disorder that are associated with the ingestion, injection, or inhalation of a substance, and the depressive symptoms persist after intoxication or when experiencing withdrawal.
Depressive disorder due to another medical condition	Prominent and persistent period of depressed mood or markedly diminished interest or pleasure in almost all activities that's due to another medical condition, such as lupus, cancer, Parkinson's disease, or stroke.
Other specified depressive disorder and unspecified depressive disorder	Clusters of symptoms that have characteristics of a depressive disorder but don't meet the criteria for any of the other depressive disorders. Symptoms cause "clinically significant distress" and/or impair your everyday functioning.

There are also specific forms of major depressive disorder, including:

• **Perinatal depression,** which is depression that begins during pregnancy (prenatal depression) or in the first year after delivery (postpartum depression). Both are characterized by feelings of sadness, anxiety, and exhaustion that interfere with maternal functioning and bonding with your baby.

- **Seasonal affective disorder (SAD)**, which is depression that occurs seasonally, typically in the fall and winter. Symptoms (such as low mood, fatigue, increased sleep, weight gain, and cravings for carbohydrates) often improve in the spring and summer.

- **Depression with symptoms of psychosis**, which is a severe form of depression that comes along with psychosis symptoms, such as hallucinations (hearing or seeing things others don't hear or see) or delusions (disturbing false beliefs).

- **Bipolar disorder** (formerly called manic depression) is a chronic mood disorder where one experiences depressive episodes (feeling sad, hopeless, worthless, indifferent, and low energy) as well as manic episodes (feeling very happy, "up," irritable, and high energy). These intense shifts in mood, behavior, and energy levels can last for hours, days, or even months.

Anxiety

Most of us have felt anxious at some point (or many points) in our lives. We may have had anxious jitters or butterflies or experienced a more extreme response that makes our breathing and heart rate quicken and maybe even prompts extreme worry or fear. Anxiety is a normal emotion, and one we can even use to our advantage. (More on the upsides of anxiety on page 485.)

Anxiety disorders, however, are something else entirely. These are a group of mental health conditions defined by excessive feelings of worry, fear, or dread that are out of proportion to the situation you're facing. While there's not one sign or symptom that marks the point where normal anxiety crosses over to an anxiety disorder, consider setting up an appointment to talk with a mental health professional if you're experiencing any of these symptoms:

- Anxiety that is interfering with your ability to function and/or do everyday activities

- Difficulty controlling your responses to situations

- Reactions (fear, worry, dread) that are out of proportion to the situation in which you find yourself, to the point where others might say you're overreacting

- Restlessness, feeling on edge, irritability, difficulty concentrating, muscle tension, sleep disturbances, and/or being fatigued more days than not for the past six months or more

» THE TYPES OF ANXIETY

As with depression, there are several types of anxiety disorders. Here's how the American Psychiatric Association classifies them in the *Diagnostic and Statistical Manual of Mental Disorders*, 5th edition (DSM-5), including some of the symptoms of each.

ANXIETY DISORDER	SYMPTOMS
Separation anxiety disorder	Excessive fear or anxiety about being separated from a loved one or home that exceeds what's considered developmentally appropriate.
Selective mutism	Failure to speak in certain situations where there's an expectation to speak (at school, for example) due to fear or anxiety. This is most common in young children but can persist into adolescence and adulthood.
Specific phobia	Intense or severe fear or anxiety about a specific object or situation. There are hundreds of different types of phobias.
Social anxiety disorder (aka social phobia)	Marked or intense fear or anxiety of social situations; intense and ongoing fear of being scrutinized by others and negatively evaluated.
Panic disorder	Recurrent panic attacks (an abrupt surge of intense fear or intense discomfort that reaches a peak within minutes) that are unexpected, meaning there's no obvious cue or trigger at the time of the attack.
Agoraphobia	Intense fear or anxiety triggered by the real or anticipated exposure to a wide range of situations, including using public transportation, being in open spaces, being in enclosed spaces, standing in line or being in a crowd, or being outside of the home alone.
Generalized anxiety disorders (GAD)	Excessive fear, worry, and/or a constant feeling of being overwhelmed where the intensity, duration, or frequency of the anxiety and worry is out of proportion to the actual likelihood or impact of the anticipated event. If you have GAD, you might find it difficult to control your worry or keep it from interfering with your everyday activities or tasks.

ANXIETY DISORDER	SYMPTOMS
Substance/medication-induced anxiety disorder	Anxiety or panic that develop during or soon after substance intoxication or withdrawal, or after exposure to a medication, and symptoms are judged to be due to the effects of a substance (for example, a drug, medication, or a toxin exposure).
Anxiety disorder due to another medical condition	Clinically significant anxiety that is judged to be best explained as a psychological effect of another medical condition.
Other specified anxiety disorder and unspecified anxiety disorder	These are anxiety or phobias that don't meet the criteria for any other anxiety disorder but that cause "clinically significant distress" and/or impair everyday functioning.

There are other mental health conditions that have similar symptoms and share other features with anxiety disorders, including:

- **Obsessive-compulsive disorder (OCD),** which is characterized by getting caught in a cycle of unreasonable thoughts and fears that can become all-consuming and interfere with everyday life. Those with this disorder have recurring, persistent, unwanted thoughts and urges (obsessions), and they feel driven to repeat behaviors or thoughts (compulsions) in response to the obsessions.

- **Post-traumatic stress disorder (PTSD),** which is a condition that usually surfaces within three months after a person experiences a traumatic event, though in some cases it can surface many years later. It's important to know that women are twice as likely as men to develop PTSD after a traumatic event,[4] and we often experience a longer duration of symptoms.[5] Symptoms may include intrusive thoughts, nightmares, and/or flashbacks related to the traumatic event(s); avoidance; anxiety; and/or angry outbursts.

- **Acute stress disorder,** which is similar to PTSD in that it can happen in response to a traumatic event or set of circumstances. The difference is that in acute stress disorder, symptoms occur between three days and one month after the incident.

- **Complex post-traumatic stress disorder (CPTSD),** which is similar to PTSD but can be caused by recurring or long-term traumatic events, such as childhood abuse, domestic violence, or war. It may also include feelings of worthlessness, shame, and guilt; difficulty connecting with other people; and relationship issues, including trouble keeping friends and partners.

Trauma

At some point in our lives, nearly all of us will be exposed to what experts call a potentially traumatic event. In fact, nearly 90 percent of U.S. adults report exposure to at least one potentially traumatic event in their lifetime.[6] The result can be trauma, which is an emotional, psychological, or physical response to a distressing or harmful event. There are many different types of trauma and understanding what they are can help when it comes to your own healing, supporting others in their healing process, and helping to create an informed, compassionate community. Ultimately, recognizing trauma as a broad spectrum of experiences helps normalize it and reduces the stigma that so often rides along with it.

Here are some of the most common types of trauma.

TYPE OF TRAUMA	WHAT IT IS
Acute trauma	Results from a single, sudden, and unexpected event
Chronic trauma	Stems from repeated or prolonged exposure to a distressing situation
Complex trauma	Involves exposure to multiple (often interpersonal and invasive) traumatic events that typically occur during childhood
Secondary trauma	Occurs when someone indirectly experiences trauma through exposure to another person's traumatic experiences
Developmental trauma	Relates to traumatic experiences that occur during critical stages of childhood development and can impact social, emotional, and cognitive development
Medical trauma	Can happen after medical procedures, serious illnesses, or prolonged hospitalization
Intergenerational trauma	Trauma that's passed down through generations, often stemming from systemic oppression, slavery, or genocide

There are multiple trauma-related conditions that can surface. We've already discussed depression, anxiety, PTSD, and acute stress disorder;

other mental health conditions that can surface as a result of trauma include eating disorders, substance abuse and addiction, self-harm, and suicidal thoughts.

So Why the Sex Differences in Depression, Anxiety, and Trauma?

The unsatisfying truth is that experts don't yet know exactly why women are vulnerable, mostly because sex and gender differences have been historically under-studied.[7] But here's what we *do* know:

- **Our sex hormones are likely a factor.** Before puberty, rates of depression and anxiety are similar in boys and girls. After puberty, about twice as many women as men experience both disorders.[8] One widely accepted theory for this is that fluctuations in estrogen may trigger anxiety and depression. It turns out sex hormones may play a role in how we respond to trauma, too. Research shows that progesterone, which plays a role in memory formation, may have memory-enhancing effects at the time of trauma, making women more vulnerable to PTSD, particularly during times of the menstrual cycle when progesterone is high (around day twenty-one of a twenty-eight-day cycle).[9]

- **Differences in how we respond to psychological distress may play a part.** Research shows that men tend to "externalize" what they're dealing with by directing their action outward. (Translation: They may process what they're feeling or distract themselves from it by doing something else, like playing video games or sports or watching TV.) Women, on the other hand, are more likely to "internalize" our emotional regulation—say, by ruminating about a negative event or writing about it. This isn't to say one is better than the other, or that the behavior of all women and men will fall under these generalizations. But it may explain why women are more likely to deal with "internalizing disorders," such as depression and anxiety, whereas men experience higher rates of "externalizing disorders," such as conduct disorder and substance abuse.[10]

- **Gender-normative expectations may impact who reports depression and who doesn't.** Socially reinforced female coping styles (think things like emotional expressiveness and a willingness to ask for help) may prompt more women than men to seek help for their depression—and may make us more likely to receive a depression diagnosis. On the flip side, typical masculine coping styles (like emotional inexpressiveness and not seeking help) as well as a social expectation for men to be "tough" might make them reluctant to express symptoms of depression—and lead to mild to moderate depression going underdiagnosed and undertreated in men. The data supports this: Women are more likely to report mild to moderate symptoms of depression, whereas men tend to report more severe depression and have higher rates of suicide.[11]

- **We are more likely to experience trauma.** Women are more likely to have a higher adverse childhood experiences (ACEs) score, which has been linked to a higher risk of developing anxiety later in life.[12] We're also more likely to experience interpersonal and "high-impact" trauma, such as sexual assault: One in five women and one in seventy-one men will be raped during their lifetime.[13] In fact, the World Health Organization estimates that one in three women have been subjected to physical and/or intimate partner violence or nonpartner sexual violence in their lifetime.

Our Kids' Mental Health Crisis Is Gendered, Too

Most of us are worried about our kids' mental health these days, and for good reason. Teenage depression and anxiety are at record highs, and girls are especially susceptible. One survey given to more than seventeen thousand adolescents at high schools across the U.S. found that nearly three in five teenage girls felt persistent sadness—almost double the rate of boys.[14] That same survey found that nearly one in three girls seriously considered attempting suicide, and just over one in five teens who identified as lesbian, gay, bisexual, questioning, or another nonheterosexual identity or who had any same-sex sexual partners reported attempting suicide in the previous year.

There's a growing consensus that the rise in social media use is having negative effects on young women's mental health: Rates of depression, anxiety, and self-injury among adolescent girls have surged since social media platforms have proliferated, and research shows this has affected girls more than boys. Among girls in particular, those who spend more hours a day on social media are more likely to experience symptoms of depression. One study found that Instagram was the biggest culprit, with teens scoring it as the most harmful when asked how social media platforms affect their anxiety, loneliness, body image, and sleep, among other factors.[15] Another study found that when young women were randomly assigned to use Instagram, use Facebook, or play a video game, those who used Instagram (but not Facebook) showed decreased positive affect and body satisfaction.[16]

What's a concerned parent or caregiver supposed to do with this information? For starters, understand that this is happening on a massive scale. This knowledge alone might help you better interpret signs your child might be suffering, rather than just brushing it off as normal teenage moodiness.

Curbing social media use may be tough, especially as kids get older, but it's worthwhile to attempt. For young kids, don't let them sign up for these platforms until they hit a certain age. Most experts recommend age thirteen at the earliest. Download social media blocker apps to enforce when and for how long young ones can be on these platforms. (You might do this for yourself while you're at it!) Most important, say something if you're noticing changes in your child's mood or affect, have a conversation about it, and seek out the support they need to feel better and stay safe.

Addiction: Understanding How It Impacts Women

Years ago, addiction research mostly focused on the effects of drugs and alcohol on men. And while for most age groups, men still have higher rates of substance use than women, women are equally susceptible when it comes to developing a substance use disorder. What's more, research shows that when it comes to substance use disorders, we may be more likely to experience cravings and relapse—two key phases that keep people stuck in the addiction cycle.[17]

Here's a look at some of the most common substances that pose a risk to women's health, how our physiology may put us at an especially high risk for complications, and the new thinking on how to treat addiction.

Alcohol

For many years, men outnumbered women three to one when it came to binge drinking and alcohol use disorder. These days, the ratio of risky drinking habits in men versus women is now closer to one to one globally, and rates of alcohol use disorder have increased in women by 84 percent in recent years, compared with a 35 percent increase in men.[18] The trends among young women are especially concerning. One study found that alcohol-related deaths among women in the U.S. increased 2.5-fold.[19]

Many addiction experts say this narrowed gender gap in drinking habits is likely due to changing attitudes about women's alcohol consumption, and how it's now more socially acceptable for women to drink. Marketing campaigns and social media messaging that normalize drinking among women of reproductive age has also led to "Mommy drinking" culture, where #mommyjuice is seen as a way to deal with the stressors of parenthood and the overwhelming mental load that women typically carry.

Yet while it may be more acceptable—and even expected—for women to drink these days, the truth is that our bodies process alcohol very differently from men's. Women have lower amounts of alcohol dehydrogenase, the enzyme needed to break down alcohol in the body. The result? We can't metabolize alcohol as quickly as men and are left with higher, more concentrated levels of alcohol in our systems for a longer period of time. This can be toxic to our organs and is likely why research shows that women suffer serious health consequences of alcohol (such as liver disease, heart disease, and an increased risk of cancer) more quickly than men.[20]

Especially concerning is that even though women are dealing with alcohol use and abuse in record numbers, we're less likely than men to enter treatment. Reasons for this may relate to children: *Who will take care of the kids if I go into treatment? Will my kids be taken from me if I admit I have a problem?* There's also the fact that many women begin abusing alcohol to deal with the impact of a crisis—such as a divorce, the stress of caregiving, or kids growing up and leaving the house—which can be tough to acknowledge and discuss and, as a result, can keep many women from seeking help.

» IS YOUR DRINKING A PROBLEM?

The National Institute on Alcohol Abuse and Alcoholism has a questionnaire that can help you spot the symptoms of alcohol use disorder.[21] If you answer "yes" to two or three of these questions, you're considered to have a mild problem; if you answer "yes" to four or five, it's considered moderate; if you answer "yes" to more than six, you have a severe disorder.

In the past year, have you . . .

- Had times when you ended up drinking more, or longer, than you intended?

- More than once wanted to cut down or stop drinking, or tried to, but couldn't?

- Spent a lot of time drinking? Or being sick or getting over other aftereffects?

- Wanted a drink so badly you couldn't think of anything else?

- Found that drinking—or being sick from drinking—often interfered with taking care of your home or family? Or caused job troubles? Or school problems?

- Continued to drink even though it was causing trouble with your family or friends?

- Given up or cut back on activities that were important or interesting to you, or gave you pleasure, in order to drink?

- More than once gotten into situations while or after drinking that increased your chances of getting hurt (such as driving, swimming, using machinery, walking in a dangerous area, or unsafe sexual behavior)?

- Continued to drink even though it was making you feel depressed or anxious or adding to another health problem? Or after having had a memory blackout?

- Had to drink much more than you once did to get the effect you want? Or found that your usual number of drinks had much less effect than before?

- Found that when the effects of alcohol were wearing off, you had withdrawal symptoms, such as trouble sleeping, shakiness, restlessness, nausea, sweating, a racing heart, dysphoria (feeling uneasy or unhappy), malaise (general sense of being unwell), feeling low, or a seizure?

If you are struggling with substance abuse and need help, you can call the Substance Abuse and Mental Health Services Administration (SAMHSA) National Helpline at 800-662-4357 for free and confidential information.

Smoking

Despite the fact that fewer women than men smoke—and women who do smoke tend to smoke fewer cigarettes per day and do not inhale as deeply as men—smoking poses greater health risks for women than for men. For example, female smokers have a higher risk of experiencing health conditions associated with smoking, including heart disease and osteoporosis. Women are also more likely to become dependent on nicotine more quickly and with less nicotine exposure than men, and we tend to be less successful at quitting.

Opioids

This class of pain-relieving drugs is highly addictive—so much so that the U.S. continues to struggle with an ongoing opioid epidemic that was initially fueled by widespread opioid prescriptions in the 1990s. These drugs are primarily used for pain relief: They work by interacting with opioid receptors (involved in feeling pain) on cells in the brain, spinal cord, white blood cells, and gastrointestinal tract. Given that women tend to experience more acute and chronic pain (across a range of conditions) than men, it's not surprising that women are about twice as likely as men to be prescribed opioids. (For more on pain and the many ways to treat it, flip back to chapter 12.)

How to Help a Loved One (or Yourself) Get Treatment for Addiction

Whether it's you or a family member or friend who's struggling with a substance use disorder, talking about the issue and potential treatment options can feel daunting at best and downright impossible at worst. In part, it's because substance use disorders are still highly stigmatized, says Carrie Wilkens, PhD, cofounder of the Center for Motivation & Change. "Those with substance use problems typically walk around with so much shame," she says. "And research shows family members are often seen to be part of the problem because they haven't been able to 'fix' it, and they often feel judged, too."

So how can we collectively work to destigmatize this issue and better help those with substance use disorders? Dr. Wilkens suggests starting here:

- **Try to understand how the behavior makes sense**. For better or for worse, substances work in some way; otherwise people would not continue using them. They can distract us from the stuff we don't want to look at. They help numb our physical pain and help us reduce anxiety. The reasons people use substances are endless. Instead of thinking that you or someone you love is weak or selfish for relying on substances, try to understand how the substance is providing something meaningful. "Once you understand how a behavior makes sense, you can work on *that*—and figure out if there's something else that can meet that need in another, healthier way," says Dr. Wilkens.

- **Remember that all change is hard**. Think about anything you've tried to change in the past—your diet, your exercise habits, your social media scrolling. In these instances, it's easy to admit that change is hard. But when it comes to addiction, we want fast results and tend to get mad when our loved one's or our own efforts to quit don't stick. "Substance abuse is just like any other behavior—except it also influences your physiology, making you potentially physically and emotionally dependent on the substance you're abusing," explains Dr. Wilkens. "You're not only asking someone to give something up. You're asking someone to give something up that their body may be physically dependent on, making it more difficult."

  What's more, when you stop relying on a substance, you'll have to learn a whole host of new behaviors—how to be in relationships, how to manage stress, how to deal with emotions, how to sleep, eat, and take care of your body. "We don't give people who are trying to change their relationship with a substance enough credit for how hard it is to learn all the new things they have to learn to not return to the substance use," says Dr. Wilkens. "The time it takes is often compounded by the reality that many relationships have been hurt, and it may take some time to come back from that hurt."

- **Know that there's no one "right" way to treat addiction**. Going cold turkey may work for some and not others. Staying at a treatment facility might be exactly what one person needs to start to heal, whereas another may prefer to go to self-help meetings or start to meditate. "Every single person with a substance use problem gets into it for different reasons and gets out of it in different ways," says Dr. Wilkens.

- **Avoid labeling those with substance use disorders**. The words we use really do matter when it comes to how we might collectively move the needle on the stigma that exists around substance use disorders. If someone self-identifies as an alcoholic, that's very different from *you* calling someone an alcoholic, says Dr. Wilkens. There are also many terms tossed around when it comes to discussing addiction and treatment—things like *hitting rock bottom* or someone needing an *intervention* or even *codependency*—that aren't as constructive as they might seem because they can be stigmatizing and make the person struggling feel judged. "Instead, try to come from a place of curiosity and compassion," adds Dr. Wilkens.

- **Practice compassion (and self-compassion).** Self-compassion is a powerful practice that involves showing kindness to ourselves during difficult times and understanding that our struggles are shared by others and don't make us broken. Research has shown that developing self-compassion can help people persist in learning new things while facing discomfort, as it softens the harsh inner critic that is likely saying, *You can't do this; you might as well give up.* Dr. Wilkens says, "Self-compassion is the ultimate antidote to the shame and stigma associated with substance use problems. It helps people, and their families, see that others struggle in the same way and helps them bring kindness and compassion to the hard moments that inevitably occur when trying to learn new things."

How to Improve Your Emotional Health: Therapies and Treatments to Consider

Improving our mental health often involves learning how to manage our difficult emotions. Thankfully, there are a variety of approaches that can help. Here, psychotherapist Katherine Morgan Schafler, LMHC, gives us an overview of some of the most popular types of therapy. Keep in mind it's always a good idea to talk to a healthcare provider about any mental health symptoms you're experiencing, as certain conditions may benefit most from a combination of therapy *and* medication.

Psychotherapy (aka Talk Therapy)

What it is: This encompasses a variety of techniques that aim to help people identify how emotions, thoughts, and behaviors might be related to certain situations. It takes place with a trained, licensed mental health professional and can happen in individual or group settings.

    Used to treat . . . relationship issues, grief, adjusting to transitions, stress, and a number of other situations.

Cognitive Behavioral Therapy (CBT)

What it is: This is one of the most widely researched and most common forms of psychotherapy, which focuses on helping people identify and, over time, rewrite negative thought patterns and behaviors that contribute to emotional distress. By addressing these patterns and behaviors, a therapist can help clients develop better coping strategies.

    Used to treat . . . depression, anxiety disorders, PTSD, and a range of other mental health conditions.

Dialectical Behavior Therapy (DBT)

What it is: This offshoot of CBT is a type of talk therapy that focuses on helping people identify and change unhelpful behaviors. It's used in individual therapy sessions as well as "skills training" group sessions. In a group setting, participants practice specific skills drawn from four areas: mindfulness (awareness of the present moment without judgment); distress tolerance (learning to tolerate crises without making things worse); emotion regulation (learning to identify, understand, and modulate intense emotions); and interpersonal effectiveness (learning assertiveness, communication skills, and boundary setting).

    Used to treat . . . mental health conditions characterized by emotional dysregulation, impulsivity, and interpersonal difficulties.

Psychoanalysis

What it is: This style of therapy, based on the principles of psychoanalytic theory developed by Sigmund Freud, explores how unconscious thoughts, emotions, and past experiences influence current behavior and relationships. Therapists might ask open-ended questions and use free association to make connections between a client's current beliefs and past experiences. The goal is to help clients understand how unresolved conflicts might be getting in the way of feeling better.

Used to treat . . . relational difficulties and long-standing patterns of behavior.

Mindfulness-Based Therapies

What it is: These typically involve incorporating mindfulness practices, such as meditation or breathing techniques, into the therapeutic process to cultivate more awareness of the present moment, acceptance, and nonjudgmental observation of thoughts and feelings.

Used to treat . . . stress, anxiety, depression, chronic pain.

Eye Movement Desensitization and Reprocessing Therapy (EMDR)

What it is: This approach involves moving your eyes in a specific way while processing traumatic memories, with the goal of helping to reduce the emotional intensity of traumatic memories.

Used to treat . . . PTSD and other trauma-related conditions, as well as depression, anxiety, phobias, and panic disorder.

Exposure Therapy

What it is: This is a type of CBT in which a trained mental health professional creates a safe environment in which to expose you to whatever triggers your anxiety or fears (whether it's a situation, an object, an activity, or a memory). The goal is to reduce your fear and anxiety by showing you that you're capable of confronting your fears, and to learn strategies to help you cope with them going forward.

Used to treat . . . anxiety disorders, phobias, and PTSD.

Ask an Expert

I'm interested in psychedelic drugs to help treat my depression. What do I need to know as I consider this option? There's a growing body of research showing that psychedelics—psilocybin (aka magic mushrooms), LSD (aka acid), and MDMA (aka ecstasy or molly), among others—may be beneficial when it comes to treating certain mental health conditions. There's also been a big change in attitudes about using them. However, it's important to know that most psychedelics aren't legal in the majority of states, which makes it crucial to know what the laws are in your state before pursuing this treatment. If you're considering trying one of these medicines, here's what I recommend you keep in mind:

- **Know the contraindications.** Untreated or severe heart disease, uncontrolled blood pressure, a high risk of stroke, epilepsy, or another seizure disorder all raise red flags, because some psychedelic medicines can cause an increase in blood pressure and heart rate. If you have a personal or family history of psychosis, your provider will need to evaluate whether the risk of taking a psychedelic medicine is too high for you. All good providers would do both a full medical and a psychiatric evaluation.

    Another risk of some of these medicines is something called serotonin syndrome, a drug-induced condition caused by too much serotonin in the brain's synapses that can happen if you take a psychedelic while on an antidepressant or antianxiety medication that's already stimulating your serotonin pathways.

- **Prepare for the experience**—and have a plan to handle what may arise. You've probably heard a lot about how crucial it is to take these medicines when you're in the right mindset (aka set) and in the right physical and social environment (aka setting). These medicines are being studied with proper preparation, guided and safe use, and integration afterward. It's crucial to think through things like: Who will be with you (or in the next room, or on call) to help support you if needed? Who's going to help you process a past trauma that may come up? If what comes up is racial trauma, is your guide someone you feel safe processing that with? Do you have internal resources, like a meditation or breathing practice, that will help you navigate difficult emotions that may surface during your journey? Who will help you integrate afterward? These are important questions to answer before you try these medicines.

- **Trust your intuition.** As women, we are often made to believe that our intuition is a soft resource and not a provider of the concrete data we need. When we're talking about psychedelics, we're talking about very vulnerable spaces—and there are people who take advantage of that. I think it's crucial that all of us, and especially women, ask: What do I need to feel safe during this experience? Is it a different guide? Is it having someone else in the room? Advocating for yourself in this space is crucial, and the best way to do this is to trust your intuition and make sure you feel safe.

- **Remember that this wisdom came from Indigenous peoples.** In every piece of this work, it's important to hold reciprocity for where this came from. Our ability to sit with people in altered states of consciousness and use that as healing comes straight from Indigenous wisdom. And I believe that your intention for using these medicines can be amplified by having gratitude and reciprocity for the fact that this is centuries-old wisdom, and that we as humans have been healing in this way for a long time.

> When you feel that power of the global, ancestral collective, it helps you realize, *I'm not taking this medicine to cure me. I'm taking in this medicine to facilitate my inner healing to be at its greatest capacity.* Because these medicines are not a quick fix. They are more like catalysts that bring up what needs to be brought up, which then allows us to do the work that needs to be done to heal.
>
> —Tanmeet Sethi, MD, integrative family medicine physician specializing in trauma, complex mental health, and guided psychedelic medicine and author of *Joy Is My Justice: Reclaim What Is Yours*

How to Ease Everyday Anxiety—and Even Use It to Your Advantage

Even if you don't have clinical anxiety or a diagnosed anxiety disorder, you will undoubtedly feel anxious at many points of your life. At its core, anxiety is an emotion, which means it has a wide range of expression: It can feel manageable or completely overwhelming. Regardless of what's prompting your anxiety or how severe (or not) it feels, anxiety is generated in the same place in your body: the sympathetic nervous system, which is what prompts your "fight-or-flight" stress response.

This is *protective*. We experience anxiety in order to take action, says Wendy Suzuki, PhD. When you feel anxious, many things happen. The brain's fear and threat-detection center (located in the amygdala) gets activated, and high levels of the stress hormone cortisol are released by your adrenal glands, which then head straight for your brain. When that burst of cortisol rushes into your brain, it makes you alert and hypersensitive. It also gives you the power to get out of harm's way—fast.

This is a great thing when we *need* to be alert to a potential danger. When anxiety isn't debilitating, it also helps us identify what it is we value. Anxious about that big work deadline or first date? It means you really care about how it goes. You can see this as an upside of anxiety, says Dr. Suzuki. "There's an energy that comes from how anxiety makes us feel, but the key for many of us is learning how to turn down the volume," she says. Here's where Dr. Suzuki recommends starting.

Move your body. The quickest and most effective way to decrease anxiety and give yourself a quick mood boost is by moving your body in some way, says Dr. Suzuki, who has studied the benefits of exercise on the brain for more than a decade. Take a walk. Run up and down a flight of stairs. Hop on your bike and take a spin around the block. Even just ten minutes of movement has been shown to have a significant and immediate effect on lowering anxiety levels.

Practice box breathing. This style of breathwork involves breathing in for a count of four, holding the top of the inhalation for a count of four, breathing out for a count of four, and holding the bottom of the exhalation for a count of four. It works quickly to activate your parasympathetic nervous system (aka rest and digest mode), which counteracts the fight-or-flight system. Practice box breathing for even just a few minutes and you'll notice a calmer feeling throughout your body.

Rx, Explained: Antidepressants and Anxiety Medications

Millions of women take antidepressants and anxiety medications. Yet despite their prevalence, there can be a lot of confusion about how they work and their side effects. Here's a look at some of the most commonly prescribed antidepressants and anxiety medications.

DRUG TYPE	COMMON NAMES	HOW THEY WORK	PRESCRIBED FOR
Selective serotonin reuptake inhibitors (SSRIs)	fluoxetine (Prozac), paroxetine (Paxil, Paxil CR, Brisdelle), sertraline (Zoloft), citalopram (Celexa), escitalopram (Lexapro)	By preventing the reabsorption of serotonin by neurons in the brain, thereby increasing levels of serotonin (a neurotransmitter that's thought to have a positive influence on mood, emotion, and sleep) in the brain	Depression, anxiety, and many other mental health conditions
Serotonin-norepinephrine reuptake inhibitors (SNRIs)	duloxetine (Cymbalta, Drizalma Sprinkle, Irenka), venlafaxine (Effexor, Effexor XR), desvenlafaxine (Pristiq), levomilnacipran (Fetzima), milnacipran (Savella)	By preventing the reabsorption of the neurotransmitters serotonin and norepinephrine in the brain, thereby increasing the amount of them in your brain	Depression, depression that is associated with pain, fibromyalgia, neuropathy, chronic fatigue, chronic pain, anxiety, and many other mental health conditions
Atypical antidepressants **(These medications don't fit into one specific class of drugs.)**	bupropion (Wellbutrin SR, Wellbutrin XL, others), mirtazapine (Remeron, Remeron SolTab), nefazodone, trazodone, vilazodone (Viibryd), vortioxetine (Trintellix), esketamine (Spravato), which is FDA approved for treatment-resistant depression and intended to be used in combination with an oral antidepressant	By affecting one or more neurotransmitters known to regulate mood	Depression, anxiety
Benzodiazepines	alprazolam (Xanax, Xanax XR, Niravam), clonazepam (Klonopin), chlordiazepoxide (Librax), clorazepate (Tranxene T-Tab), estazolam (ProSom), flurazepam (Dalmane), lorazepam (Ativan), diazepam (Valium), midazolam, oxazepam, temazepam (Restoril), triazolam (Halcion), and more	By attaching to the gamma-aminobutyric acid A (GABA-A) receptors in the brain, which slows the nerve impulses in the brain and has a calming effect	Panic disorder, short-term sleep disorders, seizures, alcohol withdrawal

How long will it take to start feeling better once I start taking an antidepressant?

It can often take four to eight weeks to see the maximum benefits from an antidepressant, such as a selective serotonin reuptake inhibitor (SSRI) or serotonin-norepinephrine reuptake inhibitor (SNRI). It's also important to remember that some medications may worsen your symptoms at first, due to the changes happening in your brain chemistry. Let someone know you've started this new medication—ideally someone who looks out for you, like a partner, licensed mental health professional, or best friend—and mention that you might be a little more on edge or more emotional than usual as the medication starts working. You might also ask that person to tell you if you start seeming better or happier. That kind of feedback can be helpful, as you may not notice the changes happening in yourself over time.

I'm experiencing side effects. Should I switch medications?

If your side effects are bearable and aren't changing your ability to function, try to ride out those first four to six weeks before judging the effectiveness of the medication. Medications that work with your brain chemistry often take several weeks to show maximum effects and level out any imbalances that may be causing side effects. Talk to your doctor or pharmacist about what you might do to combat your symptoms. For example, you might be able to take your medication with food if it's making you nauseous, or you can drink more water for dry mouth. If you're constantly switching medications, you're less likely to find what works for you.

Can I stop taking my antidepressant once I start feeling better?

It's common to want to ditch your prescription when you're in a good place, but there are a few important things to keep in mind before you do. For starters, weaning off these medications is usually advised, as stopping abruptly (aka cold turkey) can upset your brain's delicate chemistry, can greatly impact your mood, and may even be dangerous. Talk to your doctor about your desire to stop taking the medication you're on so you can come up with an expert-approved plan for tapering off use. It's also important to remember what prompted your doctor to prescribe an antidepressant in the first place. Were you dealing with situational depression—say, you lost a loved one or a job? Or have you experienced depression throughout most of your life? Be honest about why you started taking the medication and why you want to stop, and, as always, talk to a mental health practitioner about the best plan of action for your specific situation.

Will I become addicted?

It's possible to develop a physical dependence on some of these medications because they change processes in the brain. Withdrawal-like symptoms can occur, so you'll want to talk to your doctor about your long-term treatment plan. If you're taking controlled substances like benzodiazepines (prescribed for conditions like anxiety and panic disorder), physical and psychological dependence potential is higher, which means it's key to minimize their use when possible.

Will taking an antidepressant kill my sex drive?

Sexual side effects can occur with some antidepressants and anti-anxiety medications. The most common complaint women taking SSRIs have is lowered libido. There are things you can do, such as being more intentional about when you have sex and experimenting with different types of touch and stimulation, to combat these side effects. Most important: Talk to your partner about your symptoms so you're both on the same page about the medication being to blame.

—K. Ashley Garling, PharmD, pharmacist and clinical assistant professor at the University of Texas at Austin College of Pharmacy

Your Game Plan: Find the Mental Healthcare You're Looking For

Deciding it's time to talk to your doctor, a therapist, or another professional about your mental health is a great first step on the road to feeling better. Unfortunately, many women aren't getting the help they're looking for. When respondents in one survey were asked about barriers to accessing mental health services, 80 percent cited cost and 60 percent said shame and stigma as the main obstacles to care.[22] Here, psychotherapist Katherine Morgan Schafler offers tips that'll help you find support.

Talk to your primary care physician. If you're struggling with depression, anxiety, or another mental health condition—or you're wondering if the symptoms you're experiencing would be classified as a diagnosable mental health disorder—chat about how you've been feeling with the clinician who takes care of your physical health. While routine screenings for depression and anxiety are standard at your annual physical or gynecology appointment, it can be easy to brush over them given how much ground there is to cover in limited time. Make an appointment with the specific request to talk about your mental health, which will give your clinician a chance to consider your symptoms and refer you to a specialist who can best help you.

Consider working with a therapist. A psychiatrist (a medical doctor who can prescribe antidepressants and antianxiety medications), psychologist, psychotherapist, or counselor—all referred to more broadly as therapists—can provide ongoing emotional support. How can you find a therapist? Start by asking your friends if they see someone who's been helpful. You can also put your zip code into a therapist locator like the one you'll find on *Psychology Today*'s website, where you can see a list of therapists in your area and read about what they specialize in.

"You might feel bombarded with clinical jargon when you read these descriptions," says Morgan Schafler, "so you may have to make a number of calls and even have multiple conversations with therapists to get a sense of who they are and how they work."

Most therapists offer a free consultation, which can range from ten to thirty minutes. Even if you're asking pragmatic questions on these calls, like how much they charge and whether or not they take insurance, you can glean a lot about how someone engages with you and how comfortable you feel talking to them. Listen to your instincts about whom you might jive with best.

Ask about fees—and wiggle room on what you can pay if it feels cost prohibitive. While some psychotherapists accept health insurance, which can keep the out-of-pocket cost down for patients, many don't. If a therapist's fee per session feels out of your budget, tell them. Some therapists offer sliding-scale payment options, where those with lower incomes pay lower prices. "This doesn't happen in all cases, but it's definitely worth asking a therapist you want to work with if they can work with you on pricing," says Morgan Schafler.

Make sure the person supporting you feels like a good "fit." The number one factor that determines successful outcomes in therapy is something called therapeutic alliance, which means feeling mutual trust and safety within the confines of treatment. Even in moments that feel difficult, your therapist needs to be a person you can be honest with, says Morgan Schafler. That's not to say a therapist is always going to tell you what you want to hear. "A good therapist helps you understand multiple perspectives and access the internal resources you have to make the best choice for you," she adds. And just as in any relationship, things can shift over time—so it's important to continually assess how you're engaging with your therapist and how you feel around them as you work together.

Try to remember that nothing is "wrong" with you. Our mental health-care system is based on a treatment model of care. "It's built on the assumption that if we can efficiently figure out what's wrong with you, we can get you healthier faster," says Morgan Schafler. Yet trying to figure out what's "wrong" with someone can be dangerous. "It prompts mental health professionals to look for what's broken—and ignore what's whole—so we can determine what needs to be fixed," she says. This is particularly harmful for women, who are the lifelong recipients of a never-ending stream of directives about how to be *less*. How to weigh less. How to want less. How to be less emotional. "I say it's time to get *more* of what you want by being *more* of who you are," says Morgan Schafler.

What if tending to your mental health could start with accepting what's *right* with you rather than focusing on what's *wrong*? Sure, self-acceptance requires you to get vulnerable and name when you're having a hard time. It may even involve a diagnosis. Mental health disorders are real, and finding the right treatment for them can be life-changing. "No matter what you're facing, it is crucial to be gentle with yourself when you're feeling less than," says Morgan Schafler. "Remembering your capacity for greatness is also key."

· · · · ·

Your mental and emotional health is a vast, nuanced topic. The information in this chapter is meant to serve as a starting point for understanding just some of the issues that can surface throughout your lifetime and tee you up to find the support you need to feel your best.

Chapter 18

Sleep

Why It Matters for Your Health, Plus the Science Behind Getting Better-Quality Shut-Eye

> By helping us keep the world in perspective, sleep gives us a chance to refocus on the essence of who we are. And in that place of connection, it is easier for the fears and concerns of the world to drop away.
>
> —Arianna Huffington, *The Sleep Revolution: Transforming Your Life, One Night at a Time*

For something that's as crucial for our overall health as sleep, many of us aren't getting enough of it—and the sleep we are getting isn't as restorative as it could be.

In fact, only a quarter of women rate their sleep as "excellent" or "very good," even though we're more likely than men to say sleep is a high priority.[1] Those of us between ages eighteen and forty-four are nearly twice as likely as men to say we're "exhausted," according to a report by the U.S. Centers for Disease Control and Prevention.[2] And while we'd like to feel more rested, many of us view getting too little sleep as unavoidable—the price of being busy students, career women, mothers, and caretakers.

Yet there's a lot you can do to improve both the quality and the quantity of sleep you get, and the advice doesn't just involve tips you've heard a million times before (like avoiding screen time at night). The best place to start is understanding what happens in our brains and bodies when we sleep, knowing the most common sleep disorders (and why many of them are more likely to happen in women), and following the science-backed (and realistic!) advice for getting better shut-eye.

In this chapter, we'll learn . . .

- **Why we need sleep and how much of it to aim for.** Plus, we'll explore how sleep works to improve so many aspects of health, a great source of motivation for snagging more shut-eye.

- **Exactly what's going on in your brain and body to prompt you to sleep.** From the sleep stages you cycle through to your circadian rhythm, understanding these basics can help you identify the factors that may be triggering your sleep issues and set you on a path for more restful nights.

- **The reasons women have a higher risk of developing sleep problems.** We'll review the most common sleep disorders and how the big hormonal transitions we go through can impact our sleep.

- **The biggest threats to a good night's rest—and what you can do to avoid them.** Because even if you follow all the best sleep hygiene tactics, they won't help if you don't also avoid the most common sleep saboteurs.

- **Tactics proven to help you get more (and better quality) shut-eye**, so you feel better immediately while also improving your overall health for years to come.

Meet the Experts

Ilene M. Rosen, MD, MSCE, associate professor of medicine in the Division of Sleep Medicine, Perelman School of Medicine at the University of Pennsylvania

Shelby Harris, PsyD, licensed clinical psychologist specializing in behavioral sleep medicine

Jennifer L. Martin, PhD, clinical psychologist, researcher, expert in insomnia disorder, and professor of medicine at the David Geffen School of Medicine at UCLA

Emily Manoogian, PhD, staff scientist at the Salk Institute for Biological Studies who studies chronobiology and human health

Wendy Troxel, PhD, licensed clinical psychologist, senior behavioral and social scientist at RAND, and author of *Sharing the Covers: Every Couple's Guide to Better Sleep*

Why We Need Sleep:
The Health Benefits of Getting Enough Shut-eye

You've undoubtedly heard that sleep affects every organ and system in your body—from your lungs, heart, and brain to your metabolism, immune system, and mood. In fact, getting poor-quality sleep or not getting enough shut-eye on a regular basis increases your risk of many health conditions. But how, exactly, does sleep work to boost your well-being?

Let's walk through some of the biggest benefits of getting enough good-quality shut-eye.

- **It improves cognitive function.** When you sleep, your brain literally goes through a reorganization (neuroplasticity) where it forms new neural connections, eliminates weak or unnecessary ones (synaptic pruning), and consolidates short-term memories into long-term ones. The result? You're better able to learn and recall information, stay focused and efficient when you go about your everyday activities, and be creative.

- **It keeps your immune system functioning optimally.** As you sleep, your body releases cytokines, a type of protein that targets infections and inflammation, reducing your risk of conditions associated with chronic inflammation, such as arthritis, heart disease, and even certain cancers. It also activates T cells, which recognize and remember pathogens that have the potential to make you sick. In fact, just as your brain consolidates memories when you sleep, your immune system creates "memories" of pathogens and consolidates them while you snooze—which means it can launch a faster, more efficient response the next time you encounter that pathogen. Sleep is also when the body repairs and regenerates cells, including your immune cells, which helps keep your immune system in fighting form.

- **It maintains proper blood sugar regulation and balance of hunger hormones**. Blood sugar levels tend to increase at night, and sleep positively impacts a number of factors that affect how the body is able to process glucose surges. For example, we know that getting enough shut-eye keeps cortisol at healthy levels and tamps down inflammation, both of which impact glucose. Sleep also helps keep appetite and satiety where they should be by helping to keep leptin (the hormone that suppresses appetite) and ghrelin (the hormone that stimulates appetite and sends hunger signals to the brain) working optimally. If you don't get enough shut-eye, it can increase ghrelin and lower leptin, prompting you to feel hungrier during the day and eat more as a result.

- **It lowers your risk of heart disease and stroke**. During deep sleep, your blood pressure drops, giving your heart a rest. Sleep well consistently and you can maintain a healthy blood pressure even when you're awake, keeping your risk for heart disease in check.

- **It helps improve your emotional well-being**. Anyone who's ever had a bad night of sleep knows that it can really put you in a bad mood, and chronic sleep issues can lead to depression, anxiety, and an overall sense of irritability. One reason for this is because sleep helps regulate activity in the amygdala, the part of the brain involved in your emotional responses (especially fear and anger). This is why when you get enough sleep, it can make you less reactive and more capable of managing how you respond to what life throws your way. Sleep issues (like waking up very early and having difficulty falling asleep) are also closely linked with depression, and it's a bidirectional relationship: Poor sleep can lead to the development of depression, and having depression makes you more likely to get poor sleep.

- **It helps your body repair itself.** Growth hormones are essential when it comes to muscle growth and tissue repair, and your body's production of these is highest when you sleep. This is one reason why ample shut-eye is so crucial for athletes and why it's incredibly helpful for *all* of us who are moving our bodies to stay healthy. And here's the best part: The more you move, the more likely you are to get better sleep, teeing you up for a positive cycle of snagging the recommended amount of both movement and sleep needed for optimal health.

What Is Sleep? Understanding the Circadian Rhythm, Sleep Stages, and How Much Shut-eye You Really Need

Ever wonder what happens to make you feel sleepy, and then what happens after you drift off? Here's a look at the basics:

- As you go through your day, your body breaks down a molecule called **adenosine triphosphate (ATP)** to use as energy. Another compound, called **adenosine**, is released as a by-product, and it builds up in your brain throughout the day. The more adenosine builds up, the more tired and sleepy you'll feel. This adenosine buildup leads to what experts call "sleep drive"—the longer you're awake, the more pressure you'll feel to sleep. When adenosine levels get high enough, they make you feel sleepy.

- **It starts to get dark outside,** and less light hitting the retinas in your eyes signals the pineal gland in the brain that it's time to start producing melatonin. Melatonin production ramps up as the sun sets, and levels stay high all night long. This "sleep hormone" is released into your bloodstream and sends signals to your body that it's time to wind down.

- **Your body starts to relax, your heart rate slows down, and your breathing becomes more regular.** This is thanks to your parasympathetic nervous system (your rest-and-digest mode) becoming more active to prepare you for sleep.

- **Your body temperature drops slightly,** and this cooling effect helps tell your body that it's time to sleep, which in turn promotes even more drowsiness and helps you drift off. To dissipate heat and help you cool down, your body increases blood flow to your skin and extremities. This is why you might notice that your hands and feet feel warmer as you get into bed at night.

- **Your brain starts releasing certain neurotransmitters and inhibiting others to decrease your alertness and increase muscle relaxation.** For example, your brain releases gamma-aminobutyric acid (GABA), a neurotransmitter that reduces activity in the arousal centers in the brain and sends signals to relax muscles that are essential for posture and limb movements. (This is why we don't act out our dreams.) Levels of other neurotransmitters, like serotonin and norepinephrine, also decrease, which further reduces your mental and physical arousal.

- **While you're sleeping, the space between your brain cells and the blood vessels supplying them (the brain's interstitial space) expands,** allowing cerebrospinal fluid to flush out adenosine and other waste products from the brain to the liver and kidneys for further breakdown and excretion. Research shows that this waste clearance is one factor in preventing neurodegenerative diseases.[3]

- **Your brain starts transitioning from the slow waves of deep sleep to the faster waves of light sleep,** which prepares your brain for consciousness again once you wake up. (We'll go over the stages of sleep next.) As you move into the lighter stage of sleep, your brain starts to process external stimuli—such as sounds, light, and other sensory inputs—more, which can make it easier to wake up.

- **When light hits your eyes in the morning, it quashes melatonin production.** This reduction in melatonin tells your body it's time to wake up. When melatonin is working optimally—rising as the sun sets and falling as the sun rises—it helps synchronize your sleep pattern with the natural cycle of day and night.

- **Those neurotransmitters your brain inhibited to help you fall asleep (namely norepinephrine, serotonin, and dopamine) become more active,** increasing your alertness and preparing your brain to wake up. Your body also releases a surge of cortisol (known as the stress hormone), which helps you feel more awake and ready to start your day.

- **Your body temperature starts to rise,** and the warming effect tells your body it's time to wake up and be more alert.

- **Your heart rate and breathing rate gradually increase,** preparing your body for the increased activity needed when you get out of bed.

It's important to remember that falling asleep is a process. It's okay if you don't fall asleep the moment your head hits the pillow. In fact, if you do, it may be a sign that you're chronically sleep-deprived.

The Sleep Stages, Explained

A sleep cycle is characterized by three stages of non–rapid eye movement (REM) and one stage of REM sleep. Moving through these four stages of sleep (the sleep cycle) takes about 90 to 120 minutes, and ideally, you'll go through four to six cycles across the night. Early in the night, you typically spend more time in stage 3, deep sleep. As the night progresses, you spend more time in REM sleep. After your last REM cycle, you typically wake up feeling rested and alert. This progression through the different sleep stages over the course of the night is known as sleep architecture.

Here, Ilene M. Rosen, MD, MSCE, breaks down what that looks like:

Stage N1: This is the transition between wakefulness and sleep and lasts anywhere from one to seven minutes. It's a light sleep, which means it's easy to wake up during this stage. But if you're undisturbed, you can move quickly into stage 2. During this light stage of sleep, your heart rate, breathing, and eye movements slow as compared with wakefulness, and your muscles relax.

Stage N2: This is when your body temperature drops, your muscles relax even more, and your breathing and heart rate slow down further. Typically, a person spends about half their collective sleep time in N2 sleep.

Stage N3: Known as deep sleep or slow wave sleep, this is when your heart rate and breathing slow to their lowest levels, your muscles are very relaxed, and it can be difficult to wake up even if you need to. This is the most restorative stage of sleep and the one that's needed to feel refreshed when you wake up.

Stage R (REM): REM sleep is characterized by vivid dreaming, when your eyes are moving rapidly from side to side behind closed eyelids but your skeletal muscles are temporarily paralyzed to prevent you from acting out your dreams. (It's known as paradoxical sleep, because even though the brain is active, the body is in a state of deep rest.) Your heart rate and breathing become more irregular and can increase at times.

Sleep disorders, as well as certain lifestyle habits, can alter how much time we spend in each of these sleep stages. For example, drinking alcohol has been shown to suppress REM sleep early in the night and increase the amount of time you spend in the lightest stage of sleep (N1). The frequent arousals and fragmented sleep you might experience if you have sleep apnea often prevent you from spending enough time in stage 3 and REM sleep, meaning you are not getting enough deep sleep, which can lead to feeling exhausted the next day.

How Much Sleep Do You Need?

At different points in our lives, we need a little more or a little less sleep and spend varying amounts of time in each sleep stage. For example, newborns spend far more time in REM sleep than the other stages and can even enter a

REM stage as soon as they fall asleep; older adults tend to spend less time in REM.

What's more, sleep needs vary from person to person. While your best friend might genuinely function well on six or seven hours of shut-eye, you might need nine to feel your best. Here's what the National Sleep Foundation recommends.

AGE	RECOMMENDED HOURS OF SLEEP PER DAY	NUMBER OF HOURS OF SLEEP THAT MAY BE APPROPRIATE
0–3 months	14–17	11–19
4–11 months	12–15, including naps	10–18
1–2 years	11–14, including naps	9–16
3–5 years	10–13, including naps	8–14
6–13 years	9–11	7–12
14–17 years	8–10	7–11
18–25 years	7–9	6–11
26–64 years	7–9	6–10
65 and up	7–8	5–9

Source: National Sleep Foundation[4]

So how can you tell how much sleep *you* need? The next time you're on vacation (or during a stretch of five or so days when you don't have to set an alarm), go to sleep when you feel tired and wake up on your own, and keep track of how many hours of sleep you average, says Shelby Harris, PsyD, who specializes in behavioral sleep medicine. If that's not possible and you have to set an alarm clock to wake up, play around with your bedtime to see what feels best when it comes to hours of sleep. You'll know you've hit your sweet spot when you wake up refreshed and feel energized throughout your day without having to reach for coffee or another caffeinated beverage in the afternoon as a pick-me-up.

Ask an Expert

Should I track my sleep using a wearable device?

First, it's important to be clear about what sleep trackers do and *don't* measure—the most surprising being sleep. They measure how much we move around while we're sleeping, and sometimes heart rate and possibly a few other metrics, like body temperature. That information is then used to estimate whether you're asleep or awake. And while these trackers are pretty good at estimating, they're not good at knowing what type of sleep you're getting (light, deep, or REM) or how long you're staying in each sleep stage. My patients will often say things to me like "My wearable tells me I haven't had REM sleep for six weeks," and I don't believe it.

Where I think a sleep tracker is helpful is if you're wearing one for accountability. Let's say you're trying to stick to a regular sleep schedule. A wearable can really hold you accountable to your goals of going to bed and waking up at certain times. These devices can also be really helpful when it comes to giving you feedback if you're burning the candle at both ends. If you're waking up at 4:00 a.m. to go to the gym, working all day, and having dinner late at night, you're likely going to get some eye-opening data that might inspire you to change some of these habits and prioritize more rest.

The bottom line: If you're looking to use a sleep tracker to crack the minute details of your sleep, don't bother—they're not capable of doing that. If you're going to wear one to monitor behavior changes that you're trying to make in an effort to sleep better, that's useful. But if you start wearing one and your data is stressing you out and causing you to lose sleep—a condition that actually has a name, *orthosomnia*, which is insomnia caused by tracking your sleep—take it off! The goal is for these devices to help you stick to healthy sleep habits, not to mess with your quality or quantity of sleep.

—Jennifer L. Martin, PhD, clinical psychologist, researcher, expert in insomnia disorder, and professor of medicine at the David Geffen School of Medicine at UCLA

Meet Your Body Clock:
Why Your Circadian Rhythm Matters

Almost all living organisms have a clock that runs on an approximately twenty-four-hour cycle set around predictable shifts in the environment, such as light and temperature, called a circadian rhythm (*circadian* is Latin for "about a day"). Humans are no exception. In fact, we don't just have one body clock. Nearly every single *cell* in the human body has a clock that follows a twenty-four-hour rhythm, which tells it when to be active and when to perform a variety of functions.

For example, your blood pressure and heart rate are controlled by a network of biological clocks, which is why they both naturally rise in the afternoon and are lowest when you sleep. The fats circulating in your blood (called triglycerides) rise and fall based on their own clock, which is why you get a peak of these levels in the morning. (Pro tip: If you can, always schedule your checkups or get your blood drawn around the same time of the day to give you the best apples-to-apples comparison of your numbers.)

You can think of these peripheral biological clocks as an anticipatory system that helps your body's various cells and systems do what they need to do when they need to do it, says chronobiologist Emily Manoogian, PhD. But here's the catch: Your body's peripheral clocks don't talk to one another. They coordinate their work thanks to an area of your brain called the suprachiasmatic nucleus (SCN), a cluster of cells located in your hypothalamus. Dr. Manoogian likens the SCN to a symphony conductor and your body's peripheral clocks to instruments. The SCN ensures everyone is playing their parts on time, which makes the music sound good. "If you mess with your SCN, all of your body's peripheral clocks will still beat but on their own time," she says, and the resulting lack of coordination can lead to conflicting cues—and resulting health problems.

One of the primary roles of the SCN is to regulate your sleep-wake cycle. It signals the body when it's time to feel sleepy and when it's time to be alert, in part thanks to its role in releasing melatonin. It regulates those subtle body temperature fluctuations you have throughout the night to promote sleep and wakefulness (remember, your body temperature drops as sleep approaches). And, when consistent, it can improve your sleep architecture, helping you move through an ideal distribution and timing of REM and non-REM sleep throughout the night.

Our circadian rhythms tend to change as we age and move through different hormonal transitions. While young kids go to bed early and wake up with the sun, a teenager's circadian rhythm naturally shifts later, pushing bedtimes and wake times later. (This is why it can feel nearly impossible to get a teen to go to bed before 10:00 p.m., and why there's a big push among circadian rhythm experts for later start times in junior high and high schools.) As we age, our circadian rhythm shifts again, prompting us to get sleepier earlier in the evening and wake up earlier each morning. Interestingly, estrogen tends to speed up our circadian rhythm a little, shifting things so we're more likely to wake up a bit earlier.

As humans evolved, light and food were reliable cues that kept our body clocks working optimally: Light impacts the "master" clock and food impacts most of the peripheral body clocks. If all these cues are working as they should and your SCN is coordinating all your cells' clocks, your body is more likely to operate at its highest level and stay healthy. But these days, light and food are available 24-7. Jet lag, shift work, blue light exposure in the evening, and irregular sleep patterns like staying up late and sleeping in on the weekends (aka social jet lag)—all normalized aspects of modern society—also disrupt our circadian rhythms.

To stay healthy and operate at our best, we need to follow our body's natural rhythms more closely. In fact, research links mood disorders, diabetes, cardiovascular disease, immune disorders, and other chronic diseases to circadian disruption.[5]

The Best Ways to Keep Your Circadian Rhythm Functioning Optimally

So what can we do to tee ourselves up to stay on an ideal schedule?

- **Keep your body on a consistent wake-sleep schedule.** "The circadian rhythm thrives on consistency," says Dr. Manoogian. Choose a bedtime and wake-up time that work for your schedule and stick to them.

- **Get lots of bright, natural sunlight in the morning.** When the sun comes up and the brightness of dawn starts to hit your eyes, that light stops melatonin from flooding your body and gets your body clock on a healthy wake-sleep schedule.

- **Decrease light at night.** Dim or turn off lights you're not using and try to keep screen time to a minimum in the time leading up to when you plan on falling asleep.

- **Stop eating at least three hours before bedtime.** While the exact timing of your meals can vary depending on what works best for you, making sure to finish eating at least three hours before bed gives your digestive system ample time to do its job and then wind down before you drift off, which can help the rest of your body know it's time to fully rest.

- **Avoid vigorous exercise right before bed.** Intense workouts too close to when you want to wind down can raise your body temperature and adrenaline, making it harder to fall asleep. Over time, this can shift your body clock to later bedtimes and wake times. Aim to finish exercise at least three hours before you're planning to fall asleep—though keep in mind that activities like an easy walk or gentle stretching are still okay to do closer to bedtime, especially if they help you relax.

How to Support Your Body's Melatonin Production Without Taking a Supplement

Melatonin is a powerful hormone that tells the body it's time to sleep and regulates the timing of your overall sleep-wake cycle. Inexpensive and easy to find, melatonin supplements are so ubiquitous these days that it can seem as if they're harmless. Yet sleep experts warn against taking them without consulting a medical professional. That's because you can't be sure how much of the synthetic hormone you're actually getting when you buy an OTC supplement. In fact, one study found the concentration of melatonin in more than 70 percent of supplements varied widely from what the labels claimed (from 83 percent less melatonin than the amount listed to 478 percent more).[6]

Thankfully, there's a lot you can do to help your body's own production of this important sleep hormone, says Dr. Manoogian. Here's where to start:

- **Spend fifteen minutes outside in the daylight first thing in the morning.** Go outside without wearing sunglasses (and without looking at the sun!) within thirty minutes to an hour after you wake up. If you can't go outside, sit by a window. Morning light exposure can help reset your internal body clock, signaling that it's time to be awake during the day and to sleep at night.

- **Work near a window during the day, if possible.** Exposure to daylight during the daytime, even if you're not actually outdoors, can go a long way toward helping you produce the ideal amount of melatonin (and at the right time) at night. "Just keep in mind that while direct light is good, looking at a window or getting too much bright light can be hard on your eyes," says Dr. Manoogian.

- **Spend some time outside during dusk, a few hours before bedtime.** Being outside in this natural low light signals to your body that it's time to wind down and prepare for sleep.

- **Dim the lights and eliminate all exposure to blue light at least one to two hours before you want to fall asleep.** Even very low lights can suppress your melatonin secretion, which can shorten the body's perception of night and delay your production of melatonin.

- **Stick to a consistent bedtime and wake-up time, even on weekends.** Going to sleep and waking up around the same time every day helps to regulate your body's master clock, which in turn improves your melatonin production.

Sleep Disorders:
What You Can Do to Prevent and Treat Each

Sleep disorders are twice as common in women as they are in men, and women's symptoms are often overlooked, leading to missed and delayed diagnosis. Knowing some of the most common sleep disorders in women and many of their symptoms can help you identify what may be keeping you from getting enough good-quality shut-eye and know when to seek treatment.

Insomnia

This condition is characterized by difficulty falling asleep, staying asleep, or waking up too early and not being able to drift back to sleep. It often results in poor sleep quality and quantity, leaving you feeling tired, irritable, and not able to function as you'd like to when you're awake. There are two types of insomnia:

- **Acute insomnia** lasts less than three months and is often triggered by stress, big life events, or temporary disruptions in sleep patterns provoked by things like a major job or relationship change.

- **Chronic insomnia** is usually diagnosed when your insomnia occurs at least three times a week for three months or longer, and is often associated with chronic stress, psychological issues, or underlying medical conditions.

SYMPTOMS

- Difficulty falling asleep

- Frequent awakenings during the night and trouble returning to sleep after waking up

- Waking up too early in the morning and not being able to fall back asleep

- Feeling tired and not refreshed when you wake up despite having spent enough time in bed (a sign your sleep isn't restorative)

- Ongoing worries about sleep

- Assessing your sleep hygiene (more on this later) and making changes as necessary

- Cognitive behavioral therapy for insomnia (CBT-I), which is a structured program you do with a licensed CBT-I practitioner that can help you identify thoughts and behaviors that cause or worsen sleep problems and replace them with thoughts and behaviors that can help you sleep

- Relaxation techniques, such as progressive muscle relaxation and breathing exercises to lessen any anxiety you may be feeling around bedtime

- Sleep restriction, where you reduce the time you spend in bed and avoid napping during the day so you get less sleep (and ideally, you're more tired the next night)

- Over-the-counter sleep aids or prescription sleep medications, which can be used for short-term relief.

Obstructive Sleep Apnea (OSA)

With this sleep disorder, the throat muscles intermittently relax and block the airway during sleep, prompting repeated interruptions in breathing that can last from a few seconds to a minute.

It's important to note that after menopause, rates of sleep apnea rise markedly in women—likely because of hormonal changes that lead to a loss of lean muscle mass (including in the airway) and weight gain. What's more, getting a diagnosis can be challenging because our symptoms are often different from (and more subtle than) men's symptoms, says sleep psychologist Jennifer L. Martin, PhD. "Women don't go to their doctor saying, 'I'm told I snore loudly, and I fall asleep when I'm driving home from work,'" she says. "They say things like 'I'm tired all the time and have no energy' or 'I don't feel like I get good-quality sleep,' and their sleep apnea goes undiagnosed."

SYMPTOMS

- Loud snoring, which is caused by the vibration of the soft tissues in the throat as air attempts to pass through a narrowed airway

- Gasping or choking during sleep, or waking up suddenly feeling short of breath or with a choking sensation

- Frequent nighttime awakenings (which you may or may not remember)

- Daytime sleepiness, difficulty concentrating, or mood changes due to fragmented sleep

- Morning headaches, often caused by changes in blood oxygen levels

TREATMENT OPTIONS

- Lifestyle changes, including weight loss, reducing alcohol consumption, quitting smoking, and sleeping on your side

- Using a continuous positive airway pressure (CPAP) machine while you sleep, which delivers air pressure through a mask to keep your airway open and your oxygen levels optimal

- Oral appliances, including custom-fitted devices that reposition your lower jaw and tongue to keep your airway open

- Position changes and sleep aid support pillows to help you maintain a side-sleeping position (to keep you off your back, which can lead to a blocked airway)

- Surgery to remove excess tissue from the throat, reposition the jaw, or implant a device that stimulates the airway muscles to stay open

Restless Legs Syndrome (RLS)

This sleep disorder is characterized by a very strong urge to move the legs, typically during nighttime hours when a person is sitting or lying down—making it difficult to sleep. The condition is more common in women than in

Sleep

men and is especially common before menopause. One reason for this is that RLS is tied to iron deficiency, which is more common in women who are still menstruating.

SYMPTOMS

- Unpleasant sensations in the legs, such as tingling, burning, itching, or throbbing, that usually begin after you've been sitting or lying down for an extended period

- A strong compulsion to move your legs to alleviate discomfort

- Difficulty falling or staying asleep due to symptoms

- Involuntary leg jerks or twitches (aka periodic limb movements) that often happen at night and are temporarily relieved by moving

TREATMENT OPTIONS

- Maintaining a regular sleep schedule and following other good sleep habits (fatigue tends to worsen RLS symptoms)

- Regular, moderate exercise (though excessive exercise may worsen symptoms)

- Reducing or eliminating caffeine, which can worsen symptoms

- Iron supplements for those with low ferritin levels

- Medications, including dopamine agonists (which mimic dopamine's effects in the brain), anticonvulsants (which help tamp down uncomfortable sensations), opioids (used only in severe cases), and benzodiazepines (which are sometimes used for their sleep-inducing and muscle-relaxing effects)

- Alternative therapies, such as massage, warm baths, and compression devices, which can boost blood flow to the legs and help relax muscles

Periodic Limb Movement Disorder (PLMD)

This condition involves repetitive, involuntary movements of the legs and/or arms while you sleep. These movements often include toe and ankle flexing, bending at the knees and/or hips, and kicking. While these bursts of movement tend to disrupt sleep, many with PLMD don't know they have an issue until a bed partner alerts them to their symptoms.

SYMPTOMS

* Noticeable, repetitive jerking or twitching of the legs or arms during sleep

* Frequent awakenings (which you may or may not remember) or fragmented sleep due to limb movements

* Persistent tiredness or sleepiness during the day, despite spending enough time in bed, and mood changes

* Insomnia symptoms due to the frequent movements

TREATMENT OPTIONS

* Many of the same medications and lifestyle changes that are recommended for those with RLS (flip back to page 510 for the list)

* Medications to improve sleep quality by reducing the frequency of limb movements and their associated sleep disruptions

* Treating coexisting sleep disorders, such as sleep apnea

Sleep-Related Eating Disorder (SRED)

This disorder is characterized by episodes of eating during the night while fully or partially asleep, often without any recollection of the event the next morning. It's most common in women under age twenty, though the reasons aren't fully understood. (Many point to hormonal factors, but eating behaviors and higher stress levels may also be at play.) This disorder is often linked to other sleep disorders, such as insomnia and restless legs syndrome, which also tend to be more prevalent in women.

SYMPTOMS

- Recurrent episodes of nighttime eating, often with little or no memory of the eating episodes the following day
- Fragmented sleep patterns and poor sleep quality due to these nighttime awakenings
- Potential gastrointestinal issues, weight gain, and other health consequences due to nighttime consumption of food

TREATMENT OPTIONS

- Medications, including SSRI antidepressants, to help manage symptoms
- Improving sleep habits (such as by maintaining a consistent sleep schedule, avoiding stimulants before going to sleep, and creating a relaxing bedtime routine)
- Managing stress

How to Tell If You Have a Sleep Disorder and If It's Time to See a Specialist

It's normal to have some issues with your sleep every now and then. Sleep can vary from night to night and from person to person, and waking up after you've fallen asleep doesn't signal a problem. In fact, most of us wake up multiple times throughout the night—we just don't remember it later.

If you wake up but you're able to fall asleep again within fifteen minutes or so, it's generally considered okay. But if you wake up and can't get back to sleep, or if you have trouble falling or staying asleep—and this happens multiple nights a week over the course of many weeks and is impacting your ability to get through your days—it's a good idea to seek help.

Diagnosing sleep disorders often involves a combination of a few factors:

- **Your sleep history**, which makes it important to keep a sleep diary for a couple of weeks where you track your bedtimes, wake times, nighttime awakenings, and daytime naps.

- **A medical history and physical evaluation** to identify any underlying health issues that may be contributing to your sleep issues, including blood tests to identify conditions such as iron deficiency or thyroid problems.

- **Specific diagnostic tests**, such as polysomnography (which monitors your sleep stages and cycles), multiple sleep latency test (which measures how quickly you fall asleep during the day and also how quickly REM sleep begins), actigraphy (a device you wear on your wrist for a week or two that tracks movement to estimate sleep and wake patterns), and home sleep apnea testing (a portable breathing monitor you wear overnight).

It's important to bring up your sleep concerns with your primary care physician or other healthcare provider. They can refer you to a sleep medicine specialist who's able to diagnose and treat a wide range of sleep disorders and refer you to other specialists, such as a pulmonologist, neurologist, psychiatrist, psychologist, or otolaryngologist, as needed. When looking for a sleep medicine specialist, aim to see someone who is board certified in sleep medicine by an organization such as the American Board of Sleep Medicine (ABSM).

How Big Hormonal Transitions Can Impact Your Sleep

During times in our lives when we go through significant fluctuations in our reproductive hormones, our ability to get a good night's sleep can be greatly impacted. What's more, women are especially vulnerable to developing insomnia disorder during these times of hormonal upheaval.[7] Here's how the menstrual cycle, as well as disruptions in it, can impact your sleep.

» YOUR PERIOD

During the first half of the menstrual cycle (the follicular phase), estrogen levels rise, which has been linked with better sleep. After ovulation, restless sleep is more common. As estrogen and progesterone decline in the days before menstruation, the quality of the sleep you get may take a hit.[8] Some research shows that if you have premenstrual syndrome (PMS) or premenstrual dysphoric disorder (PMDD), you may be more likely to experience poor sleep in the week leading up to your period than those who don't have these conditions.[9]

» PREGNANCY

When you're expecting, fluctuating hormone levels (as well as general discomfort and other symptoms) can lead to sleep issues. In fact, up to 80 percent of women report getting poor sleep throughout their pregnancies.[10] During the first trimester, a surge of progesterone can actually make you extremely sleepy. However, the hormonal fluctuations you're going through during this time can also lead to nausea, vomiting, back pain, and an urge to urinate frequently throughout the day and night—all of which can lead to broken and lighter sleep throughout the night and an urge to nap during the day.

During the second trimester, sleep may improve as your body adjusts to the big hormonal changes it has gone through. Yet while first-trimester symptoms like morning sickness and vomiting typically resolve once you hit your second trimester, more physical discomfort starts to set in, including heartburn and leg cramps. The third trimester can be especially challenging for sleep, as the growing fetus, back pain, leg cramps, and heartburn can make it difficult to get comfortable enough to sleep well. Anxiety and excitement about the baby's arrival are also a big part of this phase of pregnancy, which can trigger sleep disturbances.

» POSTPARTUM

Many people experience poor sleep quality and get fewer hours of uninterrupted shut-eye after giving birth. Those levels of estrogen and progesterone, which were high during pregnancy, drop rapidly after childbirth, creating a sudden hormonal shift that can disrupt your circadian rhythm and affect your sleep patterns. On the upside, elevated levels of prolactin (which rise to stimulate milk production) are associated with increased sleepiness, helping you fall back asleep after nighttime feedings. That said, those frequent nighttime wakings to feed your baby lead to fragmented sleep, which can cause you to wake up feeling the opposite of refreshed.

That precipitous drop in hormones isn't the only sleep saboteur in the postpartum period: Newborns don't have a strong circadian rhythm (they need feedings around the clock to develop and grow as they should), and *you* are programmed to stay alert-ish 24-7 to make sure your baby is okay. When you consider these factors, it's easy to see how getting deep, restful sleep is often completely out of the question during the weeks after childbirth.

» THE MENOPAUSE TRANSITION

In the years leading up to menopause, estrogen and progesterone levels fluctuate wildly until they drop significantly and remain at their postmenopausal low levels. This decline can cause a number of physical and emotional symptoms that affect sleep. Lower levels of estrogen can lead to hot flashes during the night (night sweats), which are often intense enough to disrupt sleep. As estrogen wanes, your muscles lose estrogen's protective powers and muscle tone goes down—including in the muscles of the airway, which can impede breathing when sleeping and cause obstructive sleep apnea. Lower progesterone levels can lead to difficulty falling and staying asleep, as well as lighter, more fragmented sleep. Fluctuating hormone levels can also contribute to mood disorders, such as anxiety and depression, which are associated with sleep disturbances.

Ask an Expert

My significant other keeps me up at night, but it makes me sad to think about getting a "sleep divorce" and sleeping in separate bedrooms. What should we do?

Sleeping next to a close and trusted significant other can be incredibly beneficial. For many people, it can elicit many positive emotional and physiological benefits that can *help* you sleep. That said, sleeping next to someone can also lead to sleep problems. We see this most obviously when one partner is a snorer and keeps their bed partner awake. In fact, women who are partnered with a snorer are three times more likely to have insomnia compared with women who are paired with a nonsnorer.

For many years, there was no science behind shared sleep, so we just followed the *should*s. Many of us thought, *We're married, so we should sleep in the same bed. We're a couple, so we should go to bed and wake up at the same time.* Now we know better.

If you're struggling to get quality sleep when sleeping next to someone, it's important to identify what your issues are and then talk about how you can share important ritual time in bed without forcing yourselves to sleep in the same bed or at the same time. Using "I" statements is key when you have this discussion. You might say, "I'm not sleeping well, and because of that, I can't be the partner I want to be." With a statement like that, you're not blaming or nagging; you're setting the tone for how to address this as a "we" problem. And while the term *sleep divorce* has become popular, what you're really doing is creating an alliance around sleep because it's so foundational to the quality of your relationship.

In some cases, sleeping in separate bedrooms may be the answer. Or maybe one partner needs to wear a sleep mask or earplugs. Perhaps buying a new mattress that dampens the feeling of motion will help you sleep next to a restless bed partner. Maybe one of you needs to be evaluated and treated for a sleep disorder, which could be the root of the problem for both of you. Doing this kind of problem-solving with your significant other is a sign of a healthy relationship.

The bottom line: It's okay to talk to your bed partner about your sleep disturbances and work together to find strategies that are going to help you get the sleep you need to support your health and your relationship.

—Wendy Troxel, PhD, licensed clinical psychologist, senior behavioral and social scientist at RAND, and author of *Sharing the Covers: Every Couple's Guide to Better Sleep*

Your Game Plan: The Tactics That Really Work to Help You Get Better Sleep

Making sure you're getting enough good-quality sleep is crucial for your health. And yet most of us receive little education about all the things we can do to set ourselves up for the best shut-eye possible. Dr. Shelby Harris is on a mission to change that. Here, she shares exactly where to start for better, deeper sleep.

Avoid the biggest sleep stealers. Following all the best sleep hygiene practices won't be helpful if you don't avoid some of the most common sleep saboteurs, including:

- **Consuming caffeine too late in the day**, thanks to its half-life of about six hours, which means that six hours after you have that coffee, soda, or tea, only half the caffeine has been eliminated from your body.

- **Drinking alcohol or eating a meal within three hours of bedtime**, which may induce sleep but is also likely to disrupt your sleep as your body works hard to metabolize the alcohol and/or food.

- **Trying to fall asleep in a room that's too hot**, which can prevent your body temperature from naturally dropping. In fact, if you like to take a warm shower or bath before bedtime, make sure it's at least 1.5 to 2 hours before you get into bed, to give your body enough time to cool down before you drift off.

- **Noise, especially if it's loud or irregular**—like the banging of a radiator or a snoring bed partner.

- **Daytime naps that are longer than twenty minutes**, which can let out some of the "sleep pressure" that builds during the day, making it tougher to fall asleep at night.

Get choosy about your before-bed screen time. Even more important than the blue light exposure you get from the TV and other screens before bed is *what* you're looking at on those screens, says Dr. Harris. "If you're doomscrolling or watching something that's going to stress you out or keep you hooked in—like your social media feeds, which are meant to be addictive— it's more likely to keep you awake longer than if you're watching something that relaxes you."

Stick to a relatively regular bedtime and wake-up schedule. Set alarms for both bedtime and wake-up, seven days a week. This is key when it comes to optimizing your circadian rhythm, and it's especially important if you're struggling with sleep issues. "Find something that motivates you to get up in the morning, even on weekends, when you may be tempted to sleep in," says Dr. Harris. Schedule a walk with a friend. Create a coffee ritual you really look forward to.

And try to resist "revenge bedtime procrastination," a new term for an age-old scenario where you're so busy throughout your day that you get de-fiant at night, desperate to steal back some time just for you. Because many of us watch a favorite TV show during this time, Dr. Harris's favorite tip is to turn off autoplay on streaming services.

"If you turn off that function, it forces you to make a conscious decision as to whether you're going to watch the next episode, which is often enough to give you that little pause to ask yourself, 'Do I want to choose sleep, or do I want to watch another show?'" says Dr. Harris. "If you choose to watch an-other episode, that's fine every once in a while!" But that pause will help you make it the exception, not the norm.

If you're having sleep issues, focus on better *quality* sleep first, then *quantity*. It can be easy to get discouraged (and anxious) if you're experiencing acute or chronic insomnia or another sleep disorder is keeping you from getting the recommended seven to nine hours a night. But rather than trying to get more sleep by getting into bed earlier, it's better to start by improving how *well* you're sleeping—which means falling asleep within fifteen minutes or so, being able to fall back asleep quickly if you wake up in the middle of the night, and feeling refreshed when you get out of bed in the morning.

"I'd rather see you start getting six hours of *good* sleep a night than be in bed for eight hours but report feeling frustrated, anxious, or like you didn't sleep well," Dr. Harris says. It sounds counterintuitive, but spending less time in bed helps you build up sleep pressure and makes it more likely you'll fall asleep more easily and get into a deeper sleep after nighttime awakenings. If you're still having trouble sleeping well, see a sleep specialist.

Consider cognitive behavioral therapy for insomnia (CBT-I). This type of talk therapy uses a range of cognitive and behavioral techniques (like reframing negative thought patterns, practicing mindfulness, changing bedtime routines, and tracking sleep) and has been proven to improve sleep and reduce anxiety. CBT-I can be effective whether you're dealing with short-term or chronic insomnia and typically works over the course of just six to eight sessions.

• • • • •

Once you understand the many factors that can impact your ability to get a good night's rest and learn some of the evidence-based tactics proven to improve sleep, you can pinpoint the challenges getting in your way and start to implement changes that can help you get the shut-eye you need to feel your best.

Chapter 19

Exercise

How to Improve Your Health at Every Stage of Your Life Through Movement

> Women have never been given the space to test their potential and to set their own benchmarks without the weight of expectations that have been tainted by what men have accomplished or misconceptions about women's bodies. What could women achieve if they were given a blank slate and nothing to compare themselves to? What if women were given the freedom to launch an entirely different athletic trajectory than men?
>
> —Christine Yu, *Up to Speed: The Groundbreaking Science of Women Athletes*

You've probably heard many times how crucial exercise is for your health. That's because it's true. There's overwhelming evidence proving its many upsides, from boosting cardiovascular and bone health to reducing stress, increasing energy, helping you sleep and maintain a healthy weight, and so much more. The Academy of Medical Royal Colleges has even gone so far as to call exercise a "miracle cure."[1]

And while research on female athletic performance is still woefully lacking—only 6 percent of sports science studies are focused exclusively on women, and transgender athletes are largely left out of these studies[2]—there are a growing number of exercise scientists, researchers, and clinicians helping to translate the information we *do* have into actionable advice for women of all ages. That's what we'll explore in the pages that follow.

In this chapter, we'll learn . . .

- **What happens when we exercise, and why movement improves so many health outcomes.** When you know the mechanism behind the health-boosting powers of working out, you may find yourself even more motivated to start or stick to a fitness routine.

- **The inner workings of our skeletal muscle**, a highly specialized and dynamic tissue in the body that's continuously breaking down and growing anew.

- **The types of exercises you'll hear most about**, and what you should know about each. From strength training to "zone 2 cardio," we'll cover the details that'll help you translate the (often contradictory!) fitness advice you'll undoubtedly receive and apply it to your life.

- **Some of the female-specific factors that can influence exercise performance**—from your menstrual cycle to your muscle fibers—and how to work with these sex differences to optimize the time you spend moving your body.

- **How your exercise routine needs to change during big hormonal transitions**, such as puberty, pregnancy, the postpartum period, and menopause.

- **The tools you need to build a fitness foundation that'll tee you up for a lifetime of feeling good in your body.** You'll finish this chapter knowing how to create an exercise routine that'll help you achieve your goals, avoid the most common injuries in women, and fuel your workouts with the right types and amounts of food.

Meet the Experts

Mallory Boyd, ACSM, clinical exercise physiologist certified by the American College of Sports Medicine

Michelle Gray, PhD, professor of exercise science at the University of Arkansas, Fayetteville

Suzanne Steinbaum, DO, cardiologist specializing in preventive care, author of *Dr. Suzanne Steinbaum's Heart Book: Every Woman's Guide to a Heart-Healthy Life*, and founder and CEO of Adesso by Heart-Tech Health, a med-tech innovation for women's cardiovascular prevention, health, and wellness

Hannah Cabré, PhD, RDN, postdoctoral fellow at the Pennington Biomedical Research Center at Louisiana State University

Megan Roche, MD, PhD, health and performance consultant and cofounder of Huzzah, a platform that breaks down female athlete health and performance science and builds scholarships for athletes and teams

Emily Kraus, MD, sports medicine physician and clinical assistant professor and director of the FASTR Program (Female Athlete Science and Translational Research) at Stanford University School of Medicine

Katie Hirsch, PhD, assistant professor in the Department of Exercise Science at the University of South Carolina, Arnold School of Public Health

Sabrena Jo, PhD, exercise physiologist and liaison to the scientific advisory panel at the American Council on Exercise

Rx Exercise: How Movement Can Help You Stave Off Disease and Optimize Your Health

Getting regular exercise—or even simply incorporating more movement into your everyday life—is often among the top pieces of advice when it comes to improving your overall health. And here's the best part: Exercise doesn't have to mean expensive gym memberships, hiring a personal trainer, or going to an intense cardio class. Sure, it can involve lifting heavy weights at a gym. But at its heart, exercise is movement—which means activities like walking, dancing to your favorite music, and even playing with kids all count. And that's something that's accessible to all of us, doesn't have to cost a thing, and really does have health-boosting benefits.

The Biggest Benefits of Exercise, Explained

For far too long, the benefits of exercise tended to focus on one thing: looking good. Yes, exercise can help you build muscle, lose excess body fat, and "recomp" your body—a phrase increasingly being used to describe the process of losing fat while gaining muscle. But the upsides of regular exercise span way beyond the aesthetic results. Here, exercise physiologist Mallory Boyd, ACSM, walks us through what happens when we move our bodies—and the health benefits that result:

- **Your heart health improves**. Your heart rate increases in order to pump more blood to the muscles you're working so they get the oxygen and nutrients they need to fuel them for the task at hand. This prompts your blood vessels to dilate so blood flow can get to the muscles you're working—and this dilation is great for your heart's vasculature, especially if you're a woman. That's because as we age and estrogen decreases, the blood vessels in and around our heart get stiffer. With moderate-intensity exercise, the arteries can fill to their maximum capacity, which keeps them flexible and makes them less likely to develop plaque. Over time, your heart has to work less to deliver oxygen because it's able to squeeze out more blood per beat, thanks to how well the arteries dilate. This improved blood flow reduces the workload on the heart and lowers both your blood pressure and your resting heart rate—which means your heart doesn't have to work as hard when you're *not* exercising.

- **Your blood sugar works as it was intended**. As you move your body and your muscles start to contract, they need glucose for power. That glucose is stored in the muscle tissue itself. But once those stores are used up, your muscles draw the additional energy they need from glucose circulating in your bloodstream, which in turn helps to lower blood glucose levels. This is why regular exercise improves insulin sensitivity and helps cells take in glucose more effectively, ultimately reducing blood sugar levels.

- **Your brain health gets a boost.** Exercise increases blood flow to the brain, which can improve things like your memory and mental sharpness and reduce your risk of cognitive decline as you age. In fact, one large study found that cognitive decline is about twice as common among older adults who aren't active compared with ones who are.[3]

- **Your muscles get stronger.** If you're lifting weights or doing high-intensity interval training, the stress on your muscles creates microscopic tears in muscle fibers. These microtears are an intentional (and ultimately beneficial!) form of injury, which prompts your immune system to launch an inflammatory response and initiate the repair and regrowth process in those damaged muscle fibers. (This is why you feel sore after exercise—it's those proinflammatory cytokines flooding the muscles you worked so hard.) Satellite cells, a type of stem cell located on the outer surface of muscle fibers, get activated after those microtears in the muscles occur, which prompts them to multiply and fuse with existing muscle fibers to repair the damage and grow the muscle (this growth is called hypertrophy). This process is known as muscle protein synthesis (MPS). When MPS outpaces muscle protein breakdown (MPB), your muscles grow—which you feel as increased strength.

- **Your bones get stronger.** Movements that prompt your muscles to pull on your bones—such as when you lift weights—are a good type of stress: When the bone senses this pulling, the change in pressure and tension triggers a chemical reaction that activates osteoblasts (cells responsible for bone formation) and osteoclasts (which break down bone tissue to make sure bone mass is optimally distributed according to the demands placed on it). This osteoblast and osteoclast activity is like a remodeling that makes your bones stronger and denser, particularly in areas that experience frequent and intense stress. And the stronger your muscles get over time, the harder they pull on your bones—and the more bone growth you'll experience. Good muscle tone also helps stabilize the body's joints, which can improve range of motion and help keep you pain free.

- **Your immune system gets stronger.** All that increased blood flow you get when you exercise means more movement of immune cells (which travel in your blood) throughout your body. This makes your immune cells likely to detect and respond to pathogens more efficiently. Exercise also stimulates the lymphatic system, which transports immune cells and removes toxins and waste from the body.

- **You get better, deeper sleep.** Exercise helps regulate your circadian rhythm, the body's internal clock that dictates your sleep-wake cycle. When your circadian rhythm is working optimally, you're more likely to fall asleep easily at bedtime, stay asleep during the night, and wake up feeling rested and refreshed. What's more, regular exercise may help you get more slow-wave sleep (aka deep sleep), which is the most restful sleep phase and when your muscles and bones repair most efficiently.

- **You get an immediate (and lasting) mood boost.** When you exercise, your brain releases endorphins—natural mood lifters that reduce how intensely we perceive pain and induce feelings of euphoria (hence the "runner's high" you've likely heard of). Exercise also increases levels of the neurotransmitters serotonin and norepinephrine, both of which play key roles in mood regulation, and it gives you a dopamine boost as well, which improves motivation and pleasure. Turns out these immediate, happy-making effects of exercise can have a long-term impact.

A Closer Look at Your Muscles: What They Are and How They Work

Most of us tend to think of our muscles in pretty simple terms when it comes to exercise: We use them to run and jump, squat and lift, and push and pull heavy things. Yet our muscles are these incredibly specialized and dynamic tissues in our bodies that continuously break down and regrow. Knowing the basics of how they work—and how they change over time—can help you optimize your exercise of choice, prevent injuries, and maintain your independence as you age.

The first thing to know is that there are three types of muscle:

- **Skeletal muscle**, which are the muscles that attach to your bones by tendons and allow you to move. These muscles are voluntary, which means you control how and when they work. You use skeletal muscle to do things like lift your arms or take a walk.

- **Smooth muscle**, which lines your organs (except the heart), blood vessels, digestive tract, and more. Smooth muscles are involuntary, which means your autonomic nervous system controls them without your having to think about it. They help to do things like keeping your digestion working well and blood pumping throughout your body.

- **Cardiac muscle**, which makes up the entire heart and also works under involuntary control. It helps keep your heart beating without your doing anything or even knowing about it.

Skeletal muscle is what we'll look more closely at here, because it's what we try to strengthen when we exercise.

» HOW DO SKELETAL MUSCLES WORK?

Muscle cells—commonly referred to as muscle fibers—tighten (aka contract) to allow the muscle to move your bones so you can perform a vast range of movements. Each muscle is attached to a bone by a tendon, a fibrous, cord-like tissue that acts as a "mechanical bridge" to transfer muscle force to bones and joints and help muscles complete their movement.

Proteins in those muscle fibers (known as actin and myosin) slide past each other to produce muscle contractions. Your muscles are constantly turning over and remodeling muscle proteins to keep your muscles healthy (a process called muscle protein synthesis). At the same time, muscle is also continuously breaking down (a process called muscle protein degradation).

"This happens over and over in all of us—little kids, middle-aged people, older adults, all of us—every single day," says Michelle Gray, PhD, professor of exercise science. When muscle protein synthesis exceeds muscle protein breakdown, muscles grow. When the opposite is true and degradation exceeds synthesis—something that naturally happens as we age if we don't do something about it—muscles atrophy or get smaller. "The goal is for both muscle protein synthesis and muscle protein degradation to remain stable all your life," says Dr. Gray. "This doesn't happen unless we exercise and maintain proper nutrition."

» WHY WE LOSE MUSCLE AS WE AGE

Age-related loss of muscle mass and a resulting loss of strength is a condition known as sarcopenia. Why does this happen? Decline in activity, inadequate nutrition, and increased inflammation likely contribute. Changes in hormone levels can also lead to changes in how efficiently and effectively muscles contract, which can contribute to muscle loss. For example:

- Testosterone (which steadily declines as we age) plays an important role in protein synthesis.

- Estrogen (which drops precipitously during the menopause transition) is crucial in helping myosin and actin bind together to generate a strong force when muscles contract.

As these hormones decrease, skeletal muscle is greatly impacted. The antidotes?

- **Exercise that works your muscles to the point of prompting microtears in your skeletal muscle** and, as a result, muscle growth. "To maintain consistent growth of muscle, we need progressive overload, which means gradually lifting more and more weight," says Dr. Gray.

- **Eat enough protein** so your body has ample stores of this important macronutrient for your muscles to draw on for protein synthesis (and its resulting muscle growth). Pro tip: Spread out your protein intake throughout the day, especially as you get older. As we age, the digestive tract is able to process only about thirty grams of protein at a time, says Dr. Gray, so you're better off aiming to get a good amount of protein every time you eat rather than eating the majority of it later in the day.

Ask an Expert

Why is everyone talking about the importance of grip strength, and should I be focused on improving mine?

In recent years, hand grip strength has been called a key vital sign, and many healthcare professionals use it when assessing muscle function and overall physical capability—areas of health that are particularly important to stay on top of as we age. In one multi-country study of about 140,000 adults between ages thirty-five and seventy, grip strength was strongly correlated with physical health.[4]

Grip strength is measured using a handheld device called a dynamometer (aka dyno), which gives you a reading when squeezed. The average healthy grip strength for men is about seventy-two pounds, and for women it's around forty-four pounds, and research shows grip strength is a good proxy for overall health.

But the word *proxy* is key here: Grip strength is simply a measure for overall muscle strength. Improvement in grip strength alone isn't going to improve your overall health, and it's not something you need to focus on improving with specific exercises, such as the farmer's carry (where you grab a pair of dumbbells and walk with them). Your better bet: Focus on overall body strength and there's a good chance the next grip-strength test you take will improve.

If you've never had your grip strength tested but you'd like to gauge your physical function, try an at-home exercise test called the Eight Foot Up and Go. Here's how to do it: Put a straight-back chair that doesn't swivel against a wall and a cone (or other object) eight feet in front of the edge of the chair. Then sit on the front edge of the chair with your feet flat on the floor and time yourself as you get up, walk quickly (not running) around the cone, and sit back down. If you can do this in about six seconds, your physical function is optimal.

—Michelle Gray, PhD, professor of exercise science at the University of Arkansas, Fayetteville

How to Train Like a Girl: Optimize the Way You Move

There are many types of exercise—and experts agree that all movement is beneficial. Yet with so much contradictory information about the "best" way to work out, it can be tough to know where to start. Here's an overview of some of the training styles you'll hear about the most, and what to consider about each so you can figure out what your body needs in any given moment.

Zone 2 Training

What it is: Aerobic exercise (aka cardio) that's often referred to as happening at a "talking pace," where you can hold a conversation with someone while you walk, ride a bike, or do any movement that gets your heart rate up but that you can do comfortably and without being breathless. Exercising at moderate intensity increases the capacity of your heart's ventricles to fill with blood. The more easily they dilate, the more pliable they stay—and the less likely you are to suffer from cardiovascular disease, says cardiologist Suzanne Steinbaum, DO.

What women need to know: Zone 2 training is great for improving heart health (which is especially important for women, as heart disease is our leading cause of death), helping you recover from other workouts (such as strength training), and allowing you to be social while you get your movement in. High-intensity workouts can help increase cardiovascular fitness, but only after you've reached a good level of cardiovascular conditioning.

Strength Training (aka Resistance Training or Weight Training)

What it is: Exercise that involves using resistance to induce the contraction of muscles, which builds strength. It can involve the use of free weights (like dumbbells, barbells, and kettlebells), resistance machines, body-weight exercises, and/or resistance bands. By asking your muscles to push, pull, and/or lift something heavy, you make them work against a force, prompting them to contract. Gradually increasing the resistance or load forces your muscles to adapt, which leads to muscle growth and increased strength over time.

What women need to know: Estrogen plays a key role in protecting muscle in women. One way it does this is by keeping the satellite cells in your muscles—the ones that respond to the stress you put on your muscles when you push, pull, or lift heavy things—working optimally. When estrogen is reliably high (before the menopause transition), traditional strength training—say, doing three sets of eight to twelve repetitions lifting a moderately heavy weight—should lead to muscle gains. However, as estrogen goes down during perimenopause and after menopause, your muscles' satellite cells don't react as quickly and strongly to the stresses you place on them—and you start to need greater stresses (heavier weights) to get the same muscle-building results, says Hannah Cabré, PhD, RDN. For example, aim to lift a heavy enough weight that you can do just four to six repetitions with good form, and repeat that for three sets.

Need more inspiration to strength train? As you age, your body starts storing fat in your muscle cells so they have a readily available source of energy for intense or prolonged bouts of exercise. But if you're not asking your muscles to work hard (such as during strength training), the fat builds up in your muscles, which weakens them over time.

High-Velocity Resistance Training

What it is: A form of strength training where the goal is to move a moderate to low load of weight as quickly as possible during the lifting phase of a resistance exercise, when muscles shorten while under load (the concentric phase) and then lower the weight down more slowly as the muscle lengthens again (the eccentric phase). By emphasizing speed during the contraction portion of resistance exercises, you improve your nervous system's ability to recruit motor units efficiently, which improves the coordination and strength of muscle contractions. You'll also recruit fast-twitch muscle fibers, which are the ones responsible for generating high force and power but which fatigue quickly. Over time, this allows your muscles to generate maximum force in minimal time.

What women need to know: Women generally have a lower proportion of fast-twitch muscle fibers than men, and as we age our muscle loss mostly occurs in this type of muscle fiber. Adding high-velocity resistance training into your exercise routine can counter this phenomenon, helping you maintain muscle mass. If you decide to experiment with this type of training, be sure to move quickly only during the lifting, concentric phase of an exercise. Moving quickly on the muscle-lengthening eccentric phase can increase your risk for injury.

High-Intensity Interval Training, or HIIT (aka Sprint Interval Training)

What it is: A form of cardiovascular exercise that alternates between short bursts of intense movement (high-intensity intervals) and periods of lower-intensity movement or rest that should help you recover enough that you're able to do your high-intensity intervals at full intensity. During those intense intervals, you're working at a near-maximum effort for somewhere between twenty seconds and a few minutes. This induces significant stress on your heart and muscles, which prompts adaptations that boost your health over time. It also improves mitochondrial function in muscles (which improves strength and endurance) and helps improve insulin sensitivity.

What women need to know: Estrogen improves how efficiently our muscles use the glucose floating around our bloodstream. When estrogen is high before menopause, it helps make cells sensitive to insulin (which acts like a key to let glucose into your body's cells, where it can be used as energy) and enhances glucose uptake into your muscles. After menopause, this insulin sensitivity goes down—and one of the best ways to counter this is by doing short bursts of intense exercise (like HIIT).

These exercises place a big demand on your muscles, essentially prompting them to say, "Hey! I need glucose to do what you're asking me to do!" As a result, HIIT work prompts your body to use that glucose floating around your bloodstream and shuttle it into your muscles so they have the energy they need. Over time, HIIT sessions create adaptations in your muscles that improve their ability to take up glucose from the bloodstream even when you're not exercising.

Functional Training

What it is: Exercises that focus on training the body for activities performed in everyday life, which often involve building strength, coordination, balance, and flexibility. This style of training includes multijoint movements, balance and coordination, core strengthening and stability, and common movement patterns (such as lifting, reaching, twisting, pushing, pulling, and squatting). Exercises often include squats, lunges, and push-ups—which translate to movements like sitting, standing, lifting, and pushing.

By working out in a way that mimics activities of daily living, you're able to perform those tasks with more ease and efficiency, ultimately reducing your risk of injury while also building overall strength and endurance.

What women need to know: Given our increased risk of bone loss (and consequent fracture risk) as we age, functional training is particularly important and can be a great place to start if you're not already doing other forms of strength training regularly.

Jump Training (aka Plyometrics)

What it is: A type of high-intensity exercise that involves explosive movements—usually jumping or hopping movements that engage multiple muscle groups at the same time—designed to increase power, speed, and strength. By jumping, you're asking your body to generate force quickly. This explosive movement prompts your fast-twitch muscle fibers to spring into action, which strengthens them over time. It's also a good type of multidirectional stress to your bones, which stimulates osteoblasts (those cells responsible for bone formation), which can help increase your overall bone density.

What women need to know: Jumping has been shown to improve bone density, which is something women especially need to be aware of. One study of premenopausal women found that jumping ten to twenty times a day significantly improved bone density in the hips after just four months, with the biggest gains seen in those who did the most jumping.[5]

Keep in mind, however, that if you've already been diagnosed with osteopenia (lower-than-normal bone mineral density) or osteoporosis (severely reduced bone density), it's important to talk to your clinician before starting to incorporate jump training into your routine. And no matter how fit you already are, the explosive, high-intensity nature of plyometric exercises means it's crucial to do them correctly and with good form, which is why you'll want to start slowly and build up over time.

Ask an Expert

Can I maximize my workouts based on my menstrual cycle?

Cycle syncing is the idea of matching different workout styles or approaches to what phase of the menstrual cycle you're in. The thought is that hormonal fluctuations throughout your cycle can influence strength, endurance, and recovery—and that by syncing your training plan with these changes, you can optimize performance.

Yet the data we have shows no significant changes in strength, endurance, or recovery across the phases of the menstrual cycle. Plus, there are hundreds of different variables that feed into optimizing training. Did your kids wake you up in the middle of the night? Are you stressed about a big work deadline? These are part of a broader scope of variables that also have an impact on your training. If you're trying to tweak how you work out based on just *one* variable—your menstrual cycle—you risk missing the bigger picture of other things that have an impact, too.

I'm a clinician and a coach. The menstrual cycle is something I talk about with my athletes—and a lot of them *do* feel some changes during their cycle. It's always helpful to tune in to your body, and it can be empowering to track your cycle and understand it. But I also remind my athletes that if they're competing, they'll likely have to compete during all phases of their menstrual cycle, which means you want to train across all phases of the menstrual cycle so you're able to perform well no matter what your hormones are doing.

The body knows movement; it doesn't know perfection. Go ahead and track your cycle and symptoms, listen to how you feel, and let that help direct your training. If cycle syncing makes you overthink your workouts as you try to match the exact right workout style to the phase of your cycle, it could be holding you back. If it helps you sneak in some movement even if you're dealing with bad PMS symptoms, that's a win.

—Megan Roche, MD, PhD, health and performance consultant and cofounder of Huzzah, a platform that breaks down female athlete health and performance science and builds scholarships for athletes and teams

Staying Injury-Free: Preventing the Most Common Exercise Injuries in Women

Getting injured is a surefire way to keep yourself sidelined from your favorite activities. Here, sports medicine physician Emily Kraus, MD, explains some of the most common overuse injuries in women and the best ways to protect your body from each.

Knee Issues (Including ACL Tears and Kneecap Pain)

If it seems like you know more women than men who've experienced knee pain or had some sort of knee surgery, you're not imagining things: Women are up to eight times more likely than men to tear their anterior cruciate ligament (ACL).[6] We're also more likely to deal with patellofemoral pain syndrome (PFPS)—aka runner's knee—which is pain in the front of the knee and around the kneecap (aka the patella) that often intensifies when the knee is flexed or bent during weight-bearing activities.

One reason for this is that women tend to have wider hips than men, which means the angle between our quadriceps and our knees—aka the Q-angle—is greater. This makes us more prone to our knees tilting inward and our feet being pronated, which means our body weight is more on the insides of the feet rather than evenly distributed. This can cause pain and structural problems over time. Women also have less muscle mass around our knees than our male counterparts and tend to have stronger quadriceps than hamstrings, combinations that can lead to knee instability. And our often hypermobile joints also make it so that the kneecap—which protects your knee joint and supports the muscles, tendons, and ligaments in your leg—is more vulnerable to slipping out of place.

How to prevent knee injuries: A combination of strength and flexibility exercises along with proper technique can help you stabilize the knee joints. For example, exercises like dead lifts, squats, lunges, and glute bridges can strengthen all the muscles surrounding the knee, providing better support and stability. Dynamic stretching movements such as leg swings, walking lunges, and high knees can also help prepare your muscles and joints for physical activity. And learning proper technique and biomechanics (things like landing with your knees slightly bent and avoiding excessive inward knee movement), especially when doing high-impact exercises, can reduce your risk of knee pain and injury.

Bone Stress Injuries (aka Stress Reactions or Stress Fractures)

This type of injury occurs when a bone is subjected to repetitive stress over time, exceeding its ability to repair and adapt. It can range in severity from a mild injury with bone microdamage to a more severe injury with a visible fracture line on imaging. A bone stress injury often occurs due to a sudden increase in activity (or a change in the intensity, duration, or frequency of exercise), poor training techniques, inadequate equipment (such as improper footwear), or conditions that cause low bone mineral density, such as relative energy deficiency in sport. Signs of a bone stress injury include pain that develops gradually, intensifies with weight-bearing activities, and gets better with rest; swelling and tenderness; bruising; and a decreased ability to do your go-to physical activities due to your pain.

Women are more likely than men to develop a bone stress injury in our lifetime due to a combination of anatomical, hormonal, and nutritional factors. Women are subject to more hormonally induced changes to bone, especially during puberty and perimenopause. Reduced estrogen levels as we age and during menstrual cycle irregularities (especially amenorrhea) can lead to decreased bone density and an increased risk of bone stress injuries. And not getting adequate nutrition, whether due to dietary restrictions or eating disorders (common among female athletes), also increases the risk of low bone mineral density and bone stress injuries.

How to prevent bone stress injuries: Building a strong foundation in training is key. Increase the intensity, duration, and frequency of your workouts gradually over time. This gives your bones the opportunity to adapt to the increased stress. Adding variety to your workouts, where you incorporate low-impact activities (like swimming and cycling) into a routine of higher-intensity exercises (like strength training and HIIT workouts) will help you maintain your overall fitness while giving specific bones and muscles ample periods to recover. Also, make sure you're using proper technique and equipment and that you're eating enough food (and the right balance of nutrients at the right times) to support bone density and strength. Incorporating strength training into your routine is also valuable for bone health because it can strengthen the muscles that stabilize bones while also contributing to overall bone mineral density.

Ankle Sprains

This happens when the ligaments that support and stabilize the ankle stretch beyond their limits and tear, causing pain or tenderness, swelling, weakness, muscle spasms, and/or cramping. Female athletes suffer from ankle sprains more often than males, likely due to higher joint and ligament laxity of the outer side of the ankle, which can cause increased range of motion of the ankle joint; variations in hormone levels when puberty begins, which can impact ligament strength; and/or underlying biomechanical differences of the ankle joint when it moves. Translation: If you turn your ankle when walking or running or land in a way that prompts your foot to roll inward or outward even slightly, the ligaments surrounding your ankle may not be able to hold it in place, and you'll be more likely to roll it and stretch those already-lax ankle ligaments even more, possibly causing a more severe tear.

How to prevent ankle sprains: Strengthening the muscles around the ankle with things like calf raises, ankle circles, and balance exercises helps you feel more stability in your ankle joint and feet and reduces your risk of ankle sprains. Wearing the right footwear or ankle support (which, in some cases, may mean custom orthotics or an ankle brace to help correct biomechanical imbalances) can also help prevent ankle injuries.

Plantar Fasciitis

The plantar fascia is the thick band of tissue that runs along the bottom of your foot and connects your heel bone to your toes, supporting your foot's arch. If this ligament becomes inflamed due to repetitive stress and overuse, it can cause intense heel pain, especially when you take your first steps in the morning after a night's sleep or after long periods of standing or sitting.

Women tend to have higher arches than men and different foot shapes, which can influence how pressure is distributed across the foot. Wearing heels or other nonsupportive footwear can also place stress on the plantar fascia that can alter the natural biomechanics of your foot. If this happens— and then you do a high-impact activity like running, jumping, or another activity that places repetitive stress on your feet—it can make your feet more susceptible to injury.

How to prevent plantar fasciitis: Wearing shoes that provide good arch support and cushioning (both when you're exercising and in everyday life) can help distribute pressure more evenly across your feet and reduce the risk of plantar fasciitis. Strengthening the muscles of your feet and lower legs can provide better support and stability in your arches, and regular stretching of the calf muscles, Achilles tendons, and plantar fascia can improve your flexibility.

Ask an Expert

I know stretching is important, but should I do it before or after exercise—and how should I approach it?

Before you exercise, a dynamic warm-up is the best way to optimize mobility and reduce overall injury risks, especially if you've experienced an injury in the past and want to keep that potential weak spot from being painful or problematic again when you're exercising.

Here's the key: The dynamic warm-up you choose should be based on the sport or exercises you're about to do. For example, if you're going for a run, you'll want to activate the muscles you'll use when you're running, such as the quads and hamstrings. If you're doing a sport like pickleball or tennis, you'll want to do some lower-body warm-ups as well as some upper-body mobility and multidirectional movements that mimic the ones you'll do when you're on the court. It doesn't have to be rapid movements, but you want to do more than touch your toes!

After your workout, it's a good idea to do some foam rolling or a few muscle-specific movements that look similar to your dynamic warm-up, which can help improve your mobility in the muscles you've just worked the most and help jump-start the recovery process.

—Emily Kraus, MD, sports medicine physician and clinical assistant professor and director of the FASTR Program (Female Athlete Science and Translational Research) at Stanford University School of Medicine

Exercise

Fuel Your Workouts: Exactly What to Eat Before and After a Sweat Session to See the Most Gains

For years, most of us followed the (wrong) advice about eating less and exercising more in order to lose weight. The more we restrict calories—and the more calories we burn when we exercise—the more weight we'll lose and the better our bodies will look, right? Wrong, says Katie Hirsch, PhD.

"This common thought process—that if I work out after fasting, I'll burn calories without adding any calories to the equation, which will lead to a deficit that'll help me lose weight—is outdated," she says. In fact, fueling your workouts is especially advantageous for women.

Why? Like so many sex-specific differences that are finally being properly studied, the answer lies in physiological differences that can be understood from an evolutionary perspective. Male physiology favors being strong, fast, and powerful—which means being able to physically perform even in a fasted state. Female physiology favors endurance. "We were designed to survive, reproduce, and then keep ourselves and other little humans alive—and as a result, the female body is more sensitive than a man's to energy stores and nutrition availability," says Dr. Hirsch.

Translation: If you exercise after restricting calories and carbohydrates, that exercise will be even more stressful on your body than it already is, making it feel harder while you're at it *and* making it tougher for you to recover once you've finished. On the flip side, going into a workout fueled—particularly with protein and carbohydrates—gives your body what it needs to get through your workout and recover quickly. Bonus: Eating before a workout also up-regulates the amount of protein your muscle cells turn over in the hour or so after your workout (your anabolic window), which ups the ante on the "afterburn" effect of a workout and helps you continue to burn calories and oxidize fat postworkout.

So What Should You Aim to Eat Before and After Your Workouts?

A mix of protein and carbohydrates, anywhere from fifteen to thirty minutes before you exercise and as soon after your workout as possible. Why this combination of macronutrients?

- **Protein** provides an influx of amino acids that starts to stimulate your muscle to grow, replaces damaged proteins with new ones, and prepares your muscle fibers to contract strongly. Aim to get anywhere from fifteen to thirty grams before and after your sweat session.

- **Carbohydrates** are a primary fuel source for the body, especially during exercise. Anytime we need to burn more calories than it usually takes to do our activities of daily living, we rely on carbohydrates for that fuel. This means the higher the intensity or the longer the duration of your workout, the more carbohydrates you should consume. Aim to get around fifteen to thirty grams of carbs before and after your workout.

Examples of pre- and postworkout snacks that hit these protein and carb goals include Greek yogurt with berries and granola; a smoothie with protein powder; rice cakes or crackers with sliced turkey, chicken, or tuna; two eggs with a piece of toast; and overnight oats with protein powder. Exactly how much you eat—and what foods or supplements you choose for your pre- and postworkout snacks—will depend on your goals and what your gastro-intestinal system can tolerate. For example, if early-morning workouts are part of your routine, you may find it tough to stomach a bowl of yogurt and granola before you exercise. If that's the case, you might think about a protein powder that has the mix of protein and carbs you're aiming for, which will digest more quickly than solid food. If you exercise a little later in the morning, eat something light when you wake up and then eat a bigger breakfast after your workout. Are you an end-of-day exerciser? Have an afternoon snack before you work out and then bring a snack, like a protein bar or shake, to eat on the way home before you eat a well-balanced dinner, says Dr. Hirsch.

"It's clear that if you want to get the most bang for your buck when it comes to exercise, the nutrition piece is extra important for women," says Dr. Hirsch. Anytime you're in a calorie deficit—something diet culture has ingrained in women as a good thing—your protein intake needs to go up. That's because when you're not eating enough calories and carbs to burn energy, your body essentially says, "What else do we have?" And it starts burning fat *and* protein. Over time, this can lead to muscle *loss*.

"If we want to keep muscle and just lose the fat, we have to make sure we're eating enough protein to rebuild and support the muscle," says Dr. Hirsch. "It'll also help you feel better during and after your workouts, which means you'll be more likely to show up again tomorrow and be more consistent."

Your Game Plan: Create (and Stick To!) an Exercise Plan You Actually Enjoy

Many of us feel inundated with contradictory advice when it comes to exercise, which can make starting and sticking to a routine feel overwhelming. Here, Dr. Hirsch and exercise physiologist Sabrena Jo, PhD, offer ideas on how to be more consistent—and genuinely enjoy whatever movement you choose to do.

Don't overthink what you do, especially if you're just starting out. There's a lot of information and advice flying around about exercise that can be overwhelming and confusing. Your best bet is to focus on figuring out what you like to do and then moving your body most days of the week, says Dr. Hirsch. "Remember, exercise works regardless of what type you do," she says. Then, once you find the exercise style or activity you enjoy so much that you actually look forward to doing it, make it nonnegotiable by putting it on your calendar and giving it the same emphasis you would a healthcare appointment.

Strength train at least a couple of days a week. For too many years, the weight rooms in gyms across the country were filled with men while the women sweated it out on treadmills and elliptical machines in the cardio rooms. Thankfully, this has changed. Women are hearing how essential strength training is when it comes to maintaining and building muscle, especially as we get older. And here's what fitness and health experts really want us to know: Even incorporating strength work a couple of times each week can translate to big benefits.

If you're looking to get going on a strength training routine, start with a small number of functional movements that involve pushing, pulling, squatting, and deadlifting, says Dr. Jo. There's a big push for women to lift heavy weights, and that's a great goal to build up to. That said, it's important to start light to make sure you're lifting with good form. "You don't want to lift heavy weights when doing movements you're learning, as 'loading' exercises you do in poor form puts you at greater risk for injury," says Dr. Jo.

If you're not strength training, consider working in some high-intensity intervals into your go-to exercises. In an ideal world, you'd have access to a gym (or a set of free weights or kettlebells at home) so you can strength train. But if that's not feasible, adding even a little high-intensity interval training (HIIT) to your usual cardiovascular exercises is a good alternative. "That's because HIIT work stimulates your muscles more than traditional low- to moderate-intensity cardio," says Dr. Hirsch. If you're walking, pick up the pace to a power walk for a block (or one minute) and then do your usual pace for a block (or one minute), and repeat five to ten times, working up to longer and higher-intensity intervals over time. You could even just power up a flight of stairs quickly and then take it easy on the way down. When you give your muscles this big, quick stimulus to work hard, it pushes them to the edge of what they're capable of doing—which is when your body starts to adapt and get stronger, adds Dr. Hirsch.

"Just keep in mind that to get the most out of intervals, it's important that you work *hard* during each interval," says Dr. Hirsch. How do you know if you're going hard enough? After each interval, ask yourself how you feel on a scale of one to ten, with ten being exhausted. "If you aren't at an eight or above, go a little harder on your next interval," says Dr. Hirsch. "And if you finish your entire HIIT workout and you aren't at a ten, it's time to increase the intensity or duration of each interval."

Reframe what exercise is for. All too often, we think of exercise as a *should*: We should do it if we want to fit into a favorite pair of jeans or drop a few pounds in time for bathing suit season. But this sets us up to see exercise as a punishment of sorts. Dr. Jo suggests flipping the script by making a list of all of the activities you love doing the most and then assessing whether or not your exercise routine is helping you do those things. For example, do you love playing club volleyball or pickleball? You may need to work in some cross-training and dynamic stretching to ensure you're able to play these sports (and feel good while you do) for as long as possible. Is it important to you to be able to lift your kids or grandkids, sit on the floor to play with them (and be able to get up easily), and run around with them outside?

"Reminding yourself that the time you spend exercising is ultimately helping you do all of these activities can give your workouts more purpose," says Dr. Jo, making you more likely to not only prioritize exercise but enjoy it, too.

• • • • •

Only a quarter of adults meet the minimum recommended guidelines for both aerobic activity and strength training, and women tend to get less movement than men. When you understand how exercise works to keep you both optimally healthy and feeling great—and that the benefits result from any kind of movement—there's a good chance you'll be more inspired to make it a nonnegotiable part of your life.

Chapter 20

Nutrition

How to Eat to Optimize Your Health
and Feel Your Best

> *What would our lives—and our world—look like if everyone could feel worthy in their bodies? . . . What if we could eat, and live, on our terms, without apologizing or offering explanation?*
>
> —Alissa Rumsey, RD, MS, *Unapologetic Eating: Make Peace with Food and Transform Your Life*

When it comes to knowing what to eat, there's a good chance you're drowning in *should*s.

I should eat more vegetables. I should eat less sugar. I should swear off butter and red meat to lower my cholesterol. I should talk to my doctor about those drugs that slash appetite.

It's not so surprising, considering we're inundated with information on how we should be eating. Media outlets run clickbaity and often contradictory headlines about the latest nutrition trends. Millions of diet books are sold each year, many of them filled with one-size-fits-all advice. A growing

545

number of social media influencers with huge followings offer diet tips and "healthy" recipes based on personal experience rather than actual expertise.

Adrift in a sea of information, many of us are left feeling confused, anxious, and even guilty about what could be a fairly straightforward and downright enjoyable aspect of life: eating.

The good news is that researchers are continually learning more about how we can use our diet to optimize our health, and we know more than ever before about which foods to reach for—and which ones to steer clear of—to prevent and fight disease. Even better, we have more information now about how to tailor diet recommendations so they work for women, taking into account how food works in our bodies and our different nutritional needs.

In the pages that follow, you'll find clear, actionable steps that'll help you cut through all the diet-culture noise and become better able to listen to your own hunger cues.

In this chapter, we'll learn . . .

- **The straightforward facts about how we use food as fuel**, and why having a basic sense of the macronutrients and micronutrients you're eating each day can help you boost your overall health.

- **How to personalize diet advice**, and why it's important that we do.

- **How, exactly, insulin works to keep our blood sugar at healthy levels**, why women are at a greater risk of blood sugar dysregulation and diabetes, and what you can do about it.

- **What you need to know about semaglutide medications** (sold under brand names like Ozempic and Wegovy), how they work, and potential side effects to keep in mind.

- **The truth about body mass index (BMI)** and why it's not a good gauge of overall health. Plus, we'll talk about why it's possible to be healthy at a higher body weight—and how to talk about weight with clinicians in a way that feels empowering.

- **How to think about what we eat as a way of nourishing and nurturing ourselves** rather than equating a "healthy" diet with depriving ourselves of the enjoyment that can and should come with food.

Vijaya Surampudi, MD, MS, physician nutrition specialist and associate director of the UCLA Medical Weight Management Clinic

Ashley Koff, RD, nutrition director for the University of California at Irvine Susan Samueli Institute's Integrative and Functional Medicine Fellowship, founder of the Better Nutrition Program, and author of *Your Best Shot: The Personalized System for Optimal Weight Health—GLP-1 Shot or Not*

Jessie Inchauspé, biochemist and author of *The Glucose Goddess Method: The 4-Week Guide to Cutting Cravings, Getting Your Energy Back, and Feeling Amazing*

Jennifer L. Gaudiani, MD, eating disorders and weight stigma expert and founder and medical director of the Gaudiani Clinic

Madeline Breda, MD, cofounder of Medical Students for Size Inclusivity

Alissa Rumsey, RD, MS, registered dietitian and author of *Unapologetic Eating: Make Peace with Food and Transform Your Life*

Macronutrients and Micronutrients: What You Need to Know About How the Body Uses Food as Fuel

You've likely heard the term *metabolism* kicked around when it comes to how quickly or slowly our bodies process the food we eat. Being "metabolically healthy" is something more of us are talking about these days as well, especially given research showing that very few of us have optimal metabolic health.[1] But what, exactly, is metabolism—and what does it mean to be metabolically healthy?

Put simply, metabolism is the complex series of reactions that happens throughout the body and within every cell to generate energy from our food and environment. You're metabolically healthy when this process works well. And to make sure the process works well, you have to pay attention to the macronutrients and micronutrients you're consuming.

Nutrition

Meet the Macronutrients

Macronutrients (aka macros) break down into glucose and fatty acids to provide us with energy—though they're digested at different rates, and in different ways.

There are three key macronutrients: protein, fat, and carbohydrates. You'll find a lot of (often contradictory) information about the ideal ratio of macros that should make up your diet, but here's the bottom line: There's no one right answer. You get to choose what percentage of each you want to aim for based on what you know about your body as well as your short- and long-term goals.

Let's dive into more details about each of the macros and some guidelines to help you figure out how much of each you need.

Protein provides your body with essential amino acids, which help grow, maintain, and repair your body's muscles, tissues, and organs. Our bodies need twenty different amino acids, eleven of which we can produce on our own and nine of which we need to get from our food. Complete proteins contain those nine essential amino acids and are typically found in animal-based foods (think beef, chicken, fish, and dairy products). Incomplete proteins contain only some of those nine essential amino acids and are typically found in plant-based sources of protein (legumes, nuts, vegetables, and whole grains).

Proteins also have a higher "thermic effect" than fats and carbs, which means your body burns more calories digesting and absorbing them. What's more, eating foods high in protein gives you a feeling of fullness, which can help reduce hunger and keep cravings in check. This combination of high thermic and satiety effects may help you feel satisfied with smaller portions of food, making protein a great choice if you're trying to reduce your overall calorie intake to lose weight.

How much to get: Making sure you get enough protein is crucial—and this is especially true for women, who typically don't get as much of this macronutrient as we should. This may be because what we're often advised to eat—the recommended dietary allowance (RDA) of 0.36 grams of protein per pound of ideal body weight, which factors out to fifty-four grams of protein for the average 150-pound woman—is too low. In fact, there are experts who say that women need more like 1 gram per pound of ideal body weight, which for most of us means getting double the current RDA.

As we get older, eating enough protein is especially important, because the GI tract becomes less efficient at metabolizing and absorbing protein as we age, says physician nutrition specialist Vijaya Surampudi, MD, MS.

Fats are also used to fuel many of the body's functions, and they also help the body store energy. But just like carbs, not all types of fats are created equal. Unsaturated fats (monounsaturated and polyunsaturated fats) are known as "good" fats and are found in plant-based foods like nuts, seeds, fatty fish, and olive oil. Saturated fats, found in processed foods and dairy products like cheese and butter, can raise the level of LDL cholesterol (known as the "bad" kind) and increase your risk of heart disease and stroke. Artificial trans fats (aka trans fatty acids) are found in processed foods, usually as "partially hydrogenated oils."

As the most calorie-dense macronutrient and the one that plays the biggest role in energy *storage*, dietary fat often gets a bad rap. Yet this macronutrient is crucial for so many of your body's functions, from maintaining a healthy brain and cushioning your internal organs to fueling everyday activities and helping you feel full after eating.

How much to get: It's recommended you get anywhere from 20 to 35 percent of your total daily calories from fat. However, it's important to remember that the majority of your dietary fats should come from monounsaturated and polyunsaturated sources (generally, plant-based foods such as nuts, seeds, olives, avocados, and fatty fish like salmon, tuna, and mackerel) and not saturated and trans fats (such as the saturated fat in meat and dairy or the trans fat in ultra-processed foods—both of which can raise LDL cholesterol and increase your risk of heart disease and stroke).

Carbohydrates (aka carbs) include fiber, starches, and sugar, which are all broken down into glucose—the body's main source of energy. However, some carbs are better than others.

- **Complex carbohydrates** (found in vegetables, legumes, and whole grains) take longer to digest, which makes them a healthier source of carbohydrates.

- **Simple carbohydrates** (naturally found in fruit and milk products and also found in processed and refined sugars like syrups, table sugar, and soft drinks) break down quickly and spike blood sugar; they should be enjoyed in moderation.

- **Fiber** is a type of complex carbohydrate that's especially interesting because it can't be digested by the body. While most carbs are broken down into sugar molecules (called glucose), fiber passes through the body undigested. There are two main types of fiber:
  - Soluble, which dissolves in water and turns into a gel-like substance when it hits your digestive tract. It takes work to break down, which helps slow digestion and keeps you feeling fuller, longer.
  - Insoluble, which doesn't dissolve in water and, as a result, helps move food through the stomach and intestines.

How much to get: It's recommended that you get anywhere from 45 to 65 percent of your total daily calories from carbohydrates. But as with fats, the key is remembering that certain types of carbohydrates are way better than others when it comes to giving your body what'll help it run best. Whole grains, fruits, vegetables, and legumes are loaded with micronutrients and fiber and should make up the bulk of the carbs you eat each day. Simple carbohydrates (especially ones high in refined sugar) should be kept to a minimum.

Meet the Micronutrients

Micronutrients are vitamins and minerals your body needs so your cells work properly. While micronutrients don't provide energy as macronutrients do, they are essential for keeping our various body systems (digestion, brain function, hormone production) working well. Just like macros, these are found in many of the nonprocessed foods you eat—especially fruits and vegetables.

Vitamins are organic substances that are needed for normal cell function but are not produced in our bodies and must come from the food we eat. Vitamins are generally classified as either fat-soluble (which means they dissolve in fat and tend to accumulate in the body) or water-soluble (they must dissolve in water before they can be absorbed by the body, which means they can't be stored). Fat-soluble vitamins include vitamin A, vitamin D, vitamin E, and vitamin K. Water-soluble vitamins include vitamin C and the B-complex vitamins (including folate).

Minerals are inorganic compounds that are present in soil and water and are absorbed by plants or consumed by animals. Like vitamins, they're crucial players in keeping the body functioning optimally. In fact, deficiencies in certain minerals (think iodine, iron, calcium, and zinc) can lead to disease, which is why so many foods are fortified with them.

How to Personalize Nutrition Advice—and Why You Should

Advice on how to eat is often presented as a one-size-fits-all solution, which couldn't be more wrong, says Ashley Koff, RD.

"Generalized nutrition recommendations make us feel like there is a plan that works for everyone," she says. "There isn't. What *you* need to eat for optimal health will be different from what someone else needs." Here's where Koff suggests starting when it comes to evaluating the different dietary advice that comes swirling at you and deciding which pieces you want to make work for you (or not!).

Recognize what's already working in your diet and your life. All too often, we think we need to overhaul *everything* when it comes to making changes to our diet. This is especially true for women, says Koff, adding that her female patients tend to focus so intensely on what they perceive they're doing "wrong" that they completely ignore what's going well. So start by listing all of the ways your current diet is working for you. Are you drinking plenty of water and getting a few servings of vegetables every day? Do you limit the amount of ultra-processed foods you eat? There are undoubtedly things you're already doing well, and when you start with a recognition of that fact, you'll have a better mindset as you experiment with the changes you'd like to make.

Think of dietary advice as an experiment, not a rule. Let's say you read an article about intermittent fasting helping to promote weight loss. Rather than setting a new goal of following an intermittent fasting plan yourself, commit to experimenting with time-restricted eating.

"An experiment isn't right or wrong—it yields information," says Koff. This mindset helps you stay curious about what nutrition advice is working (or not) for your lifestyle and can help you make adjustments that tee you up for success.

Be wary of advice that promises fast results. We've been taught to seek out quick food or supplement fixes for whatever ails us. For example, if you're feeling constipated, go-to advice often includes adding more fiber to your diet. Yet if your constipation is actually due to poor motility in your gut, adding heaps of fiber to your system is going to compound the problem. When something is going on that you want to resolve, first ask, "Why is this happening?" rather than "What can I take to fix this?"

Understanding Blood Sugar: Why Women Are at Greater Risk for Blood Sugar Dysregulation and Diabetes—and How Your Diet Can Make All the Difference

For many years, healthcare providers and nutrition experts talked about blood glucose (aka blood sugar) like it was something only those with diabetes needed to be concerned with. These days, we hear these terms a lot more frequently, and more of us realize that problems in how our body is making and using blood sugar can lead to both short- and long-term health problems.

What Exactly Is Blood Glucose—and How Does It Work?

The food you eat is broken down into sugar—also known as glucose—which your blood carries to your body's cells to either use as fuel or store as fat. Your body carefully regulates your blood glucose levels with two hormones: insulin and glucagon.

Insulin helps glucose enter the body's cells so it can be used for energy. As glucose enters those cells, blood sugar levels decrease, and insulin also goes down. If there's more glucose in the bloodstream than the body can use, insulin sends a signal to the liver, muscles, and other cells to store that excess glucose. Some of it is stored as body fat; some is stored in the liver and muscles. When insulin is low, the hormone **glucagon** triggers your liver to convert stored glucose (called glycogen) into a usable form and release it into your bloodstream so energy is always available—even if you haven't eaten for a while. Glucagon thus increases blood sugar levels, preventing them from dropping too low.

Insulin resistance happens when a lot of blood sugar enters the blood consistently over time, which prompts the pancreas to pump out more insulin to get all that glucose into the body's cells. Eventually, cells stop responding to insulin as they should—but the pancreas keeps making more insulin to try to force the cells to respond. The result: Blood sugar and insulin keep rising, which tells the liver and muscles to store blood sugar. When they are full, excess blood sugar is shuttled to fat cells to be stored as body fat.

There's a good chance you'll hear the term *insulin sensitivity*, which refers to how well (or not) your body moves glucose from your blood into your body's cells. If you have insulin resistance, you have impaired insulin sensitivity.

Diabetes: Why Women Are at Increased Risk for Blood Glucose Dysregulation

Now that you know the basics of blood sugar, you're in a better position to understand diabetes. First, it's important to know the difference between the various types of this disease.

Type 1 diabetes is an autoimmune disease that develops when the immune system's antibodies mistakenly attack beta cells in the pancreas—which in turn means the pancreas is unable to produce adequate amounts of insulin to shuttle glucose into the cells. When too little insulin is available, blood sugar rises to dangerous levels (hyperglycemia).

Type 2 diabetes is a chronic condition where you have persistently high levels of blood sugar and you become insulin resistant as a result. When your body's cells don't respond to insulin as they should, your pancreas tries to keep up with the glucose overload in your blood by making more insulin. Type 2 diabetes can develop if your cells become too resistant to insulin and your pancreas can't produce enough to overcome it. The resulting hyperglycemia can cause serious health problems if it goes untreated. Unlike type 1 diabetes, type 2 diabetes can be prevented and even reversed with lifestyle modifications such as increasing physical activity and eating in a way that minimizes blood glucose spikes and dips (which you can read more about on page 556).

Gestational diabetes is a type of diabetes that can develop during pregnancy when blood sugar levels get too high. It happens when the hormones from the placenta block your body's ability to use or make insulin. (In fact, all pregnant women have some insulin resistance during late pregnancy.) Gestational diabetes can happen in women with no history of diabetes, and insulin sensitivity can return to normal after you give birth. However, about 50 percent of women with gestational diabetes will go on to develop type 2 diabetes,[2] so it's important to talk to your healthcare provider about the steps you can take to lower your risk.

So why are women more likely to have impaired glucose tolerance over the course of our lives? Several factors may play a role:

- **Our body fat distribution**: Compared with men of the same age, healthy women have less muscle mass and higher body fat, which could promote insulin resistance.

- **Our sex hormones**: During our reproductive years, estrogen improves insulin sensitivity. Yet when we reach menopause and estrogen declines, we're at risk of developing insulin resistance. If left unchecked, this can progress to prediabetes or type 2 diabetes, among other chronic conditions.

- **A history of gestational diabetes**: If you were diagnosed with this condition when you were pregnant, you're more likely to experience blood sugar dysregulation later on and have a higher risk of developing type 2 diabetes.

- **Sleep issues**: Women have a higher likelihood than men of suffering from sleep disturbances and insomnia, which are known causes of glucose impairment (not to mention of appetite dysregulation and weight gain, which can also lead to impaired glucose tolerance).

- **Higher levels of stress**: When we're stressed, the body prepares itself to fight or flee by ensuring there's enough blood sugar to use as energy. As stress hormones rise, insulin levels fall, and more glucose starts pumping through your body. Yet over time, if stress is chronic, it can lead to insulin dysregulation.

What to Keep in Mind If You've Been Diagnosed with Diabetes

About fifteen million women in the U.S. have diabetes—that's one in every nine adult women.[3] If you're one of them, it's important to recognize that this is a condition you must continually manage—and women have even more to monitor than their male counterparts.

- **Women with diabetes have a higher risk of developing yeast infections and urinary tract infections (UTIs).** High blood sugar levels can lead to releasing excess sugar in your urine, which encourages bacteria and yeast to grow and can cause a disruption in the balance of bacteria in the vagina.

- **Blood sugar levels may be harder to control around your period and after menopause.** Changes in hormone levels before and during your cycle can make blood sugar levels more difficult to control, which means it's recommended that you check your blood glucose levels more regularly around your period. After menopause, changes in hormone levels can trigger unpredictable ups and downs in blood sugar—and when blood sugar fluctuates, you have an increased risk of diabetes complications. Add to that postmenopausal weight gain and sleep issues, and you can see how multiple factors can add challenges to your diabetes management.

- **You may have a tougher time getting pregnant.** Diabetes that isn't well controlled can make it more difficult to conceive, and if you do get pregnant, high blood sugar increases your risk of miscarriage or stillbirth, high blood pressure during pregnancy, gestational diabetes, delivery by Cesarean section, and other complications. It's crucial to talk with your healthcare provider if you're considering pregnancy so you can get your blood sugar levels in your target range before you conceive.

Steps to Keep Your Blood Glucose Regulated

Here's the good news: You don't need a total diet overhaul to have a positive impact on your blood glucose, says biochemist Jessie Inchauspé. "Simple things really go a long way when it comes to avoiding glucose spikes and keeping your insulin sensitivity where it should be."

Here are three of Inchauspé's favorite hacks:

1. Have a savory (not sweet and starchy) breakfast. Want to help set yourself up for steady glucose throughout your day? Your first meal of the day is hugely important, says Inchauspé.

"When your stomach is empty, anything that lands in it will be digested quickly," she says. A savory breakfast, typically built around protein, fiber-rich carbohydrates, and healthy fats, will be digested more slowly than a sugar- and starch-filled meal and won't lead to a big spike in glucose.

"This has the added benefit of keeping you feeling fuller longer," Inchauspé adds. "The lower the glucose spike after breakfast, the lower the drop will be afterward, which helps keep hunger and cravings in check."

2. Eat a vegetable before at least one meal a day (and all, if you can). The fiber in veggies hits your intestine before other foods and then forms a protective mesh that reduces the absorption of any glucose you eat, reducing the overall glucose spike after your meal. You'll still get plenty of health-boosting benefits if you eat veggies with your meal, but for the biggest glucose-regulating punch, front-load your meal with those plant powerhouses.

3. Move after you eat. Every cell in your body likes to use glucose for energy—especially your muscles. So if you use your muscles after you eat, you give the glucose that's just hit your bloodstream somewhere to go immediately, says Inchauspé, which in turn will reduce that postmeal glucose spike.

"Even ten minutes of movement works," she says. "It can be a ten-minute walk, some calf raises or squats at your desk, or even cleaning your kitchen or dancing to a favorite song."

Rx, Explained: Semaglutide

Originally used as a diabetes medication, semaglutide (brand names: Ozempic, Wegovy, Rybelsus) has exploded into our culture and become synonymous with weight loss. Yet along with it have come a lot of questions about how, exactly, the medication works and what the downsides are.

What Is Semaglutide?

It belongs to a class of drugs known as glucagon-like peptide-1 receptor agonists (GLP-1 RAs), which work by mimicking the GLP-1 hormone in the body.

All of us make GLP-1 in response to eating. When food enters the stomach and moves through the digestive tract, your body releases GLP-1 in the intestine, and it travels to receptors in multiple parts of your body to trigger different actions.

- In the pancreas, GLP-1 triggers the release of insulin (the hormone that lowers blood sugar levels) and suppresses the release of glucagon (the hormone that raises blood sugar levels).

- In the stomach, GLP-1 receptors slow gastric emptying, which means food doesn't move through the digestive system so quickly and you stay fuller longer.

- In the brain, GLP-1 receptors suppress hunger and food cravings.

The most potent stimulators of GLP-1 are protein and fat, which is one reason why you tend to feel more full after eating these macronutrients than after eating carbohydrates, says Dr. Surampudi. But here's the catch: The GI tract rapidly breaks down the GLP-1 our bodies naturally make. In fact, it's broken down so quickly that it has little effect on our appetites.

Enter semaglutide medications, which stimulate GLP-1 receptors and in turn influence a number of your body's weight-management mechanisms. These injections work in a few different ways:

- They control appetite and enhance satiety, thanks to the GLP-1 receptors in the brain responsible for appetite regulation, leading you to consume fewer calories. In fact, they're thought to modulate reward pathways in the brain responsible for the pleasurable sensations we associate with certain foods, ultimately dampening the allure of high-calorie foods and dulling "food noise" (the nonstop thinking about food)—a combination that makes it easier to stick to a healthy-eating plan.

- They delay gastric emptying, leading to a prolonged feeling of fullness and satiety after you eat, which in turn prevents you from overeating.

- They increase the release of insulin when blood glucose levels are elevated, which in turn improves blood sugar levels.

- They bind to GLP-1 receptors in the pancreas and suppress the release of glucagon (the hormone that stimulates the liver to release glucose into the bloodstream), helping to lower blood sugar levels. This is why they're so beneficial for those with type 2 diabetes.

And the research shows semaglutide works. One major clinical trial of semaglutide in adults showed an average weight reduction of around 15 percent when paired with a diet and exercise routine, compared with a 2 percent weight reduction in the placebo group.[4]

Other incretin-based therapies (as we learned on page 215, incretins are hormones that stimulate insulin secretion and suppress glucagon production) include:

- Tirzepatide (brand names: Mounjaro and Zepbound)
- Liraglutide (brand names: Saxenda, Victoza)
- Dulaglutide (brand name: Trulicity)

» POTENTIAL SIDE EFFECTS—AND HOW TO MANAGE THEM

There are a number of side effects people taking semaglutide for weight loss may experience. Some of the most common include:

- Stomach issues (like nausea, vomiting, pain, and/or bloating)
- Gastrointestinal issues (like diarrhea, constipation, and/or gassiness)
- Dizziness
- Fatigue
- Headache

Another side effect that Dr. Surampudi frequently sees at her clinic is malnutrition.

"I see a lot of patients who aren't eating enough protein because of the GI side effects they're experiencing, or they're not drinking enough water because they're not hungry or thirsty," she says. "If these medications are preventing you from getting all the nutrients and hydration your body needs, you'll want to have a conversation with your clinician and potentially reduce the dose or reevaluate the pros and cons of being on the medication."

Dr. Surampudi recommends that everyone on a GLP-1-based medication keep a food diary so your healthcare provider can see at a glance what nutrients you might not be getting enough of, run lab tests to confirm any deficiencies, and offer suggestions on how to address them. And while you may be focused on the number on the scale dropping when you're on one of these medications, you'll want to make sure you're not losing too much muscle—a metabolically active organ that is crucial for overall health—along with the fat. This is where a body-composition analysis (in addition to tracking your weight on a traditional scale) is helpful.

"The goal is to have your percent body fat go down, with as much muscle weight maintenance as possible," says Dr. Surampudi. The key to doing this is to eat adequate protein and make sure you're doing some form of resistance training (such as lifting weights or doing exercises that use your body weight as resistance) a few times a week.

The bottom line: There are multiple considerations when it comes to

Nutrition

understanding if you're a candidate for a semaglutide, and it's important to talk through your health history with your care team when discussing whether this medication is right for you.

Rethinking Fatness: Why BMI Is Bogus, and How to Navigate Our Weight-Centric Healthcare System

When you live in a larger body, healthcare visits can feel especially charged. Whether you're at a routine exam or a visit for a specific ailment or concern, conversations about your health and treatment for various symptoms often center around one thing: reaching a "healthy" weight. But here's the kicker: While society and even many healthcare providers would have us believe that thin is "healthy" and fat is "unhealthy," weight is not a good gauge of someone's health status.

So what's the best way to navigate our weight-centric healthcare system? It starts with understanding why body mass index (BMI) is flawed, the science-backed truth about how it *is* possible to be fat* and healthy, and knowing how to talk to clinicians about your weight.

The Truth About Body Mass Index (BMI)—and Why It's Not an Acceptable Measure of Health

When you go to most healthcare appointments, there's a good chance you'll be weighed. That number on the scale, combined with your height, may be used to calculate your BMI—a screening tool that estimates the amount of body fat you have. If your number is 25 or higher, you fall into the "overweight" category; if it's 30 or higher, you're "obese."

BMI has been used for decades to assess disease risk and how someone's weight may be impacting their health. However, there are a number of flaws with the BMI calculator—so many, in fact, that in 2023, the American Medical Association (AMA) characterized it as an imperfect measure of health.[5]

*The term *fat* is used here and throughout this section as a neutral adjective to describe body size, similar to descriptors like *short* or *tall*.

The Problems with BMI

So what's wrong with this still commonly used calculation?

- **It wasn't intended for medical use—or for individual assessment.** The formula for BMI was created in 1832 by a Belgian mathematician (not physician) in order to figure out the average body size among men. Translation: It was designed to be a reflection of how much a group of (mostly white) men weigh on average, not what one person *should* weigh for optimal health.

- **It's sexist and racist.** BMI weight categories are the same regardless of your age or sex, which is problematic. Extrapolating data from predominantly white men to create norms and expectations for women and people of color is simply bad science.

- **It doesn't take body composition into account.** BMI doesn't differentiate between fat, muscle mass, and bone density—all key factors when it comes to your overall health. Because bone and muscle are denser than fat, a person with strong bones, good muscle mass, and low fat could have a high BMI. You can see how this would be an issue for muscular athletes, who are often labeled "overweight" when they are actually healthier than "normal-weight" individuals with lower muscle mass. It's also an issue for older people, who are considered healthy when they have a "normal" BMI when really, age-related muscle loss (sarcopenia)—which increases mortality risk—might be going undetected.

- **It is often used as shorthand for "healthy" or "unhealthy."** However, a higher BMI doesn't necessarily correlate with significant unhealthy health markers—and you can have multiple markers for disease even if your BMI is in a "healthy" range. In fact, these "healthy" and "unhealthy" labels based on BMI can blind clinicians to a patient's *actual* medical conditions. For example, women in larger bodies often don't get screened for eating disorders, despite symptoms like significant weight loss, signs of malnutrition, and even reported eating disorder behaviors. Women with eating disorders are often seen as being healthy—and certain assumptions are made and important questions aren't asked—because of a "healthy" BMI.

The American Medical Association recommends that BMI be used in conjunction with other measures, including visceral fat (which is found deep within the abdomen, around the internal organs) and body composition (the percentage of bone, muscle, and fat). These measurements, along with an assessment of metabolic and genetic risk factors, should be taken into consideration when getting a picture of someone's health.

Can You Be Fat *and* Healthy?

For generations, most of us have gotten the message that weight and health are crucially connected. If you're thin, you must be healthy. If you're fat, not so much. Yet here's the truth: You can be healthy at a higher body weight.

"I see patients all the time who are in larger bodies due to higher fat and they are equally healthy in all measurable ways to patients who are thinner," says Jennifer L. Gaudiani, MD, an eating disorders and weight stigma expert. How is this possible, given the prevailing belief that carrying excess fat puts you at higher risk for all sorts of disease? Here are some of the science-backed reasons why associating a large body with poor health is misguided—and dangerous.

Your genetics impact your health regardless of your weight. In the same way that all of us have a unique genetic tolerance to different exposures, we also have unique responses to carrying extra weight.

"It's similar to how a person who drinks heavily for five years may end up with cirrhosis at age thirty-five while another might toast her ninetieth birthday with a pink, healthy liver despite drinking heavily all her life," says Dr. Gaudiani. "Asking if fat people can be healthy is like asking if old people can be healthy. There are some really old people who are really healthy, and there are some who have age-related illnesses. Should we look down on those people because they dared to get sick as a result of age?"

Losing weight doesn't always lead to better health outcomes. With our collective emphasis on the importance of losing weight for better health, you'd think *all* the evidence would point to improvements in health outcomes when the number on the scale drops. But that's not the case. One review of nearly two dozen studies found "no clear relationship" between weight loss and meaningful improvements in health measures like blood pressure, cholesterol levels, and diabetes risk.[6] Another large, yearslong study found that weight loss did not reduce the incidence of cardiovascular events like heart attack or stroke in overweight and obese people with type 2 diabetes.[7]

Healthy habits matter more than how much you weigh. Evidence points to the importance of turning our focus and efforts from weight loss to the addition of healthy behaviors. Eating more vegetables and plant-based food. Moving your body, even if you start by walking just a few days a week. Getting a good night's sleep and a handle on your stress. These are things that can improve health no matter your size and whether or not they change the number on the scale, says Dr. Gaudiani.

A focus on weight loss via diet and exercise can do more harm than good. Dieting often leads to stress, which, ironically, can cause your body to deposit fat in your belly region, where it's associated with a greater risk of disease.

It's not that weight doesn't matter at all when it comes to health. Dr. Gaudiani says it's reasonable to acknowledge that fatness can contribute to certain disease processes. Look at animal research, for example, where mice are forced to gain weight and the ones who gain more fat do go on to develop certain diseases. However, Dr. Gaudiani is quick to add that this doesn't mean weight loss should be the go-to recommendation for people with excess fat. The better approach: Treat the health conditions you have and also have a conversation with your clinician about getting out of the dieting loop, eating good food that's relatively balanced consistently throughout the day, and moving your body. In some ways, it doesn't matter if it's possible to be healthy and fat, says Dr. Gaudiani.

"As soon as my fat patients who have been metabolically healthy develop diabetes, hypertension, or blood sugar problems, they often have this crisis of conscience, like 'I'm no longer the poster child for *good* fat people,'" she says. "What's most important is for everyone, at every body size, to feel worthy."

Talking About Weight with Our Healthcare Providers: How to Feel More Empowered

When you live in a larger body, it can feel like weight is the only marker of your health that really matters to clinicians. In one study of nearly 2,500 women characterized as overweight or obese, 69 percent said they experienced weight stigma from a doctor.[8] Unfortunately, the implicit bias (when you aren't conscious of your attitudes, preferences, or prejudices) and explicit bias (when you're aware of your prejudices) that have led to our current weight-centric healthcare system don't seem to be going anywhere anytime soon—and in fact, implicit bias is getting worse.[9]

So what can we do to fight the weight stigma that's so prevalent in medical settings? Madeline Breda, MD, cofounder of Medical Students for Size Inclusivity, offers advice.

When making healthcare appointments, ask questions. In an ideal world, all of us would be able to see weight-inclusive providers at fat-positive clinics (healthcare offices with features like armless chairs in the waiting room, appropriately sized blood pressure cuffs and robes, and exam tables that are low to the ground to make them easier for those in larger bodies to get on and off). When you're searching for a new provider, try using the keywords *weight neutral*, *weight inclusive*, and *HAES* (short for the organization Health at Every Size).

You can also call a healthcare provider's office ahead of your appointment and get a sense of how the practitioner you'd like to see approaches weight and health. Ask questions like "I'm looking for a doctor who provides weight-neutral care, which means treating me without weight-loss advice. Do you have a provider who can do this?" If a friendly receptionist answers the phone, you might even ask which clinician at the practice has the best bedside manner or is most beloved by patients, which could lead you to an empathetic provider with whom you'll feel comfortable discussing your history of weight stigma and how you'd rather not have your weight be the focus of your visits.

Request to not be weighed. This is completely within your rights as a patient, says Dr. Breda, who acknowledges that even she used to put off going to the doctor for checkups because she didn't want to get weighed. Now she provides an estimate of her weight at healthcare visits. Another tactic is to request to step on the scale at the end of your appointment, so any angst you have about that moment doesn't overshadow the rest of your visit.

In some cases, it may be necessary to get weighed. For example, during pregnancy your provider will want to make sure you're gaining enough weight to keep you and the baby healthy; you may also need to get weighed if your clinician is prescribing a medication that's dosed based on weight.

Get a sense of how your clinician has come to their diagnosis and treatment plan. If the reason for your diagnosis and discussion about how to treat what ails you veer to your weight or diet and exercise habits, Dr. Breda recommends asking the clinician, "What other options have you worked through before coming to your conclusion about my diagnosis and best course of treatment?" Asking your clinician to walk through this answer can help you understand how they're thinking about your care, says Dr. Breda. And if your weight comes up but it's not a conversation you want to have, ask for treatment options beyond diet, exercise, and weight loss.

"You could say something like 'I know we both want what's best for my health, and I'd love to focus on the many things I can do to support my health—which may or may not include weight loss,'" she suggests.

Bring a friend with you into the exam room. It can be incredibly difficult to respond to weight stigma in a clinician's office, given the power differential between you and the provider, as well as the years of fatphobia you've likely experienced in other doctors' offices and in everyday life. What's more, if you ask questions or advocate for a weight-neutral approach, there's a chance you'll be met with irritation or defensiveness, which can lead to worse care. So ask an ally to join you, particularly someone who can speak up for you to help ensure your appointment stays focused on what you need and want to cover.

Your Game Plan: How to Think of Eating as a Way of Nourishing and *Nurturing* Yourself

We're bombarded with so much advice on how to eat—confusing and often conflicting directives on what foods are "good" versus "bad"—that somewhere along the way, many of us pick up this idea that eating "healthy" means depriving ourselves of the enjoyment that can and should come with food. It's time to claim something different for ourselves, says registered dietitian Alissa Rumsey, RD, MS. Here's where to start.

Recognize the outside forces that have been influencing you and messing with your inherent trust in yourself. Those of us who are socialized as women can't escape the messages about how our bodies *should* look—and how we can control what we eat to achieve that ideal. We get these messages implicitly, thanks to the diet culture that's still so pervasive in our society. And sadly, we also get these messages explicitly through family, friends, and even many healthcare practitioners. The basic gist of these messages: *Thin is best*. And so we try to shrink ourselves by monitoring and restricting what we eat.

"This breeds a distrust in ourselves—a disconnection from our bodies that prevents us from knowing what foods we like or what, when, or how much to eat," says Rumsey. "And it creates this cycle of feeling like we have to rely on those external rules and other people telling us what we should eat." Simply being aware of this is the first step in starting to think about food as a source of both nourishment and enjoyment.

Ask yourself: What does hunger—and satisfaction—feel like in your body? When Rumsey poses this question to her clients, they often find it easy to explain what ravenous hunger feels like. But outside of that stomach-growling "I have to eat now" sensation, what does hunger feel like? What does satisfaction feel like? (And remember, there's a difference between "my stomach is stuffed" *fullness* and "I really enjoyed that meal" *satisfaction*.) How do you know when you're deeply satisfied by food you've just eaten?

Once you're able to answer these questions, start experimenting. Think of what you eat for lunch. Is it something you're eating because you want to—or because you feel you should? There are no wrong or right answers—asking is simply a way of gathering information and exploring choices. And if the answer is "I'm only eating a salad because I feel I should," then you might ask: "What *does* sound delicious to me right now?" And just once this week, eat that meal that sounds delicious.

"Be extra gentle with yourself when you do this, and show yourself a lot of self-compassion," says Rumsey. "It can be so hard to trust your body when you've been told for so long that you can't."

Eat for physical *and* emotional satisfaction. Too often, we get stuck in binary thinking when it comes to our food choices. We think, "Either I have the blueberry muffin for breakfast and know I'll love it but then be hungry again an hour later, or I have the scrambled eggs with veggies and avocado." If you're wanting to learn how to really enjoy your food, try to find a middle ground by opting for a meal that'll feel emotionally satisfying and also help you feel physically full and energized until lunchtime. A great way to do this is to ask yourself what you can add to that emotionally satisfying food you want that'll give you some more nutrients and keep you feeling satisfied. For example, can you have some Greek yogurt or a cheese stick and fruit along with the muffin so you're also getting some satiating protein, fat, and fiber?

"Rather than focusing on what you have to avoid or remove from your diet to eat 'perfectly,' think about what you can add to a meal so that you're having carbs, protein, and fat along with the taste satisfaction," says Rumsey. This is an important piece when it comes to really embracing the concept that food is something we're allowed to enjoy.

Notice when you want to explain to yourself or others why you're eating something—and try to stop yourself from doing it. So often we feel the need to justify why we're choosing to eat certain foods: "I'm going to order the bread basket with dinner because I'm really hungry and did a tough workout earlier today," when really, you want the bread because the focaccia is mind-blowingly delicious. This is especially common when we're eating with others, who might say something about our food choices. What woman hasn't sat at a restaurant where another woman has said something like "The bread is so tasty here, but that's too many carbs for me"?

Eating what you want without explanation or justification can be really challenging, especially at first. And if you're living in a larger body, it can feel downright impossible, because you're working with not just your own internal messaging but also external weight stigma. That's why Rumsey suggests starting by noticing when you have the urge to offer an explanation about what you want to eat and then eating it anyway if it feels safe for you to do so—which may not be out at a restaurant. If someone around you makes a comment (or your own internal dialogue starts piping up in a judgy tone), change the topic.

"Not only can this help you practice clueing in to your body and its hunger cues, but it can also plant seeds for the people around us to do the same, too," says Rumsey.

• • • • •

While we may be contending with diet culture and weight stigma for the foreseeable future, there is a way to think of food as something that can help us feel deeply nourished and satisfied, and even as a way to care for ourselves.

Chapter 21

Health in an Ever-Evolving Digital Age

Stay Informed, Avoid Misinformation, and Use Technology to Optimize Your Health

> *Feminism demands bodily autonomy, and that can be achieved only with facts. You cannot make an empowering decision about your health when the information you have been given is false.*
>
> —Jen Gunter, MD, *Blood: The Science, Medicine, and Mythology of Menstruation*

We live in an era when smartwatches and other wearables can give us incredible data—from the number of steps we take and number of hours we sit versus stand to the amount of sleep we're getting at night. Thanks to lightning-fast search engines, we can get health information on demand, our search results opening the way to countless sources of information. Some of us are even having conversations about our health woes with ChatGPT and other artificial intelligence platforms.

Yet with all this technology also comes information overload, a growing volume of misinformation, and health data privacy issues. How can you trust the answers an AI chatbot provides when you know these bots often produce plausible-sounding yet totally inaccurate responses? Is it even possible to make sense of the pages of legal text we're expected to read through before clicking the "agree" button on those health tech apps we all use? And what might the repercussions be if we Google our most private health concerns or speed-scroll through legalese without reading the fine print?

These are very real dilemmas with few black-and-white answers. Enter this chapter on something previous health books could skip, filled with practical advice on how to optimize your health in our exciting, if a little scary, digital age.

In this chapter, we'll learn . . .

- **How clinicians themselves use the internet to answer their questions about your health,** and how to apply the same tactics they use to your own internet health searches, too.

- **Why your favorite chatbot has a terrible habit of giving you false health information.** Plus, how to use AI to its potential when searching for answers to questions about your well-being.

- **The simple, practical ways to spot health misinformation** and how to do your part to stop it from spreading.

- **How to read and understand a scientific study,** as well as some of the key things to keep in mind as you're reading research to tell the difference between quality studies and ones you should ignore.

- **Some of the issues that can surface as we increasingly rely on websites and apps to help us manage our health**—and how to keep your health data safe.

Meet the Experts

Nina Shapiro, MD, author of *Hype: A Doctor's Guide to Medical Myths, Exaggerated Claims and Bad Advice—How to Tell What's Real and What's Not* and *The Ultimate Kids' Guide to Being Super Healthy*

Katy Byron, former director of the Poynter Institute's MediaWise, a media literacy initiative aimed at teaching Americans how to use fact-checking skills to spot misinformation online

Marzyeh Ghassemi, PhD, associate professor at MIT, whose research focuses on developing machine-learning algorithms to inform healthcare decisions

Dina Burstein, MD, MPH, project director for the Center for Community-Engaged Medicine at Tufts Medical Center and associate professor of medicine at Tufts University School of Medicine

Karen S. Rheuban, MD, associate dean for continuing medical education and external affairs at the University of Virginia and cofounder and director of the UVA Center for Telehealth

K. Ashley Garling, PharmD, pharmacist and clinical assistant professor at the University of Texas at Austin College of Pharmacy

Leah Fowler, JD, MPH, assistant professor of law at the University of Houston Law Center

How to Google Health Info Like a Doctor and Spot Misinformation

It's easy to assume your healthcare providers have all the answers—and when they don't, they must be using some sort of special medical database. Here's the truth: Clinicians often search for answers to their questions using Google and ChatGPT just as you do, says Nina Shapiro, MD.

"There's a lot of really good, factual information out there, and the key is knowing how to get to that and avoid the misinformation," says Dr. Shapiro. Here, she offers a view into some of the best practices healthcare providers use to suss out the sound from the sketchy.

- **Stick to the basics in your search question.** When you plug your keywords or question into a Google search, try to be as unbiased as possible. "You want to use terms that don't have an opinion embedded in them," says Dr. Shapiro. For example, instead of searching "megadosing vitamin C to prevent the common cold" you might plug in "vitamin C and dose recommendations." The latter should turn up search results that give you a baseline understanding of how vitamin C works and what medical experts and institutions recommend when it comes to optimal dose, which will be important background to keep in mind when the more salacious articles about the latest megadosing trend start popping up. Starting with the basics will help you more easily differentiate between the factual and the farcical.

  "Just take time to educate yourself even a little about the nuts and bolts of a topic before digging into the extremes, trends, or controversies," says Dr. Shapiro.

- **Look closely at the source of the information.** Healthcare pros look for articles posted by well-known medical centers and health institutions, such as the Cleveland Clinic or Mayo Clinic. If there's a *.org* or *.gov* at the end of the URL, that's a good sign the content was created as a public health service. Can't immediately tell if a source is trustworthy or not? Skim the content and look for links to health research, quotes from healthcare experts, and (depending on the topic) medical illustrations and images.

  "You can pretty quickly get a sense if the source's mission is to provide factual, helpful, science-backed health information or not," says Dr. Shapiro.

- **Consider who wrote the content.** If the author is listed, what are their credentials to write on the topic you've searched? Is the author a health journalist or expert in the field? (This is ideal.) Was the article reviewed by a medical expert? If there's no author, look for sources and citations for the information contained in the article, which should be linked throughout or listed at the bottom of the page.

- **Think about any potential ulterior motives for the content.** Sometimes a website or author will have a financial stake regarding the information being provided. This can be tricky to figure out, but it's worth doing a little digging. For example, does the doctor who's providing the health information sell supplements that supposedly treat that health condition? Or does the pharmaceutical company with an article on a specific condition have a drug to treat that condition? This may not make the information being provided false—but it does make it biased.

- **Look at the date the article you're reading was created, reviewed, or updated**. This information should appear near the top or bottom of the web page. Ideally, you'll want the article to be recent (created within the last year). Sure, older information can still be useful, but health information is constantly being updated and more recent articles are more likely to include current information.

- **Avoid content that's filled with dramatic claims**. When it comes to our health, we should be wary of "miracle cures," says Dr. Shapiro. Not only should a big claim make you question the credibility of the information, but it should also prompt you to wonder if there might be ulterior motives for spreading the information.

Of course, no information you find online—no matter how accurate or trustworthy—should replace seeing your healthcare provider. Do your online research at home, then bring that information to your next appointment so your healthcare provider can put it in the context of your unique situation and give you more personalized, specific advice than you'll be able to find on the internet.

How to Spot Health Misinformation and Disinformation— and Stop It from Spreading

Misinformation is on the rise in all aspects of our lives, and false news and information about our health is no exception. The ever-growing number of online places to which people go for this information—from social media and search engines to online retailers and reputable news sites—is one reason we're seeing misinformation spread faster and at a much larger scale than ever before. Add to that a growing number of bad actors intentionally spreading disinformation, as well as a decrease in patient trust in physicians and hospital systems, and we're all at a greater risk of receiving faulty health advice.

It's also important to realize that even the savviest and smartest among us are at risk of falling for fake news online. In fact, contrary to the popular belief that older generations are more likely to get duped, millennials and Gen Zers may actually be more susceptible, according to research[1]—possibly due to the fact that they're more likely to get their news from social media sites and YouTube, which often don't have the same rigorous fact-checking as more traditional media outlets.

Katy Byron, a media literacy and misinformation expert, says each of us can limit the impact of misinformation with a few simple steps.

» STEP 1: ASK YOURSELF THREE QUESTIONS WHEN READING ANY INFORMATION RELATING TO YOUR HEALTH (OR ANY ASPECT OF YOUR LIFE, REALLY)

After Stanford History Education Group (SHEG) studied the work of fact-checking journalists, they developed three key questions to help students—and really anyone—determine if the online content they are consuming is factual:

1. *Who is behind the information?* Is it a reliable, authoritative source like the Centers for Disease Control and Prevention or a major health organization like the Cleveland Clinic? Or is it a social media influencer with no health background sharing information based on their personal experience?

2. *What is the evidence?* Does the information have peer-reviewed research backing up the claims—and is that research cited throughout the article, making it easy for you to click through to it? Or is the data lacking?

3. *What do other sources say?* Do multiple experts—researchers, scientists, clinicians—agree on the information being presented? Or does what you're reading seem to be an anomaly?

» STEP 2: LEARN A FACT-CHECKING SKILL CALLED LATERAL READING

So what's the best way to answer those three important questions? As you're reading, open a new browser window (or even better, multiple windows) and start searching. Do a web search on the author of the content (if possible) and the publication. Do another search to see what other media outlets and experts say about the same topic. This is *lateral reading*, a term coined by SHEG: Instead of scrolling through one piece of content, you open up a new tab (or two or three or ten) next to it to seek out additional information.

Yes, it can feel annoying to have to do extra work. But it's an important step to ensure that the information you're getting is verified and factual.

» STEP 3: FACT-CHECK INFORMATION BEFORE SHARING IT TO YOUR OWN SOCIAL MEDIA

If you see a post on social media that makes you say "wow"—whether it's a health headline or a statistic that scares you, excites you, or riles you up in any way—it can be tempting to share it with your friends and followers immediately. But before you do that, verify that the information is accurate and coming from a reliable source.

Byron's rule of thumb when it comes to reposting health info on social platforms: If you have a physical reaction to what you're reading, that's an indicator to stop what you're doing, put your phone down for a minute, and do some of your own research and fact-checking before resharing.

"If you don't do this, you could be spreading misinformation to someone else," says Byron. "If there's no verified source attached to a social media post and you share it, you are part of the problem."

» STEP 4: BE BRAVE ENOUGH TO ENGAGE WITH YOUR FRIENDS AND FAMILY ON THE PROBLEM OF HEALTH MISINFORMATION

When you see health misinformation or disinformation spreading online, it may be tempting to ignore it and assume you won't make inroads with that person. However, starting a conversation about the topic—and listening to the person sharing the false info with empathy as you ask questions and provide alternate, factually correct explanations—can actually go a long way toward stopping the spread of misinformation, says Byron.

"The more you try to understand where someone else is coming from, the better able you'll be to have a productive conversation."

Should You Trust an AI Chatbot with Your Health Questions?

With ever-evolving technology making chat-based artificial intelligence (AI) bots more sophisticated than ever before, more of us are turning to them for medical advice. This isn't necessarily a bad thing. Just as ChatGPT can spit out a great meal plan or workout, it's also well able to answer questions about your health.

However, when you use these chatbots for the types of queries you'd typically run by your doctor—say, to find out what specific symptoms might mean, or for possible side effects of a medication you're taking—there are some things to keep in mind to optimize the results and make sure you're basing your health decisions on accurate, unbiased information. Here, MIT associate professor Marzyeh Ghassemi, PhD, whose research focuses on developing machine-learning algorithms to inform healthcare decisions, shares some of the pitfalls, plus tips on how to use this technology to its potential.

» THE DOWNSIDES

- **AI is biased against women and people of color.** Chat-based AI technology developed thanks to large language models (LLMs), which are a type of AI that's trained on text across the internet. That training enables them to predict the next word in a sequence of words in a human-like style and "talk" to us in easy-to-understand language. But keep in mind that text on the internet was initially created by real, live humans—who generate biased copy, says Dr. Ghassemi.

    "Humans' ability to generalize is one of the things that keeps us alive, but it also creates tropes and stereotypes," she says. "We're training LLMs to learn from all these examples and then generalize, so it's not surprising that these models reflect the biases of society."

Sadly, this likely means the prejudices that persist in medicine—the lack of adequate research focused on women and people of color, for example—may be perpetuated by chatbots. Scrubbing racism, sexism, and all the other isms from the internet is also impossible, which means they will likely persist to some degree in the conversations we have with these LLMs, adds Dr. Ghassemi.

- **AI can (and will) generate factually inaccurate content that disproportionately affects women and minorities.** Chatbot algorithms are based on the text they were trained on—and so far, that text includes copy scraped from the internet at large, not just reliable sources of information on the internet. This means that health information from the National Institutes of Health or a reputable medical institution such as the Cleveland Clinic is given equal weight to information posted on Facebook and pulled from widespread misinformation campaigns.

What's more, chatbots have the potential to "hallucinate," meaning they sometimes make up answers that aren't true and provide sources for those answers that are completely made up. It can be very convincing and even formatted in such a way that it's tempting to believe the chatbot is pulling factual, expert-backed information. This puts a burden on us—the users—to determine whether the chatbot's information and source citations are actually legit or not.

Why would a chatbot make up potentially harmful and even life-threatening information rather than simply stating that it can't answer your question? The answer is simple, says Dr. Ghassemi: You told it what you wanted, and it's trying to please you.

"LLMs weren't designed to evaluate the information they're providing compared to some capital-*T* objective truth," she says. "They're currently designed to give us the answers we want, and to provide some variation in the responses. I don't think end users would be as excited to use them otherwise."

How to Use AI to Its Potential

- **Ask your questions with possible biases in mind**. If there's potential that what you're asking about may contain biases, go ahead and name that in your prompt. For example, you might specify your biological sex in your query: "What are the side effects of sleep medication for females?"

- **Use AI for background research—not to diagnose yourself**. When something is wrong with us, we all want quick and accessible answers. Just as we've been consulting Dr. Google for years now, we're increasingly turning to AI to give us diagnoses and treatment recommendations. Do this with caution, urges Dr. Ghassemi. Patient symptoms are complex, and the way LLMs pull information means it's highly likely that you'll get wrong information. So save the official diagnoses and medical consults for a professional and use your favorite chatbot as you would a search engine: for information that can help educate you on what might be happening with your health and give you some basic knowledge to use as background for those discussions with your clinician.

- **Check chatbot answers against reliable sources**. It's a well-known problem that LLMs powering AI chatbots are capable of responding to user questions with plausible-sounding answers that turn out to be completely made up—not exactly what you're going for when it comes to your health concerns. While technologists are continuously at work trying to fix this, it's always a good idea to fact-check the responses you get against other sources. Have an answer to your question that sounds right? Do a quick search online to see if other, reputable sources share similar information.

- **Ask follow-up questions**. Can't understand an answer ChatGPT has just spit out? It's not you! LLMs can be excessively verbose and overuse many phrases, which can make their answers confusing and easy to misinterpret. So don't be afraid to follow up with more questions.

Ideally, ask those follow-ups in different ways, until you feel like you have a grasp of the content. And if the answers you're getting don't sound right, trust your gut.

- **Use AI to translate medical jargon.** LLMs are really good at extracting specific pieces of information from large amounts of text. Say, for example, you want to make sense of a research paper that uses scientific language you're having a tough time understanding. Copy and paste that text into your go-to chatbot and ask it to translate the information into simple, conversational language. Yet keep in mind that if you feed a chatbot personal health information—say you're looking for an explainer of all that medical lingo in your latest post-visit doctor report—it's not necessarily private or safe. (For more on health data privacy and how to keep your personal information safe, skip ahead to page 589.)

How to Read and Understand a Scientific Study: A Simple Guide for Those of Us Who Aren't Scientists

There's no denying the power of scientific research to change our lives for the better. Thanks to rigorous research into countless diseases, we have a better understanding than ever before of what causes us to get sick *and* what heals us. On the flip side, getting science wrong has the potential to do a lot of harm, whether it's a study with questionable findings that gets widely reported or sound science that gets inaccurately spun by the media for a clickbait headline.

The fact is that millions of scientific papers are published every year. Some of this research causes big shifts in the way practitioners care for their patients. More often, the results of new studies are considered food for thought—especially until the outcomes are replicated in other research. Much of this research will make headlines. Sometimes what you read about one study will seem a direct contradiction of something you read somewhere else. Given how all of us are inundated with health news these days—both accurate analysis of research from reputable and trustworthy sources and questionable takes from more nefarious players across the internet—it's more important than ever before to understand the basics of how to read and understand a scientific paper.

Even if you don't have a science background, it *is* a skill any of us can learn. Here, Dina Burstein, MD, MPH, walks us through the different types of studies and what to keep in mind when reading them.

Observational studies: In this type of research, individuals are observed or certain outcomes are measured and no attempt is made to affect the outcome. The researchers merely observe subjects, rather than manipulating different variables or assigning subjects to a treatment (as they do in experimental studies). Also in this category are case studies, which look at what's happening in very small groups of people (sometimes just one patient).

Experimental studies: In this type of research, researchers intentionally change the situation, circumstances, or experience of participants (manipulation) to see if it leads to a change in the outcome. Key features of experimental studies include use of intervention (when researchers change one or more variables to determine whether it causes a different outcome); control groups (a group of research subjects who are similar in every way to the intervention group except that they don't receive the intervention); and randomization (when study participants are randomly assigned to different groups rather than intentionally placed in one or another).

Analysis or review of studies: In this type of research, the researcher collects and evaluates multiple research studies or papers on a particular topic. The three main types of analyses are meta-analysis, scoping literature reviews, and systematic literature reviews. A meta-analysis uses statistical techniques to combine the findings from independent studies in an effort to derive conclusions about that body of research. A scoping literature review is an overview of the existing research on the topic, which involves searching for all relevant research and summarizing it with the goal of getting a broad understanding of the topic and different findings and perspectives on it. Systematic literature reviews involve formal quality ratings of the included literature.

What's important to remember about analysis or review of studies is that the significance of the results will only be as good as the studies being analyzed. Translation: If you do a review of a bunch of poorly designed experimental studies, the findings won't be as significant as a review of a bunch of well-designed studies.

Clinical trials: These are experimental research studies that test new drugs or combinations of drugs to determine their effectiveness, compare them with current standard treatments, and discover new ways a drug approved to treat one condition may be used to treat others. Drug trials are typically conducted in several phases:

- **Phase I:** Researchers test a drug or treatment in a small group of people (typically twenty to eighty) with the aim of identifying the highest dose humans can take without serious side effects. They also look at the best way to administer the drug (by mouth, injection, or infusion, for example) and identify side effects.

- **Phase II:** The new drug or treatment is given to a larger group (usually one hundred to three hundred people) to determine its effectiveness and continue to assess its safety.

- **Phase III:** The new drug or treatment is given to an even larger group (anywhere from one thousand to three thousand people) to continue to evaluate its efficacy, safety, and side effects. Phase III trials also aim to determine whether the new drug or treatment is as good as the current standard of care or similar treatments for a disease or condition.

- **Phase IV:** Also known as postmarketing trials, these studies are conducted in large populations after a drug, test, or procedure has been approved by the FDA for consumer use. They are designed to monitor the effectiveness of the approved drug in the general population, continue to collect information about any adverse side effects, and study any additional ways the drug may be used.

Because in this type of experimental study, participants are randomly assigned to either the experimental group (which receives the intervention) or the control group (which does not), which helps minimize bias and ensure that any differences in outcomes for each group are due to the intervention being studied, not other variables. If the RCT is "double-blind," that means neither the researchers nor the participants know who's receiving the intervention and who's in the control group, which can help minimize bias even more—both in how the study is conducted and interpreted.

What to Keep in Mind as You're Reading Studies

Now that you know the different types of studies, let's delve deeper into how to read and understand a scientific paper—something that's totally different from reading an article, blog post, or book about the same topic. Keep these points in mind as you dive in to be a more discerning reader of any article on health.

You may need expert help to make sense of what you're reading. If you don't have a scientific or medical background, research papers can be very difficult to fully comprehend. Even many people who do have scientific training say studies can be complex and hard to follow. So ask for help. Bring a study you've found and have questions about to your healthcare practitioner to see if they can explain what it's saying and help you decide if the results may be applicable to you.

Consider the source. Just as the outlets that run health news articles have a hierarchy when it comes to trustworthiness, scientific journals that publish research articles do, too. Studies hold more weight if they're peer-reviewed. (This is just what it sounds like: Research papers must be reviewed by a group of the scientists' peers before publication.) Also, take note of the authors, their institutional affiliations, and any disclosures they make about funding they've received, which can alert you to any potential biases.

Scan a study or article to see if the research was done on humans or animals. Animal studies are a great first step toward discovering new treatments for humans. But the fact is that we are not the same as lab mice. If you see the term *preclinical*, it's another way of saying "no human subjects."

Look for the number of study participants. When it comes to studies aiming to tell us what causes disease, the bigger the better. That's because big "cohorts" are more representative of our broader population. Small studies can still be valuable; they give researchers ideas about what needs to be further studied. However, keep in mind that small studies with exciting findings are often given lots of media attention—but that hype is often premature. Usually what the analysis in studies of small cohorts actually indicates is that there's something here worth studying in larger populations.

Ask, "Do the results replicate other research?" If study results are valid or true, other researchers should be able to get that same result, too. It's also important to keep this in mind when you read articles in the mainstream media touting new research in a way that makes it feel groundbreaking: Almost all new research builds on studies that came before it and considering that new research in relation to the other literature on the topic will give you the best perspective on what it really means.

Know the difference between correlation and causation. Correlation means that two things (say, an environmental factor and a disease) occur together more often than you'd expect by chance alone. Causation means that one thing (say, following a Mediterranean diet) led to a specific outcome (less heart disease).

Virtual Doctor Visits and Web-Based Pharmacies: What You Need to Know to Optimize Your Visits and Stay Safe

How to Get the Most Out of a Telehealth Visit

There's a good chance you're using telehealth services more than ever before—or at least, you're probably pretty open to video chatting with your healthcare provider if you're dealing with a symptom that they may not have to see in person to diagnose and treat. In 2021, 37 percent of adults polled by the CDC had used telemedicine within the previous year, and that number was higher among women (42 percent) than among men (32 percent).[2] Of course, there are times when making an in-person visit will be crucial. However, if your clinician suggests a virtual visit, Karen S. Rheuban, MD, cofounder and director of the UVA Center for Telehealth, has some tips to help you get the best care:

- **Check that your clinician is licensed to see you.** In most cases, the law requires that your healthcare provider be licensed to practice in the state in which you are physically located for your first appointment. Depending on state law, after an initial visit, your clinician may be able to treat you if you are not located in a state in which they are licensed if you have seen that provider within the prior twelve months. The provider also may not be able to prescribe medication if you are not located in a state in which they're licensed to practice. Keep in mind that some states require you to see a clinician in person for a first visit and allow telehealth appointments only after that initial in-person appointment.

  "The burden is on providers to be certain they are licensed to treat you," says Dr. Rheuban, "but it can't hurt to be clear on the requirements of the state in which you are located and make sure the clinician can see you and prescribe medication if needed when you make the appointment."

- **Make sure the technology platform you'll use is HIPAA compliant.** The Health Insurance Portability and Accountability Act of 1996 (HIPAA) is a federal law that protects a patient's sensitive health information from being shared without their knowledge or permission. Given the potential lack of security on common video-chat platforms like Zoom or FaceTime—and the rise of medical identity theft, where experts steal and sell your medical information on the black market—healthcare providers should use HIPAA-compliant tech platforms to protect you.

  "Again, your provider should state that your connection will be HIPAA compliant, but it's certainly worth talking about as part of an initial consent process," says Dr. Rheuban.

- **Check the quality of your connection before your appointment**. Many virtual appointment platforms will have a test for audio and video built into them, and they'll prompt you to do this test before your visit. This can take a few minutes, so log in to the link provided a few minutes before your scheduled appointment time. If your bandwidth isn't great, ask others in your household to avoid using the internet during your appointment, which will maximize the bandwidth for you.

- **Ask for translation services if needed**. If English isn't your first language or if you're hearing-impaired, notify your healthcare provider in advance of your visit so special translation services can be incorporated into the visit.

- **Sit in good lighting.** While it may seem like a physical exam would be impossible through a computer screen, many clinicians will check some basics—like asking you to stick out your tongue and say "ahhh" to look at your tonsils or run your fingers down your neck to pull the skin taut, which can reveal swollen lymph nodes. So, as you're getting set up for your virtual visit, choose a (quiet!) room with good natural light and make sure the light is in front of you (not behind you, which will make you appear darker on a screen and may prevent your practitioner from seeing you clearly). If natural light isn't available, sit with a lamp in front of you. If you're on your computer, have your mobile phone handy so you can use its flashlight app to shine extra light on any spots your clinician wants to take a closer look at.

- **Ask a family member to join you.** Depending on your symptoms, your clinician might ask you to hold your phone or computer camera toward an area of your body, such as your mouth or a patch of skin, for a closer look. It can be helpful to have someone with you to help you do this, says Dr. Rheuban. And if it's a consult about a worrisome health concern, having a second set of ears is always helpful—especially if they belong to someone you trust to advocate for you.

- **Have a list of medications (or your actual pill bottles) nearby.** Just as at an in-person doctor visit, your clinician will likely ask for an up-to-date list of medications as well as a general medical history and any new diagnoses.

"Sometimes patients don't think they need to prepare for a telemedicine appointment the same way they do for an in-person visit, but that's not true," says Dr. Rheuban. Be prepared to list any allergies, medications you're taking, and other pertinent information.

- **Use whatever devices you have at home to take some health stats before your visit.** If you can tell your doctor things like your blood pressure, heart rate, weight, body temperature, or oxygen saturation (using a pulse oximeter), that's great! While stats like these aren't necessary, they can be super helpful, says Dr. Rheuban.

"If you have these devices at home, ask your provider if she'd like you to take your vitals before your visit," she adds.

If your virtual visits are for remote patient monitoring—say you're dealing with a chronic condition and your clinician wants to check in regularly—there's a good chance you'll be sent electronic devices (like a scale or blood pressure machine), and when you take the measurement, your results will be automatically uploaded to your patient file.

Are Online Pharmacies Safe?

We buy everything with the click of a button these days, so it's no surprise more of us are using online pharmacies for our medications as well. However, there are a few things you should keep in mind to make sure you're ordering from a reputable source and getting the essential information you need about your prescriptions, says K. Ashley Garling, PharmD. Be sure you can answer "yes" to these questions before pressing that "purchase" button:

Q: Is there a licensed U.S. pharmacist available to answer your questions?

Talking to a pharmacist about things like dosage, storage, side effects, and any other questions or concerns you have about a prescription is crucial when it comes to ensuring you use medications correctly (like taking the medication with food or avoiding alcohol or sunlight while on it) and understand potential side effects so you're able to spot them and know what to do.

Q: Are you required to provide a prescription from your provider?

To dispense medication, a pharmacy needs a prescription from a licensed practitioner. There are no exceptions to this. If you're able to get prescription medication without this, it's a major red flag—and a sign you may not be getting the medication you need.

Q: Does the online pharmacy list a U.S. street address and telephone number?

Drugs have different names and uses in other countries, which means there's no guarantee you'll get the drug your clinician prescribed if you've ordered it from a pharmacy outside the U.S.

Q: Is the online pharmacy licensed with a state board of pharmacy?

Check the online pharmacy's license through your state board of pharmacy. The FDA has a great tool to allow you to do this easily: Visit fda.gov and search "locate a state-licensed online pharmacy" for a state-by-state database that'll help you be sure the online pharmacy you'd like to use has the appropriate licensure.

Q: Do the medications you receive look like the ones you get at your local pharmacy?

You should receive medicine that looks just like what you're used to taking, and it should arrive in packaging that's intact (not broken or damaged), is in English, and has an expiration date.

Q: Is the price too good to be true?

If a web-based pharmacy quotes you a price on a drug that's significantly less than your brick-and-mortar pharmacy says is the best price they can give you, it's a red flag.

"It's important to know that pharmacists don't benefit from you paying more for your drugs," says Dr. Garling. "It's part of our oath to make drugs accessible, and if we can find you a better price, we will." The online pharmacy should also state clearly that it will protect your personal and financial information and not sell it to other websites.

Biohacking Your Health: The Data That'll Give You the Most Helpful Information and the Best Ways to Track It

With an ever-growing number of wearable tools that give us real-time evidence of various aspects of our health, it can be tough to know what to track. Here are some metrics to consider:

- **Daily activity.** An activity tracker gives you data about how sedentary or active you really are. These days, most of us have phones with built-in activity trackers, so buying a specific wearable for this may not be necessary. That said, there are other devices that multitask when it comes to what they track—activity, sleep, and HRV—so you have a lot of choice when it comes to finding the right device for you. Pro tip: Choose one you'll actually wear. If it feels clunky or heavy, odds are it'll sit on your charger rather than your wrist or finger.

- **Your diet.** Keeping track of the food you eat in a food journal (or via a food-logging app) is a simple and free way to see exactly what you're putting into your body. Daily tracking of what you eat can help you make sure you're getting plenty of the foods that improve your overall health, as well as shine a light on the foods you're eating that may be hurting it.

- **Your blood glucose.** In an ideal world, your blood glucose level should remain relatively stable, rising only slightly after meals. When your glucose spikes and dips, it can damage your body's tissues and lead to diabetes, heart disease, and metabolic dysfunction. Wearing a continuous glucose monitor (CGM)—a small device that measures your blood glucose levels twenty-four hours a day—can help you see in real time how your blood glucose responds to the foods you eat. Over the course of even just a few weeks, this data can help you learn your reaction to foods and meal timing and use specific strategies (such as walking after meals) to keep your glucose stable.

- **Heart rate variability (HRV).** This is a measure of the variability in time between each heartbeat. It's increasingly being used as a biomarker for trends in our stress levels. If you're stressed or in fight-or-flight mode, the variation between heartbeats tends to be lower—a sign your cardiovascular system is trying to regulate your system. When you're more relaxed or in rest-and-digest mode, the variation between your heartbeats will likely be higher, signaling that your nervous system is able to be flexible and adapt easily, which is a sign of good cardiovascular fitness.

- **Sleep.** A sleep tracker can show you things like how many times you wake up each night and how much total sleep you're getting. Understanding these patterns can help you home in on specific areas to focus on, and maybe even be the push you need to see a sleep specialist.

Health Data Privacy: How to Keep Your Information Safe

If you're like most people, you download a health app on your phone and click "agree" to the terms of service without reading the fine print. You'd need a legal degree to make sense of the language describing what you're agreeing to, right? And what's the worst thing someone could do with the data you plug into your period app or fitness tracker? Send you some targeted ads that make you think your phone is spying on you?

Here's the truth: Most tech companies that make health apps aren't subject to the same privacy laws and high level of oversight as healthcare institutions and medical device companies. For example, while HIPAA is a federal law that protects your health info from being shared without your consent, it applies only to interactions with a healthcare provider, an insurance company, or their "business associates." Which means the majority of health apps aren't covered by HIPAA.

"Most of us have an intuition that when we're using an app or device that has to do with our health, the quality of the product—and the health data it captures—must be held to high standards and privacy protections," says attorney Leah Fowler, JD, MPH. "Yet in general, this isn't true."

That's not to say you shouldn't use health tech, adds Fowler.

"My opinion is that if you find a technology useful, you should use it," she says. "That said, it's always a good idea to know what type of information you are putting out in the world when you use these apps, and to then ask yourself, are you okay with other third parties having access to that info?"

Here are Fowler's top suggestions for using your favorite health trackers while also doing everything you can to protect your data:

- **Take the time to read privacy policies and terms of agreement.** Yes, these documents can be long and sometimes even tough to locate. However, most are a lot more readable than people assume, says Fowler.

    "You don't need a law degree to spend a few minutes reading about how an app will store and share your data," she says. Good news for consumers: Many apps are moving toward making their privacy policies and terms of agreements more readable, even using images to help people understand how data is shared with third parties and why the app does this. Also, these apps tend to use similar policies—so spending time reading one policy may help you skim others.

    "To the extent that you care about how your data is being used, you'll want to give these a read to know things like what rights you have and whether or not you can delete your data if you want to."

- **Email the customer service people to clarify anything in the privacy policy or terms of agreement you don't understand.** Most of us assume customer service is there to help us troubleshoot issues like payment snafus or issues that pop up when we're using these health apps or devices. However, Fowler says it's totally reasonable to ping customer service if you have questions about what the language in their terms of agreement means or if something feels especially opaque.

"I think it's okay to be as annoying as necessary to the customer service people if you have questions about a privacy policy," says Fowler. "Email them and ask for the clarification you need."

- **Consider what data you're tracking and how it might be used.** How important it feels to you to protect your data is a subjective evaluation. You may have a different risk tolerance and interest in how your health info is used than another person. That said, there's a common sentiment Fowler often hears when she talks to people about health data privacy, which goes something like this: *I don't care about what I share! I have nothing to hide!* This may be the case when it comes to what kind of sandwich you had for lunch, but what about tracking your monthly periods on an app that freely shares data when you live in a state where abortion is illegal?

"You have nothing to hide until you do," says Fowler, "which means it's important to think about what you're tracking and how that information could be used."

- **Treat your health data like the valuable information it is.** We live in a world where we're increasingly leaving robust data trails, thanks to all the technology we use. If someone were to aggregate information about you based on the tech you use, there's a good chance your purchasing patterns, your Google search history, and even health information like your fitness patterns, food consumption, and monthly menstrual cycles would paint a pretty detailed picture about you and your health.

"Everything reveals everything," says Fowler. Knowing this, it's a good idea to audit the apps on your phone every so often and even re-read their policies, which app companies are free to adjust at any time (and aren't obligated to let you know when they do). Then, says Fowler, trust your gut.

"If something doesn't sit right with you, listen to that rather than ignore it," she says.

Your Game Plan: How to Cut Through Health Hype and Get the Health Info You Need

With an ever-growing amount of misinformation lurking within articles and social media posts—essentially advertisements filled with big promises about wellness fixes and health cures—it's increasingly important to know how to distinguish between exaggerated claims and evidence-based solutions. Here, Dr. Shapiro shares her top tips.

Be wary of anything that sounds too good to be true. Information that falls at one extreme or another should toss up a red flag, says Dr. Shapiro. Think about it this way: When was the last time you heard your doctor or another medical professional use terms like *miraculous* or *groundbreaking*? Clinicians tend to be more measured than this because they know how complicated human bodies are, says Dr. Shapiro.

"We are complicated beings with a lot of moving parts, and what works for one person may not work for another," she says. Try to remember this the next time you read or hear health information that sounds like the be-all and end-all advice.

Remember that science evolves. It's frustrating when health advice changes. None of us can avoid the steady flow of often contradictory new studies and facts doled out by our favorite news sites and social media feeds. (Coffee is good for you—no, wait, it's not! Walking is the only exercise you need to do—scratch that, it's weight lifting!) But as long as the new information and advice is coming from a reputable source, it's important to keep an open mind, says Dr. Shapiro.

"Health recommendations change, usually for the better, because science is always evolving," she says. "This doesn't mean the original advice was necessarily wrong or fake. It's just that we have more access to information as time goes on."

We see this happen when big, respected medical associations change their opinions on various health statements. For example, the North American Menopause Society has updated its position statement on the use of menopause hormone therapy multiple times, based on new research. Cancer screening guidelines also change frequently, given our ever-emerging knowledge about who is getting diagnosed and when.

"These updates are a good thing," says Dr. Shapiro. "They are proof that science is happening—proof that nothing you read or hear, no matter how big the study, is the final word."

Think critically when you read or hear health information—and run it by a healthcare pro you trust. Check your sources and listen to your gut. If you're basing health decisions on scientific studies, know what a study is (flip back to page 579 for the basics) and also remember that while X can cause Y in a lab, it may have no significant health impact on *you*—a real, live human moving through the world with a lot of factors the scientists may not have been able to account for in the lab. Search for health information using questions that are specific yet not embedded with an opinion and stay on the lookout for answers that seem biased.

"Remember, there's no 'peer review' for information on the internet, which means opinions and misinformation get lumped together with facts," says Dr. Shapiro. "This makes it incredibly important to be discerning when reading information—and to have a trusted healthcare practitioner you can talk to about the information you find as it relates to your care."

• • • • •

We're living in an ever-evolving digital world where all aspects of our lives—including the ways we think about our health and care for ourselves—are becoming more technologically advanced. This is making it more crucial than ever to know how to suss out the facts, spot health misinformation and disinformation, and keep technology's potential downsides in mind so we can use it to our advantage.

Chapter 22

Your Playbook for Optimal Health and Managing Disease

Everything You Need to Chart a Path Forward That

Helps You Feel Empowered and Supported

> *It is important for a woman to be the best advocate that she can be for her health. Women are so often the caretakers of their family, putting the health of others before their own. But wives, mothers, and daughters need to make sure that their health needs are met in order to be there for others.*
>
> —Janine Austin Clayton, MD, "Seven Diseases That Affect Your Health, and What You Can Do" in *Imagining: A Journal*

All of us want to feel like we're being truly cared for by the experts we see to keep us healthy and help us heal when we're sick. In a dream scenario, you'd have a posse of healthcare providers who really know you and your specific health risks—clinicians with excellent bedside manner who make you feel like they have all the time in the world to talk through your symptoms and do a thorough physical exam when needed.

The reality is that many of us don't see the same provider year after year. We may feel rushed through appointments—or, worse, dismissed when we bring up our health concerns. We also get very little information about how to navigate the healthcare system so many of us find ourselves in at some point in our lives, whether it's knowing how to handle medical bills that seem shockingly high or navigating the implicit bias baked into every aspect of our care. What's the best way we can remedy the gaps in our knowledge and be our own best advocates? The information you'll find in the pages that follow is a start.

In this chapter, we'll learn . . .

- **The nuts and bolts of lining up your healthcare team**—from finding the best healthcare practitioners for you based on the health issues you're dealing with to understanding what to look for (and what to avoid) in a patient-doctor relationship.

- **How to make the most of your healthcare visits**, including information on how to create a personal and family medical history that'll give your healthcare team the information they need to assess your risk of disease and hatch a plan for the screenings you need.

- **How to decode any medical bill** so you're in a prime position to know what you can negotiate, to help you prevent medical debt.

- **The details you need about clinical trials**—what they are, how to find them, smart questions to ask before signing up for one, and what to know if you decide to participate.

- **Why females and people of color are more likely to have their health symptoms dismissed or not treated appropriately** by healthcare practitioners. When you know what medical gaslighting looks like, you can be more aware of it when it's happening and find a different provider.

- **How to create an action plan that'll help you face a medical diagnosis**, the treatment that follows, and your future medical care with a sense of control.

Meet the Experts

Kathy Giusti, two-time cancer survivor, founder and board member of the Multiple Myeloma Research Foundation, and author of *Fatal to Fearless: 12 Steps to Beating Cancer in a Broken Medical System*

Shilpi Agarwal, MD, family medicine physician at Georgetown University and author of *The 10-Day Total Body Transformation: A Doctor's Guide to Getting Leaner, Cleaner, and Happier in Just 10 Days!*

Emily Bernstein, CEO and lead patient advocate of Wheelhouse Health, which helps patients and their caregivers understand, access, and afford healthcare

Jayne Morgan, MD, cardiologist, vice president of medical affairs at Hello Heart, and former executive director of the largest healthcare system in Georgia

Karen Lutfey Spencer, PhD, professor at the University of Colorado Denver

Lining Up Your Healthcare Team: The Most Important Things to Keep in Mind When Looking for Practitioners

In an ideal scenario, your healthcare practitioners will feel like true partners in your care. You will feel comfortable talking about your symptoms with them, and they will ask the kinds of questions that ensure no potential health issues get overlooked. They will make you feel safe, seen, and heard. This is especially crucial when you're managing a chronic disease, given the number of doctor visits you'll likely have and the importance of feeling confident in your plan for care.

So what's the best way to go about finding the physicians and other healthcare professionals who'll feel like exactly the right members of your healthcare team? Kathy Giusti, two-time cancer survivor and author, offers a step-by-step guide:

- **Step 1: Get referrals**. Get a handful of recommendations from the clinician who diagnosed you for practitioners who specialize in treating your condition. You might ask, "If I was your sister, who would you want me to see for treatment?" You can also get referrals from your insurance company and friends who either have faced your same diagnosis or know someone who has.

- **Step 2: Ask the practical questions.** Once you've narrowed down your list of practitioners you'd like to consider seeing, confirm who accepts your health insurance (if you'll be using it) or what your costs will be if a practitioner is out of your insurance network. You'll also want to consider each practitioner's location and the convenience of their office. While it might be tempting to see the "best" doctor, if she's a three-hour drive away from your house and you'll be seeing her regularly, that might come to feel like a deal-breaker over time. This step will likely whittle down your list to a handful of specialists.

- **Step 3: Start making appointments and really clue in to how you feel during and after each visit.** Assess the practitioner's communication style and how you feel as you talk through your diagnosis and treatment options. Is the clinician really listening to your concerns and answering your questions? Do you feel rushed? Building a good rapport with a clinician you'll see repeatedly is incredibly important, so trust your instincts on this front and, if possible, bring someone with you to these appointments so you can talk through any concerns you might have after your visit and gut-check your initial reactions.

- **Step 4: Request names of other specialists who work in the same field.** While it might seem awkward, asking one specialist for a referral to another is a great way to broaden your provider search and confirm you've landed on the right team for you. Try to remember you're not asking for referrals to the "competition" but rather to *colleagues*, and most specialists will be more than happy to share those colleagues' names with you. (In fact, if someone bristles at the question or gets frustrated, it's a sign you might want to work with someone else.)

The Importance of Second (and Third) Opinions

After you receive an initial diagnosis, it can be tempting to make all of your decisions with a sense of urgency. It's sensible—and oftentimes necessary—to create a treatment plan as quickly as possible. However, it's also a good idea to confirm your diagnosis by getting other medical opinions.

Medical conditions can be complex, and different healthcare practitioners may have varying interpretations of your symptoms and test results. This is true for chronic conditions that are notoriously tricky to diagnose (think polycystic ovary syndrome and some autoimmune diseases as well as certain cancers). In fact, if you had a biopsy that showed a cancer diagnosis, you can actually request that your tissue sample be sent to another lab for further analysis to confirm that your diagnosis is accurate.

Second and third (and possibly even more) opinions are also a great way to make sure you're exploring all of your treatment options and verifying that certain procedures (like surgery) are necessary, as different providers may have different approaches to treating the same condition. Once you have a sense of all the options available to you (or, quite possibly, your lack of options), that broader perspective can give you greater peace of mind and confidence as you decide on your plan of action.

As for any fears you may have that seeing other physicians will make the ones you've already seen feel slighted, drop them. You can approach the process of getting more medical opinions with honesty and respect for your primary healthcare provider, who will likely understand and support your decision to seek additional perspectives.

"You won't piss off a doctor by looking elsewhere," says Giusti. "This is your life! Second and third opinions are essential to your survival and your quality of life along the way."

How to Make the Most of Doctor Visits:
The Best Ways to Prepare

Given that the average length of the time you see a doctor during a visit is under twenty minutes, there's a good chance you'll feel rushed—or leave your appointment feeling like you didn't cover everything you wanted to tackle.[1] The antidote? Being as prepared as possible *before* your appointment. Here's what medical professionals wish more patients knew about how to use your time with them so you can both make the most of every appointment.

Creating Your Personal and Family Health History: What to Include and Where to Start

Every clinician, whether they're a general practitioner or a specialist, will want a personal and family medical history—and it's best to create this before you're in the doctor's office waiting room so you can make it as accurate and detailed as possible.

Yes, this can feel like a daunting project. Yet the payoff is huge when it comes to helping your healthcare practitioners understand your risk of disease and create a plan for early detection and prevention of diseases that run in your family. Documenting your family medical history is a gift that'll benefit future generations, too. Another bonus: Do this once, print it out, and you can speed through that section of the paperwork at all future doctor visits.

Here's where to start:

- **Write down your personal medical history.** Create a document with the following info (skipping over what doesn't apply):
    - *Medical conditions you've been diagnosed with, both past and present.* This includes chronic conditions, surgeries or other procedures you've undergone, hospitalizations or emergency room visits, and any noteworthy acute illnesses (think pneumonia that prompted you to be out of school or work for multiple weeks versus a cold you managed with over-the-counter medicines at home).

- *Pregnancies you've had*, as well as any pregnancy-related health conditions you were diagnosed with and any miscarriages you may have had.

- *Menstrual cycle information*, including what age you were when your period started, the number of days you bleed, the approximate timing between periods, and any symptoms you experience during your cycle.

- *Menopause*, including what age you were when you went through it and what your symptoms were like during the menopause transition.

- *Medications you currently take*, including prescription drugs, over-the-counter medicines, and supplements (including vitamins and herbal remedies). When you make this list, snag the bottles of everything you're taking and record the dose, how frequently you take it, and the reason for taking each.

- *Allergies and adverse reactions you've experienced in response to medications*. Get specific about the type of reaction you had and when you had it.

- *Immunization record*, including vaccinations, boosters, and the dates they were administered.

- *Medical tests and screenings*—including mammograms, colonoscopies, and even things like blood pressure readings and cholesterol levels—and the date you had each done as well as the results. You can usually get this information pretty easily from your healthcare system's online portal or by calling doctors' offices or hospitals for your medical records.

- *Dates of checkups and doctor visits*, including things like when you had your last comprehensive physical exam, and appointments with specialists like a cardiologist, an eye doctor, and even your dentist.

- **Make a list of your relatives and as much of their medical histories as you know (or can gather, if they're still alive).** First-degree family members include your mother, father, and siblings and children if you have them. Second-degree family members include your grandparents, aunts, uncles, and grandchildren.

Write down the following information for each of these family members:

- Place and year of birth (and year of death, if someone has passed away)

- Ethnicity (because some genetic diseases are more common in certain ethnic groups)

- Diseases they were diagnosed with and age at diagnosis

- Their chronic conditions or patterns of poor health, including things like allergies, addiction, and even chronic coughing

If you don't have a full picture of all the health challenges your relatives have faced, that's okay. Most clinicians will want to know primarily about some of the conditions with strong genetic components, including cancer, heart disease (including high blood pressure and cholesterol), stroke, diabetes, migraines, and autoimmune disorders.

Ask an Expert

What do you love to see patients do to help optimize a short appointment?

Healthcare visits are shorter than ever, which can be frustrating for both patients *and* providers. Patients are understandably frustrated if they feel rushed, and doctors often feel torn between providing good care and not running two hours behind schedule. However, there's a lot you can do to make the most of the time you do get with your healthcare providers.

I always tell patients to prepare for a healthcare visit by writing down a list of all your concerns and questions. Then comes a key next step: Prioritize that list. If you have a handful of symptoms or issues that are bothering you, list them in order of what you find most challenging. Then, at the start of your appointment, say something like, "These are the three things I've been struggling with that I'd like to talk about, but I understand you may not have time to address all of them today. This is the one that feels most pressing to me." Saying something along those lines creates a bridge between you and your clinician. It lets us know that you realize we have limited time, and it also gives us the information we need to give you the best possible care in the time we *do* have.

If you have a specific concern, it also helps to think about the following questions:

- When did this symptom begin?

- How long has it been going on?

- What makes it better or worse?

- What home remedies or OTC medications have you tried?

- Are there any other symptoms you think are related?

These are the questions that clinicians ask to land on a diagnosis and treatment plan. If you've given some thought to your answers, it can help you lay out your issue efficiently, which helps your provider come up with a diagnosis and treatment plan.

Finally, if you have a big concern you'd like to discuss, schedule an appointment strictly for that issue rather than trying to squeeze it into your annual physical or gynecologic exam—and talk about a plan for follow-up care. You might ask your provider if they do follow-ups via telehealth, which can be a great way to tackle your concerns without waiting several weeks for another in-person appointment. Think about it this way: You'd never go to your hairstylist for a cut and then expect them to tack on a color appointment to cover your grays. The same is true for healthcare appointments. If you're scheduled for a physical, there's a lot your clinician has to cover to give you the preventive care you need—from performing a physical exam and discussing lifestyle habits like diet, exercise, and sleep to making sure you're scheduled for cancer screenings you need. If you try to tackle another problem, you may not actually get the thorough physical you need.

The bottom line: Set realistic expectations about what you can go over in one visit and make it clear to your provider that you know you won't be able to talk about every health concern you have. This can go a long way toward helping you get the care you need and deserve.

—Shilpi Agarwal, MD, family medicine physician at Georgetown University and author of *The 10-Day Total Body Transformation: A Doctor's Guide to Getting Leaner, Cleaner, and Happier in Just 10 Days!*

Understanding—and Negotiating—Medical Bills

A sobering fact: About 40 percent of Americans in the U.S. have some sort of debt due to medical bills.[2] Yet there are steps all of us should take before we pay those bills, says patient advocate Emily Bernstein. Here's her advice.

Before You Pay Any Medical Bill . . .

- **Know that you don't have to pay the bill immediately.** As urgent as the hospital or medical office will make your bill seem, you should never pay a medical bill right away. Worried about an outstanding amount you owe hitting your credit report? According to current federal laws, debt under $500 is never reported and debt over $500 will get sent to collections after three to six months (depending on the provider and institution) and will usually get reported to credit bureaus after one year. This should give you plenty of time to figure out if your bill is accurate and whether you qualify for financial assistance, or to set up a payment plan if you can't pay in full. (More details on all of that to follow.)

- **Ask for an itemized bill.** This will list Current Procedural Terminology (CPT) codes for any medical procedures and/or services you received.

- **Do an internet search for each of the CPT codes on your bill to find out what they stand for.** As tedious as this can be, it's crucial. Mistakes happen and medical bill errors are more common than you'd think. This is your chance to fact-check and make sure you actually had each of the procedures and/or treatments for which you're being charged.

  "It's not fair that we have to do this work to make sure we're being accurately billed, but the more people who do this, the more we hold these hospitals and medical offices accountable," says Bernstein.

- **Dispute anything that seems like an error.** Let's say there's a code for a procedure or treatment on your bill that you did not receive. Call the hospital billing office to say you'd like to dispute a charge, and ask for the email and/or mailing addresses where you can send your dispute. Keep this call short. The person who answers your call may make it sound like you have no chance of disputing your medical bill. If this happens, don't engage. Just get the info you need on where to send your dispute and end the call.

- **When you call about your bill, state what you need right away and ask, "Are you the right person to help with this?"** This can save you a lot of time and will tee you up to talk to the person who has the best shot of actually helping you with your request. And when you do reach the person who can help you, take notes: Write down whom you talked to, on what date, and what was said.

- **Ask the billing department to put your claim on hold if you're disputing a bill.** This will put the timeline on hold—or at least restart the clock—on when they can send your bill to collections.

  "Consumer protections state that collections agencies aren't allowed to collect on bills that are being disputed, especially if they can't verify what you owe or if you're fighting a charge for a service you didn't receive," says Bernstein. "It's crucial to let the hospital know that you're disputing the bill because of X, Y, and Z and request they put the claim on hold while you figure it out."

- **Find out if you're eligible for financial assistance, which is sometimes called charity care.** Federal law requires nonprofit hospitals to provide free or reduced-fee care to patients within a certain income range. Most for-profit hospitals will also have some sort of financial assistance program, though it's not regulated by law. Every hospital has its own application and process for applying. To track down your hospital's policy and application, do an internet search that includes the hospital name and "financial assistance."

- **Ask for a reasonable payment plan.** If your bill is accurate, there's not much room for negotiation. At this point, you can work with the billing office to come up with an agreed-upon, interest-free payment plan.

- **Recruit help from a friend, loved one, or patient advocate.** The fact that you've received a medical bill means you or a loved one has had some kind of medical issue or emergency, which was likely stressful in and of itself. Then, when you're still going through treatment or recovering, the bills begin to arrive—and taking the steps outlined here may feel like an insurmountable task. If that's the case, enlist help. Ask a friend or loved one you think will be particularly good at this task to skip the casserole drop-off and help you negotiate your medical bills instead. There are also a growing number of qualified medical billing advocates who can take the reins on the frustrating task of negotiating your bills. Some (but not all) patient advocates will do this work as well.

"When you tap out and focus on taking care of yourself or your loved one, it's a huge relief—and your advocate can be more strategic and levelheaded as she works with the hospital to help you get the best outcome," says Bernstein.

Clinical Trials 101: Why They Can Help You Get Top-Notch Healthcare and How to Sign Up for One

Women and people of color are still highly underrepresented in research.[3] But the good news is that, collectively, we have the power to change that. And it sometimes comes with a bonus, especially if you're managing a chronic disease: Participating in a trial has the potential to get you excellent, comprehensive care (for free!) with multiple healthcare visits and more health monitoring and wellness checks than you'd have received if you weren't enrolled in the study.

Here, cardiologist Jayne Morgan, MD, shares her thoughts on why all of us should consider participating in research and exactly how to get involved, plus the questions to ask if you're thinking about joining a trial.

Five Truths About Clinical Trials Most People Don't Realize

There's a lot of confusion about joining a research trial—which leads a lot of people to count themselves out when actually, it could be a great way to get free, personalized care. Here's what too many of us don't realize when it comes to participating in clinical trials.

Truth No. 1: You can participate—even if you don't have a rare or life-threatening disease. Oftentimes, when we think of medical research, we think it must involve novel and sometimes moon-shot treatments for diseases like cancer. And while these types of trials do exist and can improve the prognosis of many patients, it's important to realize there are plenty of other studies looking at almost every imaginable disease state, health habit, and so much more.

Truth No. 2: You may get free, individualized care that improves your health before you start participating in a trial. The scientists and clinicians running clinical trials are almost always on the hunt for study participants—so much so that if you don't qualify to participate in a study because of a chronic medical condition like diabetes or high blood pressure, they'll often help you improve these health conditions so you qualify to participate. Translation: You get personalized care from top-notch healthcare professionals that'll improve your health *and* help you feel better, all at no cost to you other than your time.

Truth No. 3: Your healthcare practitioner should be able to tell you about clinical trials you might qualify to participate in. One of the reasons women—and particularly women of color—are less likely than men to participate in research is because we aren't asked, says Dr. Morgan. The most common way to find out about research you may qualify for is through your practitioner, and you'll be more likely to be told about trials if your practitioner is conducting the study.

"Given the fact that most clinical trials are led by white males, it's easy to see why the research gap still exists," says Dr. Morgan. Until this changes, get proactive. Tell your healthcare provider that you're interested in enrolling in a trial. Your clinician should be able to reach out to medical centers and other practitioners, or even search the federal database of trials (clinicaltrials.gov) to help you find options for which you might qualify.

Truth No. 4: You have a right to know all the details about what's involved in a study before you sign up for it, including what will be expected of you. It's crucial to understand the ins and outs of the trial you're considering joining, including the treatment you'll take, any potential side effects, what'll be expected of you through the duration of the trial and possibly even after it ends, and more. This is called informed consent. (For a checklist of questions to ask before you join a study, see page 609.) Ask anything you like of the people running the trial so you have all the info you need to decide if enrolling is right for you and about what to expect if you sign up to participate.

Truth No. 5: Just because you join a study doesn't mean you have to stick it out if it's not working for you. Clinical trials are voluntary, which means if something comes up and you're unable to complete the study or follow through on what you signed up for, that's okay. Ideally, you'll have regular check-ins with the study facilitators, who can help you troubleshoot any issues that come up in the process of your participation. But at the end of the day, it's your call whether to be in the study or not.

What to Ask Before Joining a Clinical Trial

Once you know what participating in a study will require of you—whether it's showing up for various doctor appointments, getting lab work done at regular intervals, weathering potential side effects of a new medication, the list goes on—it's a good idea to discuss the pros and cons with a clinician you trust. The scientists conducting the study can also help you put the potential upsides and downsides in a context that'll help you make a decision.

Here are some questions to ask:

- What treatment is being tested?

- Why are you recommending this specific clinical trial for me?

- What is involved in the treatment being tested, and what will be expected of me throughout the course of the trial?

- Who will be in charge of my care while I'm participating in the trial?

- How will my doctor know whether the treatment is working?

- How does the treatment being tested differ from the current standard of care?

- Are there any known side effects or risks of the treatment being tested? If yes, how do they compare to those of the current standard of care?

- What phase of the trial will I be participating in? (For more info on what the different phases of a trial involve, flip back to page 581.)

- Has this treatment been tested before? If yes, what were the results of those earlier studies?

- Will there be a placebo (or inactive treatment) arm of the study? (If the answer is yes, consider whether it feels okay that you may be randomly selected to receive the placebo rather than the new drug or procedure being tested.)

- Will I be compensated for participating in the study? Will certain costs (like travel, medical care, or childcare needed to make it to appointments) be reimbursed?

- Will there be long-term follow-up care after the trial ends?

- When will I be notified about the trial's results?

- Who is sponsoring or funding the trial?

Medical Gaslighting: How to Spot the Signs and Ask the Questions That'll Get You the Care You Deserve

It's a far too common scenario: You go to the doctor and report symptoms that feel serious, only to be dismissed—told your concerns are the result of being tired, stressed, or overweight. There's a term for this feeling of being brushed off by your healthcare provider: *medical gaslighting*. And there is research proving it happens to women and people of color more frequently than other groups.

What Exactly Is Medical Gaslighting?

To gaslight someone means to manipulate that person into doubting themselves, their experiences, or their understanding of events, according to the American Psychological Association. The term comes from an old play called *Gas Light* about a husband's attempt to drive his wife insane so he could steal from her.

Yet while many patients describe the dismissal of their symptoms as truly maddening, the word *gaslighting* implies intentionality in a way that is unfair to many providers, says professor Karen Lutfey Spencer, PhD. Her research shows that some of the most common reasons why a healthcare provider may dismiss or misdiagnose their patients are a lack of certainty about what the diagnosis is (possibly due to a lack of research on women and people of color) and increasing demands on providers that can lead to burnout and increase their cognitive load (which may make them more likely to make decisions biased by racism).

How to Take Control

When you're not feeling your best or are dealing with symptoms that none of your doctors can figure out, it's hard enough. Getting the brush-off from a healthcare provider on top of that can be downright devastating. So what can you do if this happens to you?

- **Know the signs that could indicate medical gaslighting.** If your doctor doesn't really listen to you, interrupts you frequently, dismisses your symptoms as not serious, or suggests that what you're dealing with is purely psychological, take note. Another big red flag: not conducting a thorough examination and investigation into what you're experiencing and what might be causing your symptoms.

- **Make subjective symptoms (like pain or fatigue) as concrete as possible.** Keep a diary of your symptoms so you can be super specific. When your symptom happens, what do you do that makes it worse or better, and what brought it on? You should also track how it's interfering with activities of daily living, such as work, caring for your family, and everyday tasks like showering or grocery shopping.

- **Have an honest conversation with your healthcare provider about what's working—or not—about your care.** You can even acknowledge that you've learned about the differences in the way pain is treated in men versus women, for example, and outright ask: "Is my treatment plan specific to my age, gender, and ethnicity?" Name the fact that you feel dismissed if a clinician talks over you or doesn't answer your questions.

- **Bring a friend or family member with you to medical visits.** And empower the person accompanying you to speak up on your behalf. That person can offer additional context for the symptoms you're describing and the extent to which they're abnormal for you. Having someone with you also sends a message to your healthcare provider that someone else is invested in your care.

- **Get a second (or third) opinion.** If you feel you're being dismissed or your concerns aren't being taken seriously, find another provider. It's not right that the onus is on you to compensate for a system that's sexist and racist. But it's important to realize that sometimes it can take a lot of legwork to find clinicians who truly feel like they're on your team.

Your Game Plan: How to Create an Action Plan That'll Help You Take Charge of Any Diagnosis

It's common and completely understandable if you feel utterly overwhelmed in the days after a health diagnosis. Whether it's a chronic condition you'll have to manage over the long haul or a cancer diagnosis that'll require you to make some big, potentially life-altering decisions, it's a lot to take in. Once you've given yourself some time to wrap your head and heart around the news, it's crucial to start plotting how to face your disease and what you need to do so.

"In today's world, where science is moving so quickly, it's important to be your own advocate," says Kathy Giusti. Here, she shows us where to start.

Be specific when you search for information and discerning when you see the results. In an ideal world, our easy access to information would leave us feeling more informed, empowered, and clear on the best course of action. In reality, most internet searches for diagnoses like cancer leave us daunted and overwhelmed. You'll get the best information by using specific words that state the following: where you are in your disease journey (i.e., newly diagnosed, waiting for results, or starting treatment); the stage of your diagnosis if that applies; and as many specifics as possible about your type of disease.

When you get Google's list of results, scan for sites you can trust and don't even click on results from less reputable sources. For example, when it comes to cancer, the leading sites are cancer.org and cancer.gov. You'll also find great information on sites for hospitals and clinics that specialize in your disease. (For a lot more detail on how to suss out information you can trust online and spot misinformation, flip back to page 571.) It's also a good idea to find disease-specific organizations that tailor their information to specific types of cancer or other diseases, such as fightcolorectalcancer.org, the Multiple Myeloma Research Foundation (themmrf.org), and the Rheumatoid Arthritis Foundation (helpfightra.org).

Learn more about your insurance coverage. Once a medical diagnosis is confirmed, you'll want to start making calls and asking for referrals for second (and third) opinions. But first, it's important to contact your health insurance provider and learn more about your coverage. Find out what centers, doctors, and procedures are covered so you can get a sense of which hospital systems and doctors are in network versus out of network and what your out-of-pocket costs might be.

Get honest about your needs and wants. When you're staring down a big, life-changing (and potentially life-threatening) diagnosis, you'll want to focus on your immediate needs first—things like making calls to your insurance company and doctors' offices, going to appointments, lining up childcare, and figuring out how much time you'll need to take off from work and possibly even who will cover for you while you're out. But once the ball is in motion on these crucial steps, spending some time with these two questions can help you adjust to this new, unwanted journey you're on.

1. What do I *need* right now in addition to my medical care? The answers here might include things that'll help you ease your treatment journey, whether it's friends bringing you dinners each week so you don't have to think about cooking or a therapist for your kids who can help you track and manage their fears and emotions. It might also include what you need to give up—and mourn—while you focus on getting healthy.

2. What do I *want* throughout—and on the other side—of this journey? Answering this question will help you name what Giusti calls your north star, or the guiding light that'll help you continue to remember what's most important to you as you fight for your health. When Giusti battled multiple myeloma and then breast cancer, what she wanted was clear: to keep her family safe and happy and to build memories that would last. No matter how you answer this question for yourself, Giusti recommends writing it down, reading your answer every day, and sharing it with someone you trust who can remind you of your north star if times get tough.

Recruit your personal support team. Once you've considered some of the ways your treatment plan will impact your life, it's a good idea to build out your team of loved ones who can play a role in supporting you. This is a great time to think about the family members, friends, and other people in your life who can do things like accompany you to doctor visits, help you manage your medications, talk over treatment options with you as you make important decisions, and offer emotional support as you go through the inevitable ups and downs of the treatment process. Once you've lined up your dream team, have radically honest conversations with them about your diagnosis and treatment plan and exactly how you're hoping they'll help, and gauge their availability.

As you have these conversations, try to remember that your caregivers will have needs, too, which are also important to talk through.

"Your personal support team needs to know you understand *their* needs as much as you need them to understand *your* needs," says Giusti.

While none of us really wants to consider the possibility that we'll receive a scary medical diagnosis, the reality is that this might happen—even if you've spent years taking all the right steps to stay healthy. Facing illness is an inevitable part of being human. Yes, this reality can feel like a big buzzkill. But it can also prompt you to take action. Because one of the best things you can do—especially if you're healthy right now—is to consider how you'll handle disease if it strikes.

· · · · ·

After so many years of women being ignored in scientific studies, we are finally at an inflection point of change. And along with the advances in medical research and this newfound knowledge about women's health, we're also making giant strides in how we can look after ourselves—and one another—and create the conditions that set us up to flourish at every stage of our lives. The best part? It'll help everyone around us thrive, too.

Acknowledgments

This book wouldn't be if it weren't for Maria Shriver, who suggested I use my women's health journalism experience to take a big swing at the topic in book form. Maria, working with you and the rest of *The Sunday Paper* team, and being an Open Field author, is a true honor. Your fierce women's health advocacy is undoubtedly moving humanity forward.

This book wouldn't be what it is if it weren't for all the amazing experts I interviewed—doctors, nurses, anatomists, researchers, and other women's health clinicians and advocates—who graciously shared their time and expertise to help me deliver evidence-based information. Women have been under-studied and overlooked for far too long. We deserve better. These experts are on a mission to bring us better.

To the incredible team at The Open Field, especially my editors Nina Rodríguez-Marty and Cassidy Graham: You made this book better in so many ways.

Carrie Frye, having your hands and heart in my early drafts helped the copy take shape and transformed my overwhelm into confidence. You are a magic worker. Bonnie Solow, your insights and advice throughout this process have been essential. I'm also grateful to Katherine Wessling and Jensen Wheeler, who fact-checked this book to help me make sure I got it right.

While I spent countless hours writing and revising by myself, I didn't really write this book alone thanks to my great luck of having the most supportive people in my world.

Brian, your calm nature, analytical thinking, and awe-inspiring organizational skills are the reason I finished this project and stayed sane (sort of). Every writer should be so lucky to have a Brian to make them spreadsheets and sprint boards. To be loved and supported by you is one of my life's greatest gifts.

To my English teacher father and original writing coach, your lessons are always in my mind and heart. To my mom: "This is possibility!" you told me, pointing to the New York City skyline in the tiny bedroom I rented after landing my first job in publishing. It was all possible because of you and Dad.

To my little sister and first and forever best friend, Maureen, and to my sister friends—especially Jill, Maren, Jess, and Jackie—your endless support via calls, cards, crystals, candles, and so much more kept me feeling held throughout this wild ride.

To Maeve, McKenna, and Sydney, being your Aunt Meggie is my favorite. You were all top of mind as I worked on this book. My hope is that you have more information about your health than any generation before you, and that it'll inspire you to pick up the torch and empower the ones who come after you.

That is my hope for all of us. Because the more we know about our bodies and our health, the more empowered we'll be to take care of ourselves, speak up for ourselves, and ultimately love ourselves. And that is how all of us will thrive.

Notes

Introduction

1. "One-Fourth of Adults and Nearly Half of Adults Under 30 Don't Have a Primary Care Doctor," KFF, February 8, 2019, https://www.kff.org/other/slide/one-fourth-of-adults-and-nearly-half-of-adults-under-30-dont-have-a-primary-care-doctor.

2. Katherine A. Liu and Natalie A. DiPietro Mager, "Women's Involvement in Clinical Trials: Historical Perspective and Future Implications," *Pharmacy Practice* 14, no. 1 (March 6, 2016): 708, https://doi.org/10.18549/pharmpract.2016.01.708.

3. "NIH Policy and Guidelines on the Inclusion of Women and Minorities as Subjects in Clinical Research," National Institutes of Health, last updated October 21, 2024, https://grants.nih.gov/policy/inclusion/women-and-minorities/guidelines.htm.

4. "Item of Interest: NICHD Announces Gynecologic Health and Disease Research Themes and Scientific Vision," National Institutes of Health, June 8, 2018, https://www.nichd.nih.gov/newsroom/news/060818-GHDB.

5. Urtė Fultinavičiūtė, "Sex and Science: Underrepresentation of Women in Early-Stage Clinical Trials," *Clinical Trials Arena*, October 17, 2022, https://www.clinicaltrialsarena.com/features/underrepresentation-women-early-stage-clinical-trials.

6. Kerri Smith, "Women's Health Research Lacks Funding—These Charts Show How," *Nature*, May 3, 2023, https://www.nature.com/immersive/d41586-023-01475-2/index.html.

7. Donna L. Hoyert, "Maternal Mortality Rates in the United States, 2021," National Center for Health Statistics, last reviewed March 16, 2023, https://www.cdc.gov/nchs/data/hestat/maternal-mortality/2021/maternal-mortality-rates-2021.htm.

CHAPTER 1:
Essential Anatomy

1. Andreas Kalampalikis and Lina Michala, "Cosmetic Labiaplasty on Minors: A Review of Current Trends and Evidence," *International Journal of Impotence Research* 35, no. 3 (October 18, 2021): 192–95, https://doi.org/10.1038/s41443-021-00480-1.

2. Ellen Laan et al., "Young Women's Genital Self-Image and Effects of Exposure to Pictures of Natural Vulvas," *Journal of Psychosomatic Obstetrics & Gynecology* 38, no. 4 (September 20, 2016): 249–55, https://doi.org/10.1080/0167482x.2016.1233172.

3. Margaret A. McNulty, Rebecca L. Wisner, and Amanda J. Meyer, "NOMENs Land: The Place of Eponyms in the Anatomy Classroom," *Anatomical Sciences Education* 14, no. 6 (November/December 2021): 847–52, https://doi.org/10.1002/ase.2108.

CHAPTER 2:
Puberty

1. Kaitlin R. Taibl et al., "Newborn Metabolomic Signatures of Maternal Per- and Polyfluoroalkyl Substance Exposure and Reduced Length of Gestation," *Nature Communications* 14, no. 1 (May 30, 2023): https://doi.org/10.1038/s41467-023-38710-3.

2. Mickey Emmanuel and Brooke R. Bokor, "Tanner Stages," StatPearls, December 11, 2022, https://www.ncbi.nlm.nih.gov/books/NBK470280.

3. Frank M. Biro et al., "Onset of Breast Development in a Longitudinal Cohort," *Pediatrics* 132, no. 6 (December 2013): 1019–27, https://doi.org/10.1542/peds.2012-3773.

4. "Your Menstrual Cycle," Office on Women's Health, U.S. Department of Health and Human Services, last updated January 13, 2025, https://womenshealth.gov/menstrual-cycle/your-menstrual-cycle.

5. Sarah J. Clark et al., "Parents' Perception of Their Child's Body Image," *Mott Poll Report* 41, no. 5 (September 2022): https://mottpoll.org/sites/default/files/documents/091922_BodyImage.pdf.

6. Ciara Mahon and David Hevey, "Processing Body Image on Social Media: Gender Differences in Adolescent Boys' and Girls' Agency and Active Coping," *Frontiers in Psychology* 12 (May 21, 2021): https://doi.org/10.3389/fpsyg.2021.626763.

7. Anna Brown, "About 5% of Young Adults in the U.S. Say Their Gender Is Different from Their Sex Assigned at Birth," Pew Research Center, June 7, 2022, https://www.pewresearch.org/short-reads/2022/06/07/about-5-of-young-adults-in-the-u-s-say-their-gender-is-different-from-their-sex-assigned-at-birth.

CHAPTER 3:
Sexual Health

1. David A. Frederick et al., "Differences in Orgasm Frequency Among Gay, Lesbian, Bisexual, and Heterosexual Men and Women in a U.S. National Sample," *Archives of Sexual Behavior* 47, no. 1 (February 17, 2017): 273–88, https://doi.org/10.1007/s10508-017-0939-z.
2. Maria Uloko, Erika P. Isabey, and Blair R. Peters, "How Many Nerve Fibers Innervate the Human Glans Clitoris: A Histomorphometric Evaluation of the Dorsal Nerve of the Clitoris," *Journal of Sexual Medicine* 20, no. 3 (January 30, 2023): 247–52, https://doi.org/10.1093/jsxmed/qdac027.
3. Csaba Erdős et al., "Female Sexual Dysfunction in Association with Sexual History, Sexual Abuse and Satisfaction: A Cross-Sectional Study in Hungary," *Journal of Clinical Medicine* 12, no. 3 (January 31, 2023): 1112, https://doi.org/10.3390/jcm12031112.
4. William C. E. Berry et al., "Associations Between Gynecologic Clinician Type and Routine Female Sexual Dysfunction Screening," *Journal of Sexual Medicine* 20, no. 10 (August 8, 2023): 1235–40, https://doi.org/10.1093/jsxmed/qdad106.
5. "U.S. STI Epidemic Showed No Signs of Slowing in 2021—Cases Continued to Escalate," CDC Newsroom, Centers for Disease Control and Prevention, April 11, 2023, https://www.cdc.gov/media/releases/2023/s0411-sti.html.
6. "Sexually Transmitted Infections Treatment Guidelines, 2021," Centers for Disease Control and Prevention, accessed April 7, 2025, https://www.cdc.gov/std/treatment-guidelines.
7. K. C. Basile et al., "The National Intimate Partner and Sexual Violence Survey: 2016/2017 Report on Sexual Violence," Atlanta: National Center for Injury Prevention and Control, Centers for Disease Control and Prevention (2022), https://cdc.gov/nisvs/documentation/nisvsReportonSexualViolence.pdf.

CHAPTER 4:
Gynecology

1. Adejoke B. Ayoola, Gail L. Zandee, and Yenupini J. Adams, "Women's Knowledge of Ovulation, the Menstrual Cycle, and Its Associated Reproductive Changes," *Birth* 43, no. 3 (May 9, 2016): 255–62, https://doi.org/10.1111/birt.12237.

2. "Genital HPV Infection—CDC Fact Sheet," National Center for HIV/AIDS, Viral Hepatitis, STD, and TB Prevention (U.S.), Division of STD Prevention, January 23, 2014, https://stacks.cdc.gov/view/cdc/26043.

3. "Cervical Cancer: Screening," U.S. Preventive Services Task Force, August 21, 2018, https://www.uspreventiveservicestaskforce.org/uspstf/recommendation/cervical-cancer-screening.

4. Tim J. Palmer et al., "Invasive Cervical Cancer Incidence Following Bivalent Human Papillomavirus Vaccination: A Population-Based Observational Study of Age at Immunization, Dose, and Deprivation," *Journal of the National Cancer Institute* 116, no. 6 (January 22, 2024): 857–65, https://doi.org/10.1093/jnci/djad263.

5. "Cancer Facts for Lesbian and Bisexual Women," American Cancer Society, last revised February 1, 2024, https://www.cancer.org/cancer/risk-prevention/understanding-cancer-risk/cancer-facts/cancer-facts-for-lesbian-and-bisexual-women.html.

6. "What's the Cervical Mucus Method of FAMs?," Planned Parenthood, accessed April 7, 2024, https://www.plannedparenthood.org/learn/birth-control/fertility-awareness/whats-cervical-mucus-method-fams.

7. "Unintended Pregnancy," Reproductive Health, Centers for Disease Control and Prevention, May 15, 2024, https://www.cdc.gov/reproductive-health/hcp/unintended-pregnancy/index.html.

8. Britt K. Erickson, Michael G. Conner, and Charles N. Landen, "The Role of the Fallopian Tube in the Origin of Ovarian Cancer," *American Journal of Obstetrics and Gynecology* 209, no. 5 (April 10, 2013): 409–14, https://doi.org/10.1016/j.ajog.2013.04.019.

9. Rachel K. Jones, "An Estimate of Lifetime Incidence of Abortion in the United States Using the 2021–2022 Abortion Patient Survey," *Contraception* 135 (April 2, 2024): 409–14, https://doi.org/10.1016/j.contraception.2024.110445.

10. Ashley Kirzinger et al., "Abortion Knowledge and Attitudes: KFF Polling and Policy Insights," KFF, January 22, 2020, https://www.kff.org/womens-health-policy/poll-finding/abortion-knowledge-and-attitudes-kff-polling-and-policy-insights.

11. Katherine Kortsmit et al., "Abortion Surveillance—United States, 2021," *CDC Surveillance Summaries* 72, no. 9 (November 24, 2023): 1–29, https://www.cdc.gov/mmwr/volumes/72/ss/ss7209a1.htm.

12. Ushma D. Upadhyay et al., "Effectiveness and Safety of Telehealth Medication Abortion in the USA," *Nature Medicine* 30, no. 4 (February 15, 2024): 1191–98, https://doi.org/10.1038/s41591-024-02834-w.

CHAPTER 5:
A Guide to Gynecologic Conditions

1. Sara Berg, "What Doctors Wish Patients Knew About Endometriosis," American Medical Association, December 6, 2024, https://www.ama-assn.org/delivering-care/population-care/what-doctors-wish-patients-knew-about-endometriosis.

2. Parveen Parasar, Pinar Ozcan, and Kathryn L. Terry, "Endometriosis: Epidemiology, Diagnosis and Clinical Management," *Current Obstetrics and Gynecology Reports* 6, no. 1 (January 27, 2017): 34–41, https://doi.org/10.1007/s13669-017-0187-1

3. "Polycystic Ovary Syndrome," Office on Women's Health, U.S. Department of Health and Human Services, last updated February 22, 2021, https://womenshealth.gov/a-z-topics/polycystic-ovary-syndrome; Melanie Gibson-Helm et al., "Delayed Diagnosis and a Lack of Information Associated with Dissatisfaction in Women with Polycystic Ovary Syndrome," *Journal of Clinical Endocrinology & Metabolism* 102, no. 2 (February 1, 2017): 604–12, https://doi.org/10.1210/jc.2016-2963.

4. Divya Prasad et al., "Suicidal Risk in Women with Premenstrual Syndrome and Premenstrual Dysphoric Disorder: A Systematic Review and Meta-analysis," *Journal of Women's Health* 30, no. 12 (August 20, 2021): 1693–707, https://doi.org/10.1089/jwh.2021.0185.

5. Yumna Riaz and Utsav Parekh, "Oligomenorrhea," StatPearls, last updated July 31, 2023, https://www.ncbi.nlm.nih.gov/books/NBK560575.

6. Betsy Foxman, "Epidemiology of Urinary Tract Infections: Incidence, Morbidity, and Economic Costs," *American Journal of Medicine* 113, no. 1, supplement 1 (July 8, 2022): 5–13, https://doi.org/10.1016/s0002-9343(02)01054-9.

7. "Urinary Tract Infections," Office on Women's Health, U.S. Health and Human Services, last updated February 22, 2021, https://womenshealth.gov/a-z-topics/urinary-tract-infections.

8. "Recurrent, Uncomplicated Urinary Tract Infections in Women: AUA/CUA/SUFU Guideline (2022)," American Urological Association, 2019, https://www.auanet.org/guidelines-and-quality/guidelines/recurrent-uti.

9. "Diabetes and Polycystic Ovary Syndrome (PCOS)," Diabetes, Centers for Disease Control and Prevention, May 15, 2024, https://www.cdc.gov/diabetes/risk-factors/pcos-polycystic-ovary-syndrome.html.

10. "Overview: Ovarian Cysts," National Library of Medicine, last updated April 21, 2022, https://www.ncbi.nlm.nih.gov/books/NBK539572.

11. "Uterine Fibroids," Office of Women's Health, U.S. Health and Human Services, last updated February 28, 2025, https://womenshealth.gov/a-z-topics/uterine-fibroids.

12. Quaker E. Harmon, Ky'Era V. Actkins, and Donna D. Baird, "Fibroid Prevalence—Still So Much to Learn," *JAMA Network Open* 6, no. 5 (May 10, 2023): e2312682, https://doi.org/10.1001/jamanetworkopen.2023.12682.

13. "Endometriosis," World Health Organization, March 24, 2023, https://www.who.int/news-room/fact-sheets/detail/endometriosis.

14. Barbara A. Goff, "Frequency of Symptoms of Ovarian Cancer in Women Presenting to Primary Care Clinics," *JAMA* 291, no. 22 (June 8, 2004): 2705, https://doi.org/10.1001/jama.291.22.2705.

15. "Hysterectomy," Office of Women's Health, U.S. Health and Human Services, last updated February 27, 2025, https://womenshealth.gov/a-z-topics/hysterectomy.

16. NCI Staff, "Many Ovarian Cancers May Start in Fallopian Tubes," National Cancer Institute, November 15, 2017, https://www.cancer.gov/news-events/cancer-currents-blog/2017/ovarian-cancer-fallopian-tube-origins.

CHAPTER 6:
Fertility and Pregnancy

1. Allen J. Wilcox et al., "Preimplantation Loss of Fertilized Human Ova: Estimating the Unobservable," *Human Reproduction* 35, no. 4 (March 22, 2020): 743–50, https://doi.org/10.1093/humrep/deaa048.

2. American College of Obstetricians and Gynecologists, "Female Age-Related Fertility Decline: Committee Opinion No. 589," *Obstetrics & Gynecology* 123 (2014): 719–21, https://www.acog.org/clinical/clinical-guidance/committee-opinion/articles/2014/03/female-age-related-fertility-decline.

3. "Infertility and Fertility," Eunice Kennedy Shriver National Institute of Child Health and Human Development, accessed April 7, 2025, https://www.nichd.nih.gov/health/topics/factsheets/infertility.

4. "Infertility: Frequently Asked Questions," Centers for Disease Control and Prevention Division of Reproductive Health, May 15, 2024, https://www.cdc.gov/reproductive-health/infertility-faq/index.html.

5. "How Common Is Male Infertility, and What Are Its Causes?" Eunice Kennedy Shriver National Institute of Child Health and Human Development, last reviewed November 18, 2021, https://www.nichd.nih.gov/health/topics/menshealth/conditioninfo/infertility.

6. Sarah Druckenmiller Cascante et al., "Fifteen Years of Autologous Oocyte Thaw Outcomes from a Large University-Based Fertility Center," *Fertility and Sterility* 118, no. 1 (May 18, 2022): 158–66, https://doi.org/10.1016/j.fertnstert.2022.04.013.

7. Mahvash Zargar et al., "Pregnancy Outcomes Following In Vitro Fertilization Using Fresh or Frozen Embryo Transfer," *JBRA Assisted Reproduction* 25, no. 4 (October 4, 2021): 570–74, https://pubmed.ncbi.nlm.nih.gov/34224240.

8. Panagiotis Cherouveim et al., "The Impact of Cryopreserved Sperm on Intrauterine Insemination Outcomes: Is Frozen as Good as Fresh?" *Frontiers in Reproductive Health* 5 (May 30, 2023): https://www.frontiersin.org/journals/reproductive-health/articles/10.3389/frph.2023.1181751/full.

9. Anna Lena Zippl et al., "Predicting Success of Intrauterine Insemination Using a Clinically Based Scoring System," *Gynecologic Endocrinology and Reproductive Medicine* 306 (September 7, 2022): 1777–86, https://link.springer.com/article/10.1007/s00404-022-06758-z.

10. "IVF Success Estimator," Assisted Reproductive Technology (ART), Centers for Disease Control and Prevention, December 10, 2024, https://www.cdc.gov/art/ivf-success-estimator.

11. "What Is IVF?" Planned Parenthood, accessed April 11, 2025, https://www.plannedparenthood.org/learn/pregnancy/fertility-treatments/what-ivf.

12. Hagai Levine et al., "Temporal Trends in Sperm Count: A Systematic Review and Meta-regression Analysis," *Human Reproduction Update* 23, no. 6 (June 28, 2017): 646–59, https://doi.org/10.1093/humupd/dmx022.

13. E. Angel Aztlan-James, Monica McLemore, and Diana Taylor, "Multiple Unintended Pregnancies in U.S. Women: A Systematic Review," *Women's Health Issues* 27, no. 4 (March 9, 2017): 407–13, https://doi.org/10.1016/j.whi.2017.02.002.

14. "Prenatal Care Checkups," March of Dimes, last reviewed June 2017, https://www.marchofdimes.org/find-support/topics/planning-baby/prenatal-care-checkups.

15. "Prenatal Tests," March of Dimes, last reviewed September 2020, https://www.marchofdimes.org/find-support/topics/planning-baby/prenatal-tests.

16. "Miscarriage," March of Dimes, last reviewed October 2024, https://www.marchofdimes.org/find-support/topics/miscarriage-loss-grief/miscarriage.

Childbirth and Postpartum Health

1. "Cesarean Birth: Frequently Asked Questions," American College of Obstetricians and Gynecologists, last reviewed November 2023, https://www.acog.org/womens-health/faqs/cesarean-birth.

2. Meghan A. Bohren et al., "Continuous Support for Women During Childbirth," *Cochrane Database of Systematic Reviews* 2017, no. 7 (July 6, 2017), https://doi.org/10.1002/14651858.cd003766.pub6.

3. Kathleen Knocke et al., "Doula Care and Maternal Health: An Evidence Review," U.S. Department of Health and Human Services, Office of Health Policy, issue brief no. HP-2022-24, December 13, 2022, https://aspe.hhs.gov/sites/default/files/documents/dfcd768f1caf6fabf3d281f762e8d068/ASPE-Doula-Issue-Brief-12-13-22.pdf.

4. "Working Together to Reduce Black Maternal Mortality," Office of Women's Health, U.S. Department of Health and Human Services, April 8, 2024, https://www.cdc.gov/womens-health/features/maternal-mortality.html.

5. Kelly M. Hoffman et al., "Racial Bias in Pain Assessment and Treatment Recommendations, and False Beliefs About Biological Differences Between Blacks and Whites," *Proceedings of the National Academy of Sciences* 113, no. 16 (April 4, 2016): 4296–301, https://doi.org/10.1073/pnas.1516047113.

6. Marian Jarlenski et al., "Association of Race with Urine Toxicology Testing Among Pregnant Patients During Labor and Delivery," *JAMA Health Forum* 4, no. 4 (April 14, 2023): e230441, https://doi.org/10.1001/jamahealthforum.2023.0441.

7. Saraswathi Vedam et al., "The Giving Voice to Mothers Study: Inequity and Mistreatment During Pregnancy and Childbirth in the United States," *Reproductive Health* 16, no. 1 (June 11, 2019): 77, https://doi.org/10.1186/s12978-019-0729-2.

8. "March of Dimes Position Statement: Doulas and Birth Outcomes," March of Dimes, January 30, 2019, https://www.marchofdimes.org/sites/default/files/2023-04/Doulas-and-birth-outcomes-position-statement-final-January-30.pdf.

9. Wanda Barfield, "Matte Article: Recognizing Urgent Pregnancy-Related Warning Signs," HEAR HER Campaign, U.S. Centers for Disease Control and Prevention, May 15, 2024, https://www.cdc.gov/hearher/news-media/article-urgent-warning-signs.html.

10. "Postpartum Depression," March of Dimes, last reviewed March 2019, https://www.marchofdimes.org/find-support/topics/postpartum/postpartum-depression.

11. H. Woolhouse et al., "Perinatal Mood and Anxiety Disorders Fact Sheet," Postpartum Support International, 2014, https://www.postpartum.net/wp-content/uploads/2014/11/PSI-PMD-FACT-SHEET-2015.pdf.

12. "Baby Blues after Pregnancy," March of Dimes, last reviewed May 2021, https://www.marchofdimes.org/find-support/topics/postpartum/baby-blues-after-pregnancy.

13. Fanie Collardeau et al., "Maternal Unwanted and Intrusive Thoughts of Infant-Related Harm, Obsessive-Compulsive Disorder and Depression in the Perinatal Period: Study Protocol," *BMC Psychiatry* 19 (2019): 94, https://dspace.library.uvic.ca/items/8687ca58-cb21-46b5-873c-ec3840589b49.

14. Sara Berg, "What Doctors Wish Patients Knew About Breastfeeding," American Medical Association, August 12, 2022, https://www.ama-assn.org/delivering-care/population-care/what-doctors-wish-patients-knew-about-breastfeeding.

15. "Breastfeeding Report Card," Breastfeeding Data, Centers for Disease Control and Prevention, February 24, 2025, https://www.cdc.gov/breastfeeding-data/breastfeeding-report-card/index.html.

CHAPTER 9:
The Menopause Transition

1. Juliana M. Kling et al., "Menopause Management Knowledge in Postgraduate Family Medicine, Internal Medicine, and Obstetrics and Gynecology Residents: A Cross-Sectional Survey," *Mayo Clinic Proceedings* 94, no. 2 (January 30, 2019): 242–53, https://doi.org/10.1016/j.mayocp.2018.08.033.

2. Alexis Reeves et al., "Systematic Exclusion at Study Commencement Masks Earlier Menopause for Black Women in the Study of Women's Health Across the Nation (SWAN)," *International Journal of Epidemiology* 52, no. 5 (June 29, 2023): 1612–23, https://doi.org/10.1093/ije/dyad085.

3. Julie K. Bower et al., "Black–White Differences in Hysterectomy Prevalence: The CARDIA Study," *American Journal of Public Health* 99, no. 2 (September 20, 2011): 300–7, https://doi.org/10.2105/ajph.2008.133702.

4. Brian W. Whitcomb et al., "Cigarette Smoking and Risk of Early Natural Menopause," *American Journal of Epidemiology* 187, no. 4 (August 10, 2017): 696–704, https://doi.org/10.1093/aje/kwx292.

5. D. Stock et al., "Rotating Night Shift Work and Menopausal Age," *Human Reproduction* 34, no. 3 (February 12, 2019): 539–48, https://doi.org/10.1093/humrep/dey390.

6. Yashvee Dunneram et al., "Dietary Intake and Age at Natural Menopause: Results from the UK Women's Cohort Study," *Journal of Epidemiology & Community Health* 72, no. 8 (2018): 733–40, https://doi.org/10.1136/jech-2017-209887.

7. K. L. Szegda et al., "Adult Adiposity and Risk of Early Menopause," *Human Reproduction* 32, no. 12 (October 25, 2017): 2522–31, https://doi.org/10.1093/humrep/dex304.

8. "Pregnancy, Breastfeeding May Lower Risk of Early Menopause," National Institutes of Health, January 22, 2020, https://www.nih.gov/news-events/news-releases/pregnancy-breastfeeding-may-lower-risk-early-menopause-nih-study-suggests.

9. Albert A. Opoku, Mandy Abushama, and Justin C. Konje, "Obesity and Menopause," *Best Practice & Research Clinical Obstetrics & Gynaecology* 88 (June 2023): https://doi.org/10.1016/j.bpobgyn.2023.102348.

10. Sabrina J. G. C. Welten et al., "Age at Menopause and Risk of Ischemic and Hemorrhagic Stroke," *Stroke* 52, no. 8 (June 3, 2021): 2583–91, https://doi.org/10.1161/strokeaha.120.030558.

11. "Menopause Topics: Hot Flashes," The Menopause Society, accessed April 12, 2025, https://menopause.org/patient-education/menopause-topics/hot-flashes.

12. Ellen W. Freeman et al., "Associations of Hormones and Menopausal Status with Depressed Mood in Women with No History of Depression," *Archives of General Psychiatry* 63, no. 4 (April 1, 2006): 375, https://doi.org/10.1001/archpsyc.63.4.375.

13. Anita H. Clayton and Philip T. Ninan, "Depression or Menopause? Presentation and Management of Major Depressive Disorder in Perimenopausal and Postmenopausal Women," *Primary Care Companion to the Journal of Clinical Psychiatry* 12, no. 1 (February 18, 2010): e1–e13, https://doi.org/10.4088/pcc.08r00747blu.

14. Nancy E. Avis et al., "Duration of Menopausal Vasomotor Symptoms Over the Menopause Transition," *JAMA Internal Medicine* 175, no. 4 (2015): 531–39, https://doi.org/10.1001/jamainternmed.2014.8063.

15. Rebecca C. Thurston et al., "Menopausal Vasomotor Symptoms and Risk of Incident Cardiovascular Disease Events in SWAN," *Journal of the American Heart Association* 10, no. 3 (January 20, 2021): https://doi.org/10.1161/jaha.120.017416; Rebecca C. Thurston et al., "Trajectories of Vasomotor Symptoms and Carotid Intima Media Thickness in the Study of Women's Health Across the Nation," *Stroke* 47, no. 1 (November 18, 2015): 12–17, https://doi.org/10.1161/strokeaha.115.010600.

16. Rowan T. Chlebowski et al., "Persistent Vasomotor Symptoms and Breast Cancer in the Women's Health Initiative," *Menopause* 26, no. 6 (December 28, 2018): 578–87, https://doi.org/10.1097/gme.0000000000001283.

17. Rebecca C. Thurston et al., "Menopausal Vasomotor Symptoms and White Matter Hyperintensities in Midlife Women," *Neurology* 100, no. 2 (October 12, 2022): e133–e141, https://doi.org/10.1212/wnl.0000000000201401.

18. Pauline M. Maki and Rebecca C. Thurston, "Menopause and Brain Health: Hormonal Changes Are Only Part of the Story," *Frontiers in Neurology* 11 (September 23, 2020), https://doi.org/10.3389/fneur.2020.562275.

19. M. S. Hunter, "Cognitive Behavioral Therapy for Menopausal Symptoms," *Climacteric* 24, no. 1 (July 6, 2020): 51–56, https://doi.org/10.1080/13697137.2020.1777965.

20. Florence A. Trémollieres et al., "Persistent Gap in Menopause Care 20 Years After the WHI: A Population-Based Study of Menopause-Related Symptoms and Their Management," *Maturitas* 166 (August 11, 2022): 58–64, https://doi.org/10.1016/j.maturitas.2022.08.003.

21. Barbara Sibbald, "US Estrogen Plus Progestin HRT Trial Stopped Due to Increased Risk of Breast Cancer, Stroke and Heart Attack," *Canadian Medical Association Journal* 167, no. 3 (August 2022): 294, https://pmc.ncbi.nlm.nih.gov/articles/PMC117494.

22. Diana S. M. Buist et al., "Hormone Therapy Prescribing Patterns in the United States," *Obstetrics and Gynecology* 104, no. 5, part 1 (November 1, 2004): 1042–50, https://doi.org/10.1097/01.aog.0000143826.38439.af.

23. Usha Menon et al., "Decline in Use of Hormone Therapy Among Postmenopausal Women in the United Kingdom," *Menopause: The Journal of the North American Menopause Society* 14, no. 3 (January 19, 2007): 462–67, https://doi.org/10.1097/01.gme.0000243569.70946.9d; C. Clanget et al., "Patterns of Hormone Replacement Therapy in a Population-Based Cohort of Postmenopausal German Women. Changes After HERS II and WHI," *Experimental and Clinical Endocrinology & Diabetes* 113, no. 9 (October 19, 2005): 529–33, https://doi.org/10.1055/s-2005-865802.

24. Howard N. Hodis and Wendy J. Mack, "Menopausal Hormone Replacement Therapy and Reduction of All-Cause Mortality and Cardiovascular Disease," *Cancer Journal* 28, no. 3 (May–June 2022): 208–23, https://doi.org/10.1097/ppo.0000000000000591; Leslie Cho et al., "Rethinking Menopausal Hormone Therapy: For Whom, What, When, and How Long?" *Circulation* 147, no. 7 (February 13, 2023): 597–610, https://doi.org/10.1161/circulationaha.122.061559.

CHAPTER 10:
Breast Health

1. "Benign Breast Conditions," Brigham and Women's Hospital, accessed February 26, 2025, https://www.brighamandwomens.org/surgery/breast-surgery/benign-breast-conditions.

2. I. den Tonkelaar, P. H. M. Peeters, and P. A. H. van Noord, "Increase in Breast Size After Menopause: Prevalence and Determinants," *Maturitas* 48, no. 1 (December 12, 2003): 51–57, https://doi.org/10.1016/j.maturitas.2003.10.002.

3. Shadi Azam et al., "Hormone Replacement Therapy and Mammographic Density: A Systematic Literature Review," *Breast Cancer Research and Treatment* 182, no. 3 (June 22, 2020): 555–79, https://doi.org/10.1007/s10549-020-05744-w.

4. Michael C. Perry, "Breast Lump," in H. K. Walker, W. D. Hall, and J. W. Hurst, eds., *Clinical Methods: The History, Physical, and Laboratory Examinations*, 3rd ed. (Butterworths, 1990): 804, https://www.ncbi.nlm.nih.gov/books/NBK279.

5. Maleeha Ajmal, Myra Khan, and Kelly Van Fossen, "Breast Fibroadenoma," StatPearls, October 6, 2022, https://www.ncbi.nlm.nih.gov/books/NBK535345.

6. "Symptoms of Breast Cancer," U.S. Centers for Disease Control and Prevention, September 25, 2024, https://www.cdc.gov/breast-cancer/symptoms/index.html.

7. "Dense Breasts: Answers to Commonly Asked Questions," National Cancer Institute, last updated December 9, 2024, https://www.cancer.gov/types/breast/breast-changes/dense-breasts.

8. "Dense Breasts," National Cancer Institute.

9. "NCCN Guidelines for Patients: Breast Cancer Screening and Diagnosis," National Comprehensive Cancer Network Foundation, 2022, https://www.nccn.org/patients/guidelines/content/PDF/breastcancerscreening-patient.pdf.

10. Jennifer L. Caswell-Jin et al., "Analysis of Breast Cancer Mortality in the US—1975 to 2019," *JAMA* 331, no. 3 (January 16, 2024): 233, https://doi.org/10.1001/jama.2023.25881.

11. "Health-Related Social Needs Can Keep Women from Getting Lifesaving Mammograms," Centers for Disease Control and Prevention, June 18, 2024, https://www.cdc.gov/vitalsigns/mammograms.

12. David R. Williams, Selina A. Mohammed, and Alexandra E. Shields, "Understanding and Effectively Addressing Breast Cancer in African American Women: Unpacking the Social Context," *Cancer* 122, no. 14 (February 29, 2016): 2138–49, https://doi.org/10.1002/cncr.29935.

13. Jessica Brown, "The Alcohol and Breast Cancer Connection," Breast Cancer Research Foundation, accessed April 12, 2025, https://www.bcrf.org/about-breast-cancer/alcohol-breast-cancer-risk.

14. "Breast Cancer Risk Factors You Can't Change," American Cancer Society, last revised December 16, 2021, https://www.cancer.org/cancer/types/breast-cancer/risk-and-prevention/breast-cancer-risk-factors-you-cannot-change.html.

15. Shuai Xu et al., "Breast Cancer Incidence Among US Women Aged 20 to 49 Years by Race, Stage, and Hormone Receptor Status," *JAMA Network Open* 7,

no. 1 (January 26, 2024): e2353331, https://doi.org/10.1001/jamanetworkopen .2023.53331.

16. Jessica Brown, "5 Facts About Breast Cancer in Younger Women," Breast Cancer Research Foundation, accessed April 12, 2025, https://www.bcrf.org/about -breast-cancer/breast-cancer-young-women.

17. "Triple-Negative Breast Cancer," American Cancer Society, last revised March 12, 2023, https://www.cancer.org/cancer/types/breast-cancer/about/types-of -breast-cancer/triple-negative.html.

18. Jessica Brown, "Breast Cancer Stages and What They Mean," Breast Cancer Research Foundation, November 21, 2024, https://www.bcrf.org/blog/breast-cancer -stages.

19. "Paget Disease of the Breast," National Cancer Institute, reviewed April 10, 2012, https://www.cancer.gov/types/breast/paget-breast-fact-sheet.

20. "Key Statistics for Breast Cancer in Men," American Cancer Society, last revised January 16, 2025, https://www.cancer.org/cancer/types/breast-cancer-in -men/about/key-statistics.html.

21. "Key Statistics for Breast Cancer," American Cancer Society, last revised January 22, 2025, https://www.cancer.org/cancer/types/breast-cancer/about/how -common-is-breast-cancer.html.

CHAPTER 11:
Your Immune System

1. Sabra L. Klein and Katie L. Flanagan, "Sex Differences in Immune Responses," *Nature Reviews Immunology* 16, no. 10 (August 22, 2016): 626–38, https://doi.org /10.1038/nri.2016.90.

2. Vanessa L. Kronzer, "Why Women Have More Autoimmune Diseases Than Men: An Evolutionary Perspective," *Evolutionary Applications* 14, no. 3 (November 2020): 629–33, https://doi.org/10.1111/eva.13167.

3. Katie L. Flanagan et al., "Sex and Gender Differences in the Outcomes of Vaccination Over the Life Course," *Annual Review of Cell and Developmental Biology* 33, no. 1 (October 2017): 577–99, https://doi.org/10.1146/annurev-cellbio-100616-060718.

4. DeLisa Fairweather and Noel R. Rose, "Women and Autoimmune Diseases," *Emerging Infectious Diseases* 10, no. 11 (November 1, 2004): 2005–11, https://doi .org/10.3201/eid1011.040367.

5. Fariha Angum et al., "The Prevalence of Autoimmune Disorders in Women: A Narrative Review," *Cureus* 12, no. 5 (May 13, 2020): e8094, https://doi.org/10 .7759/cureus.8094.

6. Bilal A. Paray et al., "Leaky Gut and Autoimmunity: An Intricate Balance in Individuals Health and the Diseased State," *International Journal of Molecular Sciences* 21, no. 24 (December 2020): 9770, https://doi.org/10.3390/ijms212 49770.

7. Maunil K. Desai and Roberta D. Brinton, "Autoimmune Disease in Women: Endocrine Transition and Risk Across the Lifespan," *Frontiers in Endocrinology* 10 (April 2019): 265, https://doi.org/10.3389/fendo.2019.00265.

8. Ljudmila Stojanovich and Dragomir Marisavljevich, "Stress as a Trigger of Autoimmune Disease," *Autoimmunity Reviews* 7, no. 3 (December 5, 2007): 209–13, https://doi.org/10.1016/j.autrev.2007.11.007.

9. Jörg J. Goronzy and Cornelia M. Weyand, "Immune Aging and Autoimmunity," *Cellular and Molecular Life Sciences* 69, no. 10 (2012): 1615–23, https://doi.org/10.1007/s00018-012-0970-0.

10. "Tips for Getting a Diagnosis of an Autoimmune Disease," Autoimmune Association, accessed January 17, 2025, https://autoimmune.org/resource-center/di agnosis-tips.

11. "Ten Threats to Global Health in 2019," World Health Organization, accessed May 5, 2025, https://www.who.int/news-room/spotlight/ten-threats-to-global -health-in-2019.

12. Niharika Arora Duggal et al., "Major Features of Immunesenescence, Including Reduced Thymic Output, Are Ameliorated by High Levels of Physical Activity in Adulthood," *Aging Cell* 17, no. 2 (March 8, 2018): e12750, https://doi .org/10.1111/acel.12750.

CHAPTER 12:
Pain

1. Jacqueline W. Lucas and Inderbir Sohi, "Chronic Pain and High-Impact Chronic Pain Among U.S. Adults, 2023," National Health Interview Survey, Centers for Disease Control and Prevention, November 2023, https://doi.org/10.15620/cdc /169630.

2. "Women and Black Adults Waited Longer in ER for Chest Pain Evaluation," American Heart Association, May 4, 2022, https://newsroom.heart.org/news /women-and-black-adults-waited-longer-in-er-for-chest-pain-evaluation.

3. Esther H. Chen et al., "Gender Disparity in Analgesic Treatment of Emergency Department Patients with Acute Abdominal Pain," *Academic Emergency Medicine* 15, no. 5 (March 29, 2008): 414–18, https://doi.org/10.1111/j.1553-2712.2008 .00100.x.

4. eClinicalMedicine, "Gendered Pain: A Call for Recognition and Health Equity," *eClinicalMedicine* 69 (March 1, 2024): 102558, https://doi.org/10.1016/j.eclinm.2024.102558.

5. E. J. Bartley and R. B. Fillingim, "Sex Differences in Pain: A Brief Review of Clinical and Experimental Findings," *British Journal of Anaesthesia* 111, no. 1 (July 2013): 52–58, https://doi.org/10.1093/bja/aet127; Jon G. Dean et al., "Self-Regulated Analgesia in Males but Not Females Is Mediated by Endogenous Opioids," *PNAS Nexus* 3, no. 10 (October 2024): 453, https://doi.org/10.1093/pnasnexus/pgae453.

6. Kelly M. Hoffman et al., "Racial Bias in Pain Assessment and Treatment Recommendations, and False Beliefs About Biological Differences Between Blacks and Whites," *Proceedings of the National Academy of Sciences* 113, no. 16 (April 4, 2016): 4296–301, https://doi.org/10.1073/pnas.1516047113.

7. "Headache," National Institute of Neurological Disorders and Stroke, accessed May 5, 2025, https://www.ninds.nih.gov/health-information/disorders/headache.

8. Zoë Delaruelle et al., "Male and Female Sex Hormones in Primary Headaches," *Journal of Headache and Pain* 19, no. 1 (2018): 117, https://doi.org/10.1186/s10194-018-0922-7.

9. "Migraine Through a Woman's Life," American Migraine Foundation, March 21, 2019, https://americanmigrainefoundation.org/resource-library/migraine-through-a-womans-life.

10. "Migraine," Office on Women's Health, U.S. Department of Health and Human Services, last updated February 22, 2021, https://womenshealth.gov/a-z-topics/migraine.

11. Jelena M. Pavlović et al., "Sex Hormones in Women With and Without Migraine," *Neurology* 87, no. 1 (June 2, 2016): 49–56, https://doi.org/10.1212/wnl.0000000000002798.

12. Urszula Tataj-Puzyna et al., "Women's Experiences of Dysmenorrhoea—Preliminary Study," *Menopausal Review* 20, no. 3 (January 1, 2021): 133–39, https://doi.org/10.5114/pm.2021.109771.

13. Tor D. Wager, "Managing Pain," *Cerebrum*, March 2022, https://pmc.ncbi.nlm.nih.gov/articles/PMC9224345.

CHAPTER 13:
Brain Health

1. Debra J. Brody, Laura A. Pratt, and Jeffery P. Hughes, "Prevalence of Depression Among Adults Aged 20 and Over: United States, 2013–2016," National Center

for Health Statistics, February 2018, https://www.cdc.gov/nchs/products/data briefs/db303.htm; Tao Sun et al., "An Integrative View on Sex Differences in Brain Tumors," *Cellular and Molecular Life Sciences* 72, no. 17 (2015): 3323–42, https://doi.org/10.1007/s00018-015-1930-2; Maria Francesca Rossi et al., "Sex and Gender Differences in Migraines: A Narrative Review," *Neurological Sciences* 43, no. 9 (2022): 5729–34, https://doi.org/10.1007/s10072-022-06178-6.

2. "2024 Alzheimer's Disease Facts and Figures," *Alzheimers & Dementia* 20, no. 5 (May 2024): 3708–821, https://doi.org/10.1002/alz.13809.

3. Darby E. Attoe and Emma A. Climie, "Miss. Diagnosis: A Systematic Review of ADHD in Adult Women," *Journal of Attention Disorders* 27, no. 7 (2023): 645–57, https://doi.org/10.1177/10870547231161533.

4. Jim Russell et al., "Number of ADHD Patients Rising, Especially Among Women," Epic Research, March 30, 2023, https://www.epicresearch.org/articles/number -of-adhd-patients-rising-especially-among-women.

5. Robert McCrossin, "Finding the True Number of Females with Autistic Spectrum Disorder by Estimating the Biases in Initial Recognition and Clinical Diagnosis," *Children* 9, no. 2 (2022): 272, https://doi.org/10.3390/children902 0272.

6. "About Dementia," Alzheimer's Disease and Dementia, Centers for Disease Control, August 17, 2024, https://www.cdc.gov/alzheimers-dementia/about/index .html.

7. Gill Livingston et al., "Dementia Prevention, Intervention, and Care: 2024 Report of the *Lancet* Standing Commission," *Lancet* 404, no. 10452 (July 31, 2024): 572– 628, https://www.thelancet.com/commissions/dementia-prevention-intervention -care.

8. Lisa L. Barnes and David A. Bennett, "Alzheimer's Disease in African Americans: Risk Factors and Challenges for the Future," *Health Affairs* 33, no. 4 (April 2014): 580–86, https://doi.org/10.1377/hlthaff.2013.1353.

9. "Hispanic Americans and Alzheimer's," Alzheimer's Association, accessed April 13, 2025, https://www.alz.org/help-support/resources/hispanics-and-alzheimers.

10. Jennifer D. Walker, "Alzheimer's Disease and Related Dementia in Indigenous Populations: A Systematic Review of Risk Factors," *Journal of Alzheimer's Disease* 78, no. 4 (November 2020): 1439–51, https://doi.org/10.3233/jad-200704.

11. "Asian Americans and Pacific Islanders and Alzheimer's," Alzheimer's Association, accessed April 13, 2025, https://www.alz.org/help-support/resources/asian -americans-and-alzheimers.

12. K. Bibbins-Domingo and A. Helman, eds., "Policies to Improve Clinical Trial and Research Diversity: History and Future Directions," *Improving Representation in Clinical Trials and Research*, National Academies Press, May 17, 2022, https://www.ncbi.nlm.nih.gov/books/NBK584404.

CHAPTER 14:

Heart Health

1. Cedars-Sinai Medical Center, "Why The Top Cause of Death for Women Has Been Ignored," February 16, 2024, https://www.cedars-sinai.org/newsroom/why-the-top-cause-of-death-for-women-has-been-ignored.

2. Kevin A. Bybee and Tracy L. Stevens, "Matters of the Heart: Cardiovascular Disease in U.S. Women," *Missouri Medicine* 110, no. 1 (January–February 2013): 65–70, https://pmc.ncbi.nlm.nih.gov/articles/PMC6179634.

3. "Research Adds to Knowledge About Heart Disease and Stroke in Women of All Ages," American Heart Association, February 27, 2024, https://newsroom.heart.org/news/research-adds-to-knowledge-about-heart-disease-and-stroke-in-women-of-all-ages.

4. Abdullah Al Hamid et al., "Gender Bias in Diagnosis, Prevention, and Treatment of Cardiovascular Diseases: A Systematic Review," *Cureus* 16, no. 2 (February 15, 2024): e54264, https://doi.org/10.7759/cureus.54264.

5. "Women Hospitalized for a Heart Attack Are Less Likely to Receive Treatment and More Likely to Die Than Men," National Institute on Aging, September 19, 2024, https://www.nia.nih.gov/news/women-hospitalized-heart-attack-are-less-likely-receive-treatment-and-more-likely-die-men.

6. Hongwei Ji et al., "Sex Differences in Blood Pressure Associations with Cardiovascular Outcomes," *Circulation* 143, no. 7 (February 15, 2021): 761–63, https://doi.org/10.1161/circulationaha.120.049360.

7. Seth S. Martin et al., "2025 Heart Disease and Stroke Statistics: A Report of US and Global Data from the American Heart Association," *Circulation* 151, no. 8 (January 27, 2025), https://doi.org/10.1161/cir.0000000000001303.

8. Zulqarnain Javed et al., "Race, Racism, and Cardiovascular Health: Applying a Social Determinants of Health Framework to Racial/Ethnic Disparities in Cardiovascular Disease," *Circulation: Cardiovascular Quality and Outcomes* 15, no. 1 (January 18, 2022), https://doi.org/10.1161/circoutcomes.121.007917.

9. Chensihan Huang et al., "Associations of Menstrual Cycle Regularity and Length with Cardiovascular Diseases: A Prospective Study from UK Biobank," *Journal of the American Heart Association* 12, no. 11 (May 24, 2023), https://doi.org/10.1161/jaha.122.029020.

10. Michael C. Honigberg et al., "Association of Premature Natural and Surgical Menopause with Incident Cardiovascular Disease," *JAMA* 322, no. 24 (November 18, 2019): 2411, https://doi.org/10.1001/jama.2019.19191.

11. Marise M. Wagner et al., "Increased Cardiovascular Disease Risk in Women with a History of Recurrent Miscarriage," *Acta Obstetricia et Gynecologica Scandinavica* 97, no. 10 (May 28, 2018): 1192–99, https://doi.org/10.1111/aogs.13392.

12. "Unraveling How the Menopause Is Related to Cardiovascular & Heart Health in Women During and After Menopause," Study of Women's Health Across the Nation, accessed April 14, 2025, https://www.swanstudy.org/womens-health -info/cardiovascular-risk-and-heart-health-in-women-during-and-after -menopause.

13. Sameer Arora et al., "Twenty Year Trends and Sex Differences in Young Adults Hospitalized with Acute Myocardial Infarction," *Circulation* 139, no. 8 (November 11, 2018): 1047–56, https://doi.org/10.1161/circulationaha.118.037137.

14. Bashar Khiatah et al., "Cardiovascular Disease in Women: A Review of Spontaneous Coronary Artery Dissection," *Medicine* 101, no. 38 (September 23, 2022): e30433, https://doi.org/10.1097/md.0000000000030433.

15. Marysia S. Tweet, Susan N. Kok, and Sharonne N. Hayes, "Spontaneous Coronary Artery Dissection in Women: What Is Known and What Is Yet to Be Understood," *Clinical Cardiology* 41, no. 2 (February 1, 2018): 203–10, https://doi .org/10.1002/clc.22909.

16. "Stroke Symptoms, Even If They Disappear Within an Hour, Need Emergency Assessment," American Heart Association, January 19, 2023, https://newsroom .heart.org/news/stroke-symptoms-even-if-they-disappear-within-an-hour -need-emergency-assessment.

17. "Stroke Facts," Centers for Disease Control and Prevention, October 24, 2024, https://www.cdc.gov/stroke/data-research/facts-stats/index.html.

18. "New Guideline: Preventing a First Stroke May Be Possible with Screening, Lifestyle Changes," American Heart Association, October 21, 2024, https:// newsroom.heart.org/news/new-guideline-preventing-a-first-stroke -may-be-possible-with-screening-lifestyle-changes.

19. "Belly Fat Raises Risk of Heart Disease, Stroke in Older Women Despite Normal BMI," American Heart Association, March 7, 2019, https://www.heart.org /en/news/2019/03/06/belly-fat-raises-risk-of-heart-disease-stroke-in-older -women-despite-normal-bmi.

20. Steven P. Hooker et al., "Association of Accelerometer-Measured Sedentary Time and Physical Activity with Risk of Stroke Among US Adults," *JAMA Network Open* 5, no. 6 (June 3, 2022): e2215385, https://doi.org/10.1001/jamanet workopen.2022.15385.

21. Katherine E. Paterson et al., "Mediterranean Diet Reduces Risk of Incident Stroke in a Population with Varying Cardiovascular Disease Risk Profiles," *Stroke* 49, no. 10 (September 20, 2018): 2415–20, https://doi.org/10.1161/strokeaha .117.020258.

22. Anna Pasławska and Przemyslaw J. Tomasik, "Lipoprotein(a)—60 Years Later— What Do We Know?" *Cells* 12, no. 20 (October 2023): 2472, https://doi.org/10 .3390/cells12202472.

23. Jennifer Behbodikhah et al., "Apolipoprotein B and Cardiovascular Disease: Biomarker and Potential Therapeutic Target," *Metabolites* 11, no. 10 (October 8, 2021): 690, https://doi.org/10.3390/metabo11100690.

24. C. Justin Brown et al., "Assessment of Sex Disparities in Nonacceptance of Statin Therapy and Low-Density Lipoprotein Cholesterol Levels Among Patients at High Cardiovascular Risk," *JAMA Network Open* 6, no. 2 (February 28, 2023): e231047, https://doi.org/10.1001/jamanetworkopen.2023.1047.

25. Lisandro D. Colantonio et al., "Adherence to High-Intensity Statins Following a Myocardial Infarction Hospitalization Among Medicare Beneficiaries," *JAMA Cardiology* 2, no. 8 (April 19, 2017): 890, https://doi.org/10.1001/jamacardio.2017.0911.

26. "Women and Heart Disease: New Data Reaffirm Lack of Awareness by Women and Physicians," American College of Cardiology, June 22, 2017, https://www.acc.org/latest-in-cardiology/articles/2017/06/22/10/01/women-and-heart-disease-new-data-reaffirm-lack-of-awareness-by-women-and-physicians.

27. "Women and Heart Disease: New Data Reaffirm Lack of Awareness by Women and Physicians."

28. Mary Cushman et al., "Ten-Year Differences in Women's Awareness Related to Coronary Heart Disease: Results of the 2019 American Heart Association National Survey: A Special Report from the American Heart Association," *Circulation* 143, no. 7 (September 21, 2022), https://doi.org/10.1161/cir.0000000000000907.

CHAPTER 15:
Gut Health

1. Kenichi Utano et al., "Bowel Habits and Gender Correlate with Colon Length Measured by CT Colonography," *Japanese Journal of Radiology* 40, no. 3 (October 11, 2021): 298–307, https://doi.org/10.1007/s11604-021-01204-7.

2. Ricardo Santos Aleman, Marvin Moncada, and Kayanush J. Aryana, "Leaky Gut and the Ingredients That Help Treat It: A Review," *Molecules* 28, no. 2 (January 7, 2023): 619, https://doi.org/10.3390/molecules28020619.

3. Annelise Madison and Janice K. Kiecolt-Glaser, "Stress, Depression, Diet, and the Gut Microbiota: Human–Bacteria Interactions at the Core of Psychoneuroimmunology and Nutrition," *Current Opinion in Behavioral Sciences* 28 (August 2019): 105–10, https://doi.org/10.1016/j.cobeha.2019.01.011.

4. Vincenzo Monda et al., "Exercise Modifies the Gut Microbiota with Positive Health Effects," *Oxidative Medicine and Cellular Longevity* (March 5, 2017), https://doi.org/10.1155/2017/3831972.

5. Young Sun Kim and Nayoung Kim, "Functional Dyspepsia: A Narrative Review with a Focus on Sex-Gender Differences," *Journal of Neurogastroenterology and Motility* 26, no. 3 (June 30, 2020): 322–34, https://doi.org/10.5056/jnm20026.

6. Gottfried Novacek, "Gender and Gallstone Disease," *Wiener Medizinische Wochenschrift* 156 (October 2006): 527–33, https://doi.org/10.1007/s10354-006-0346-x.

7. Susrutha Puthanmadhom Narayanan, Bradley Anderson, and Adil E. Bharucha, "Sex- and Gender-Related Differences in Common Functional Gastroenterologic Disorders," *Mayo Clinic Proceedings* 96, no. 4 (April 1, 2021): 1071–89, https://doi.org/10.1016/j.mayocp.2020.10.004.

8. "Colorectal Cancer," World Health Organization, July 11, 2023, https://www.who.int/news-room/fact-sheets/detail/colorectal-cancer.

9. "American Cancer Society Releases New Colorectal Cancer Statistics; Rapid Shifts to More Advanced Disease and Younger People," American Cancer Society, March 1, 2023, https://pressroom.cancer.org/CRCFactsFigures2023.

10. Rebecca L. Siegel, Angela N. Giaquinto, and Ahmedin Jemal, "Cancer Statistics, 2024," *CA: A Cancer Journal for Clinicians* 74, no. 1 (January 17, 2024): 12–49, https://doi.org/10.3322/caac.21820.

11. "Never Too Young Survey Report 2020," Colorectal Cancer Alliance, https://colorectalcancer.org/sites/default/files/media/documents/CCAlliance_NeverTooYoung_2020SurveyReport.pdf.

12. "Screening for Colorectal Cancer," Centers for Disease Control and Prevention, October 17, 2024, https://www.cdc.gov/colorectal-cancer/screening/index.html.

CHAPTER 16:
Skin Health

1. "Skin Conditions by the Numbers," American Academy of Dermatology Association, last updated February 11, 2025, https://www.aad.org/media/stats-numbers.

2. "Chronic Spontaneous/Idiopathic Urticaria (Chronic Hives)," American College of Allergy, Asthma, and Immunology, https://acaai.org/allergies/allergic-conditions/skin-allergy/chronic-hives.

3. Sara Berg, "What Doctors Wish Patients Knew About the Shingles Virus," American Medical Association, April 28, 2023, https://www.ama-assn.org/de

livering-care/public-health/what-doctors-wish-patients-knew-about-shingles
-virus.

4. Hajira Basit, Kiran V. Godse, and Ahmad M. Al Aboud, "Melasma," StatPearls,
August 8, 2023, https://www.ncbi.nlm.nih.gov/books/NBK459271.

5. Alvaro Gonzalez-Cantero et al., "Gender Perspective in Psoriasis: A Scoping
Review and Proposal of Strategies for Improved Clinical Practice by European
Dermatologists," *International Journal of Women's Dermatology* 9, no. 4 (De-
cember 2023): e112, https://doi.org/10.1097/jw9.0000000000000112.

6. Hibah Osman et al., "Risk Factors for the Development of Striae Gravidarum,"
American Journal of Obstetrics and Gynecology 196, no. 1 (January 2007): 62.e1–e5.
https://doi.org/10.1016/j.ajog.2006.08.044.

7. Allen Gabriel et al., "Cellulite: Current Understanding and Treatment," *Aesthetic Surgery Journal Open Forum* 5 (June 21, 2023): ojad050, https://doi.org
/10.1093/asjof/ojad050.

8. "All About Sunscreen," Skin Cancer Foundation, March 11, 2025, https://www
.skincancer.org/skin-cancer-prevention/sun-protection/sunscreen.

9. "Skin Cancer," American Academy of Dermatology Association, last updated
March 25, 2025, https://www.aad.org/media/stats-skin-cancer.

10. June K. Robinson, "Skin Check Partner Assistance for Melanoma Skin Self-
Examination by At-Risk Patients: It Takes Two to Identify Melanomas," *Future On-
cology* 16, no. 16 (April 15, 2020): 1065–68, https://doi.org/10.2217/fon-2020-0265.

11. "What to Look For: ABCDEs of Melanoma," American Academy of Dermatology
Association, accessed April 14, 2025, https://www.aad.org/public/diseases/skin
-cancer/find/at-risk/abcdes.

12. Travis A. Benson et al., "Nonablative Fractional Laser Treatment Is Associated
with a Decreased Risk of Subsequent Facial Keratinocyte Carcinoma Development," *Dermatologic Surgery* 49, no. 2 (February 2023): 149–54, https://doi.org
/10.1097/dss.0000000000003672.

CHAPTER 17:
Mental and Emotional Health

1. Christine Kuehner, "Why Is Depression More Common Among Women than
Among Men? *Lancet Psychiatry* 4, no. 2 (February 2017), 146–58, https://doi
.org/10.1016/s2215-0366(16)30263-2.

2. Miranda Olff, "Sex and Gender Differences in Post-traumatic Stress Disorder:
An Update," *European Journal of Psychotraumatology* 8, sup 4 (2017), https://doi
.org/10.1080/20008198.2017.1351204.

3. "Generalized Anxiety Disorder (GAD)," PsychDB, last edited January 11, 2024, https://www.psychdb.com/anxiety/gad.

4. Olff, "Sex and Gender Differences in Post-traumatic Stress Disorder."

5. "Post-traumatic Stress Disorder," Office on Women's Health, last updated February 3, 2025, https://womenshealth.gov/mental-health/mental-health-conditions/post-traumatic-stress-disorder.

6. Joshua Feriante and Naveen P. Sharma, "Acute and Chronic Mental Health Trauma," StatPearls, August 2, 2023, https://www.ncbi.nlm.nih.gov/books/NBK594231.

7. Debra A. Bangasser and Amelia Cuarenta, "Sex Differences in Anxiety and Depression: Circuits and Mechanisms," *Nature Reviews Neuroscience* 22, no. 11 (September 20, 2021): 674–84, https://doi.org/10.1038/s41583-021-00513-0.

8. Paul R. Albert, "Why Is Depression More Prevalent in Women?" *Journal of Psychiatry and Neuroscience* 40, no. 4 (July 1, 2015): 219–21, https://doi.org/10.1503/jpn.150205.

9. Luke John Ney et al., "An Alternative Theory for Hormone Effects on Sex Differences in PTSD: The Role of Heightened Sex Hormones During Trauma," *Psychoneuroendocrinology* 109 (August 23, 2019): 104416, https://doi.org/10.1016/j.psyneuen.2019.104416.

10. Naima Z. Farhane et al., "Factors Associated with Gender and Sex Differences in Anxiety Prevalence and Comorbidity: A Systemic Review," *Science Progress* 105, no. 4 (November 12, 2023), https://doi.org/10.1177/00368504221135469.

11. Peixia Shi et al., "A Hypothesis of Gender Differences in Self-Reporting Symptom of Depression: Implications to Solve Under-diagnosis and Under-treatment of Depression in Males," *Frontiers in Psychiatry* 12 (October 25, 2021), https://doi.org/10.3389/fpsyt.2021.589687.

12. Ida Haahr-Pedersen et al., "Females Have More Complex Patterns of Childhood Adversity: Implications for Mental, Social, and Emotional Outcomes in Adulthood," *European Journal of Psychotraumatology* 11, no. 1 (January 10, 2020), https://doi.org/10.1080/20008198.2019.1708618.

13. "Statistics About Sexual Violence," National Sexual Violence Resource Center, 2011, https://www.nsvrc.org/sites/default/files/publications_nsvrc_factsheet_media-packet_statistics-about-sexual-violence_0.pdf.

14. "U.S. Teen Girls Experiencing Increased Sadness and Violence," press release, Centers for Disease Control and Prevention, February 13, 2023, https://www.cdc.gov/media/releases/2023/p0213-yrbs.html.

15. "Instagram Ranked Worst for Young People's Mental Health," Royal Society for Public Health, May 19, 2017, https://www.rsph.org.uk/about-us/news/instagram-ranked-worst-for-young-people-s-mental-health.html.

16. Renee Engeln et al., "Compared to Facebook, Instagram Use Causes More Appearance Comparison and Lower Body Satisfaction in College Women," *Body Image* 34 (June 4, 2020): 38–45, https://doi.org/10.1016/j.bodyim.2020.04.007.

17. "Substance Use in Women Research Report: Sex Differences in Substance Use," National Institute on Drug Abuse, April 2020, https://nida.nih.gov/publications/research-reports/substance-use-in-women/sex-differences-in-substance-use.

18. MacKenzie R. Peltier et al., "Sex Differences in Stress-Related Alcohol Use," *Neurobiology of Stress* 10 (February 1, 2019): 100149, https://doi.org/10.1016/j.ynstr.2019.100149.

19. Alexandra Matarazzo et al., "New Clinical and Public Health Challenges: Increasing Trends in United States Alcohol Related Mortality," *American Journal of Medicine* 138, no. 3 (November 1, 2024): 477–86, https://doi.org/10.1016/j.amjmed.2024.10.024.

20. "Women and Alcohol," National Institute on Alcohol Abuse and Alcoholism, updated February 2025, https://www.niaaa.nih.gov/publications/brochures-and-fact-sheets/women-and-alcohol.

21. "Understanding Alcohol Use Disorder," National Institute on Alcohol Abuse and Alcoholism, updated January 2025, https://www.niaaa.nih.gov/publications/brochures-and-fact-sheets/understanding-alcohol-use-disorder.

22. Lunna Lopes et al., "KFF/CNN Mental Health in America Survey," KFF, October 5, 2022, https://www.kff.org/report-section/kff-cnn-mental-health-in-america-survey-finding.

CHAPTER 18:
Sleep

1. "Casper-Gallup State of Sleep in America 2022 Report," Gallup, November 4, 2024, https://www.gallup.com/analytics/390536/sleep-in-america-2022.aspx.

2. "QuickStats: Percentage of Adults Who Often Felt Very Tired or Exhausted in the Past 3 Months, by Sex and Age Group—National Health Interview Survey, United States, 2010–2011," *Morbidity and Mortality Weekly Report* 62, no. 14 (April 12, 2013), https://www.cdc.gov/mmwr/preview/mmwrhtml/mm6214a5.htm.

3. Bart Van Alphen et al., "A Deep Sleep Stage in Drosophila with a Functional Role in Waste Clearance," *Science Advances* 7, no. 4 (January 20, 2021), https://doi.org/10.1126/sciadv.abc2999.

4. "How Much Sleep Do You Really Need?," National Sleep Foundation, October 1, 2020, https://www.thensf.org/how-many-hours-of-sleep-do-you-really-need.

5. Anna B. Fishbein, Kristen L. Knutson, and Phyllis C. Zee, "Circadian Disruption and Human Health," *Journal of Clinical Investigation* 131, no. 19 (September 30, 2021): e148286, https://doi.org/10.1172/jci148286.

6. Lauren A. E. Erland and Praveen K. Saxena, "Melatonin Natural Health Products and Supplements: Presence of Serotonin and Significant Variability of Melatonin Content," *Journal of Clinical Sleep Medicine* 13, no. 02 (February 14, 2017): 275–81, https://doi.org/10.5664/jcsm.6462.

7. Sara Nowakowski et al., "Sleep and Women's Health," *Sleep Medicine Research* 4, no. 1 (October 10, 2014): 1–22, https://doi.org/10.17241/smr.2013.4.1.1.

8. Padigela Rugvedh, Ppavani Gundreddy, and Bhushan Wandile, "The Menstrual Cycle's Influence on Sleep Duration and Cardiovascular Health: A Comprehensive Review," *Cureus* 15, no. 10 (October 18, 2023): e47292, https://doi.org/10.7759/cureus.47292.

9. Shazia Jehan et al., "Sleep and Premenstrual Syndrome," *Journal of Sleep Medicine Disorders* 3, no. 5 (August 3, 2016): 1061, https://pmc.ncbi.nlm.nih.gov/articles/PMC5323065.

10. Summer Cannon, Melanie Hayman, and Michele Lastella, "Pregnant Women's Attitudes and Beliefs Towards Sleep and Exercise: A Cross-sectional Survey," *Clocks & Sleep* 5, no. 1 (January 17, 2023): 34–44, https://doi.org/10.3390/clockssleep5010004.

CHAPTER 19:
Exercise

1. Scarlett McNally et al., "Exercise: The Miracle Cure and the Role of the Doctor in Promoting It," Academy *of Medical Royal Colleges*, February 2015, https://www.aomrc.org.uk/wp-content/uploads/2016/03/Exercise_the_Miracle_Cure_0215.pdf.

2. Emma S. Cowley et al., "'Invisible Sportswomen': The Sex Data Gap in Sport and Exercise Science Research," *Women in Sport and Physical Activity Journal* 29, no. 2 (September 21, 2021): 146–51, https://doi.org/10.1123/wspaj.2021-0028.

3. John D. Omura et al., "Cross-sectional Association Between Physical Activity Level and Subjective Cognitive Decline Among US Adults Aged ≥45 Years, 2015," *Preventive Medicine* 141 (October 6, 2020): 106279, https://doi.org/10.1016/j.ypmed.2020.106279.

4. Darryl P. Leong et al., "Prognostic Value of Grip Strength: Findings from the Prospective Urban Rural Epidemiology (PURE) Study," *Lancet* 386, no. 9990 (May 14, 2015): 266–73, https://doi.org/10.1016/s0140-6736(14)62000-6.

5. Larry A. Tucker et al., "Effect of Two Jumping Programs on Hip Bone Mineral Density in Premenopausal Women: A Randomized Controlled Trial," *American Journal of Health Promotion* 29, no. 3 (January 24, 2014): 158–64, https://doi.org/10.4278/ajhp.130430-quan-200.

6. "The Female ACL: Why Is It More Prone to Injury?" *Journal of Orthopaedics* 13, no. 2 (June 2016): A1–A4, https://doi.org/10.1016/s0972-978x(16)00023-4.

CHAPTER 20:
Nutrition

1. Joana Araújo, Jianwen Cai, and June Stevens, "Prevalence of Optimal Metabolic Health in American Adults: National Health and Nutrition Examination Survey 2009–2016," *Metabolic Syndrome and Related Disorders* 17, no. 1 (November 28, 2018): 46–52, https://doi.org/10.1089/met.2018.0105.

2. "Gestational Diabetes," Centers for Disease Control and Prevention, May 15, 2024, https://www.cdc.gov/diabetes/about/gestational-diabetes.html.

3. "Diabetes," Office on Women's Health, last updated May 31, 2022, https://womenshealth.gov/a-z-topics/diabetes.

4. Ariana M. Chao et al., "Clinical Insight on Semaglutide for Chronic Weight Management in Adults: Patient Selection and Special Considerations," *Drug Design Development and Therapy* 16 (December 1, 2022): 4449–61, https://doi.org/10.2147/dddt.s365416.

5. "AMA Adopts New Policy Clarifying Role of BMI as a Measure in Medicine," American Medical Association, June 14, 2023, https://www.ama-assn.org/press-center/press-releases/ama-adopts-new-policy-clarifying-role-bmi-measure-medicine.

6. A. Janet Tomiyama, Britt Ahlstrom, and Traci Mann, "Long-term Effects of Dieting: Is Weight Loss Related to Health?" *Social and Personality Psychology Compass* 7, no. 12 (December 2, 2013): 861–77, https://doi.org/10.1111/spc3.12076.

7. The Look AHEAD Research Group, "Cardiovascular Effects of Intensive Lifestyle Intervention in Type 2 Diabetes," *New England Journal of Medicine* 369, no. 2 (June 24, 2013): 145–54, https://doi.org/10.1056/nejmoa1212914.

8. Rebecca M. Puhl and Kelly D. Brownell, "Confronting and Coping with Weight Stigma: An Investigation of Overweight and Obese Adults," *Obesity* 14, no. 10 (October 1, 2006): 1802–15, https://doi.org/10.1038/oby.2006.208.

9. Tessa E. S. Charlesworth and Mahzarin R. Banaji, "Patterns of Implicit and Explicit Attitudes: I. Long-Term Change and Stability from 2007 to 2016,"

Psychological Science 30, no. 2 (January 3, 2019): 174–92, https://doi.org/10.1177/0956797618813087.

CHAPTER 21:
Health in an Ever-Evolving Digital Age

1. Jane Kelly, "Research Finds Gen Z, Millennials More Vulnerable to Fake News," *UVA Today*, September 6, 2024, https://news.virginia.edu/content/research-finds-gen-z-millennials-more-vulnerable-fake-news.
2. Jacqueline W. Lucas and Maria A. Villarroel, "Telemedicine Use Among Adults: United States, 2021," Centers for Disease Control and Prevention, October 13, 2022, https://doi.org/10.15620/cdc:121435.

CHAPTER 22:
Your Playbook for Optimal Health and Managing Disease

1. Debra Wood, "Average Time Doctors Spend with Patients," AMN Healthcare, June 23, 2023, https://www.amnhealthcare.com/blog/physician/locums/average-time-doctors-spend-with-patients; Hannah T. Neprash et al., "Measuring Primary Care Exam Length Using Electronic Health Record Data," *Medical Care* 59, no. 1 (November 16, 2020): 62–66, https://doi.org/10.1097/mlr.0000000000001450.
2. Lunna Lopes et al., "Health Care Debt in the U.S.: The Broad Consequences of Medical and Dental Bills," KFF, June 16, 2022, https://www.kff.org/report-section/kff-health-care-debt-survey-main-findings.
3. Barbara E. Bierer et al., "Advancing the Inclusion of Underrepresented Women in Clinical Research," *Cell Reports Medicine* 3, no. 4 (March 7, 2022): 100553, https://doi.org/10.1016/j.xcrm.2022.100553.

Index

Italicized page numbers indicate material in illustrations.

breathwork, 325, 486

Breda, Madeline, 547, 564, 565

bremelanotide, 62

Brisdelle, 247

Bristol Stool Chart, 425–26

bulb of vestibule, *7, 8, 10, 10, 53*

bulbourethral glands, 15, *16*

Burstein, Dina, 571, 580

butyrate, 417

Byron, Katy, 571, 574–76

C

Cabré, Hannah, 523, 531

caffeine, 517

calcifications, 269–70

calcitonin, 217

calcitonin gene-related peptide (CGRP), 339–40

calcium hydroxylapatite (CaHA), 456

Caldwell, Jessica, 357, 367–68, 377–79

calories, 540, 542, 548, 549, 558

cancer, 382, 496

  colon (colorectal), 427–29, 431

  gynecologic, 129–31

    breast, *see* breast cancer

    cervical, 64, 78–80, 130

    endometrial, 130, 209

    HPV-related, 64, 67, 78, 79, 130

    ovarian, 80, 98, 108, 130, 132

    uterine, 256

    vaginal, 130

    vulvar, 128, 130

  online information on, 612–13

  screening guidelines for, 592

  skin, 446, 450–54, 458

    development of, 450

    moles and, 452, 453

    precancers, 452–54

    risk of, 450, 454

    screening for, 452–54

    types and treatment of, 451

  treatments for, and heart disease, 393–94

candidiasis

  gut, 424–25

  vaginal (yeast infection), 87, 125–26, 129, 555

carbohydrates, 234, 343, 417, 540, 541, 548–50, 556, 558

  fiber, 226, 307–8, 326, 343, 413, 416–17, 419, 431–32, 550, 552, 556

cardiovascular disease, *see* heart disease

Casperson, Kelly, 45, 47, 48–50

causation versus correlation, 583

CDC (Centers for Disease Control and Prevention), 63–65, 70, 78, 79, 101, 184, 196, 272, 323, 493, 574, 584

celiac disease, 318, 414

cellulite, 445

cerebellum, *357,* 360

cerebral cortex, *357,* 358–60

cervical caps, 96

cervix, *3,* 9–10, *10*

  cancer of, 64, 78–80, 130

  mucus from, 86–87, 141

    family planning and, 97–98

  placenta previa and, 165, 174

Cesarean section, 173–75, 180, 184, 412, 423, 555

  vaginal birth after, 175

chatbots, 570, 571, 576–79

chemicals, *see* environmental toxins

Chen, Esther H., 330, 334, 335

chicken pox, 440–41

childbirth, xxii, 169–83

  baby's weight in, 393

  Black women and, 165, 180, 181–83

leaky gut, 316, 412–14, 417

leiomyomas (uterine fibroids), xix, xx, 120–22, 143, 237

leptin, 23, 207, 221, 415, 496

lesbians, 20, 33–35, 80–81, 474
  pregnancy and, 153–54

lesser vestibular glands (Skene's glands), 8
  prostate gland and, 15

levator ani, 13

Levine, Jody A., 435, 455

levonorgestrel, 99

LGBTQ+ people, 20, 31, 33, 35, 80, 474
  pregnancy and, 153–54

lipoprotein(a), 400

liraglutide, 558

liver, 221

LLMs (large language models), 576–78

lobular carcinoma in situ (LCIS), 284

lochia, 185

Lodhi, Sadaf, 109, 120

Lorde, Audre, 3

LSD, 483

lubricants, 96

lupus, 319, 414

luteal phase, 57, 57, 83, 84

luteinizing hormone (LH), 22, 57, 141, 211, 212, 364

lymphatic system, 264, 300, 324, 526
  breast cancer and, 281–83, 286
  gut and, 326

lymphocytes, 300

M

magnetic resonance imaging (MRI), 274, 282

Maltz, Wendy, 47, 70–71

mammograms, 266, 269, 270–75, 282, 284, 290–91

Manoogian, Emily, 495, 503, 504, 506

Martin, Jennifer L., 495, 502, 508

Maskatia, Zahida, 297, 311, 313

mast cells, 298, 300, 440

mastectomy, 278

mastitis, 184

masturbation, 72

Mayo Clinic, 572

McAllen, Jess, 329

McNally, Stephanie Trentacoste, 77, 103, 104, 109, 134, 135

MDMA, 483

meals
  breakfast, 556
  timing of, 505, 517

melanin, 435, 442, 446, 450

melanocytes, 446

melanoma, 451, 452, 458

melasma, 442

melatonin, 214, 227, 324, 497–99, 505
  supporting without supplementation, 505–6

meningioma, 355, 370

menopause, xxiii, 229–59, 367
  autoimmune diseases and, 316
  brain and, 363, 365–66
  breasts in, 266
  defined, 232
  early, 133, 233–34
  embracing, 249–50, 258–59
  estrogen drop in, 235–36, 343, 365, 515
    fibroids and, 120
    GI symptoms and, 412
    heart disease and, 238, 401, 402, 524
    hot flashes and, 245, 246
    immune system and, 304
    insulin resistance and, 554
    musculoskeletal system and, 343, 515, 528, 531–33, 537
    pain and, 352

providing support during, 43–44

sex education in, 3–4, *3*, 19–20, 46, 48

  girls' relationships and, 41–42

  healthy conversations, 36–41, 43

timeline of, 21–24

  early puberty factors, 22–23

  Sexual Maturity Rating, 23–24

Pudumjee, Shehroo, 357, 374

pulmonary embolism, 184

Q

Quaile, Heather, 231, 244, 254

R

raloxifene, 278

randomized controlled trials (RCTs), 582

Rankins, Nicole, 171, 175, 177, 178

rape, 70

Ravella, Shilpa, 297, 307, 409, 412

rectum, 13, 410, *411*

  bleeding from, 427

relaxin, 188

research, xxi–xxiii, xxvii, 593

  clinical trials, 581

    participating in, 607–10

    randomized controlled, 582

  reading scientific studies, 579–83

    correlation versus causation and, 583

    peer review and, 582

  types of studies, 580–81

  underrepresentation of women and minorities in, xxi–xxii, 577, 607

resistance training (strength training; weight training), 525, 531, 537, 542–43, 559

restless legs syndrome (RLS), 509–10, 512

retinoids, 438, 444, 445

Rheuban, Karen S., 571, 584–86

rheumatoid arthritis (RA), 317–18, 344, 414

Rheumatoid Arthritis Foundation, 613

Rh factor, 160

Roche, Megan, 523, 535

Roe v. Wade, 101–2

rosacea, 443

Rosen, Ilene M., 494, 499

Rosen, Stacey E., 383, 390, 404

Rumsey, Alissa, 545, 547, 566–68

Rybelsus (semaglutide), 215, 557–60

S

Sacks, Tina, 331, 336–38

Sahni, Sabrina, 263, 288

Salmon, Nicola, 139, 163

salpingectomy, 131, 132

sarcopenia, 528, 561

Saxenda, 558

Schumer, Amy, xxiii

scleroderma, 320

seasonal affective disorder (SAD), 468

sebum, 436, 438

selective mutism, 469

selective serotonin reuptake inhibitors (SSRIs), 247, 487, 488

self-compassion, 480

semaglutide drugs, 215–16, 557–60

semen, 141, 151

  sperm, 144, 149, 156–57, 211

    in artificial insemination, 151

    banks and donors, 153, 154, 156–57

    egg fertilized by, 9, 83, 86, 141–42

    intracytoplasmic injection of, 149

separation anxiety disorder, 469

urinary tract infections (UTIs), 8, 96, 113–17, 165
 diabetes and, 555
 menopause and, 114, 116–17, 240
 prevention of, 114–15
 reasons for, 113
 treatment of, 116
 in women versus men, 113–14
urticaria, 439–40
U.S. Preventive Services Task Force, 78, 165
U.S. Public Health Service Task Force on Women's Health Issues, xxi
uterine tubes (Fallopian tubes), 3, 4, 8, 10, 17, 18, 83, 141–42
 ectopic pregnancy in, 4, 143, 164
 ovarian cancer and, 132
 removal of, 131, 132
 tubal ligation, 98
uterus, 3, 4, 8–9, 10
 adenomyosis and, 124
 cancer of, 256
 endometrium, 209
  cancer of, 130, 209
  endometriosis, xxiii, 92, 108, 122–24, 130, 184, 237, 416
 fibroids in, xix, xx, 120–22, 143, 237
 layers of, 9
 in postpartum period, 185
 removal of (hysterectomy), 131–33, 412, 423
  for endometriosis, 124, 131
  for fibroids, 122, 131
  menopause following, 133, 233
  surgical options for, 132–33
  uterine tube removal in, 131, 132
  types of, 131

V

vaccines, 299, 301, 302, 321–24
 HPV, 64, 79
 shingles and, 441
 UTI, 115
Vaccine Safety Datalink (VSD), 323
vagina, 3, 6, 9, 10
 bacterial vaginosis and, 87, 125, 126, 129
 cancer of, 130
 microbiome of, 114, 126
 orifice of, 7, 7, 11, 11
 postpartum bleeding from, 185
 vaginitis, 129
 wetness and discharge from, 86–87
vaginal birth after Cesarean (VBAC), 175
valproate, 158
varicella zoster virus, 440–41
vasectomy, 99
venous thromboembolism (VTE), 184
Veozah, 247
vestibular bulbs, 7, 8, 10, 10, 53
vestibular glands
 greater (Bartholin's glands), 8, 16, 17, 18, 53, 54, 86
  bulbourethral glands and, 15
 lesser (Skene's glands), 8, 16, 86
  prostate gland and, 15
Victoza, 558
violence, partner, 81
virtual doctor visits, 583–86
vitamins, 156, 157, 305, 436, 446, 449, 550–51
vulva, 6, 7
 cancer of, 128, 130
 diversity of, 4, 12
 vulvar lichen sclerosus, 128

vulvar vestibule, 7

vulvodynia, 129

Vyleesi, 62

W

Waggel, Stephanie, 139, 159

warts, genital, 79

water, 431, 559

wearable health tracking devices and apps, 502, 588–91

Wegovy (semaglutide), 215, 557–60

weight

body mass index (BMI) and, 162–63, 560–62

gaining, 554, 555

health and, 562–63

healthcare system and, 162–64, 560–65

heart disease and, 398–99, 401

losing, 540, 542, 561–63

semaglutide drugs for, 215–16, 557–60

overweight and obesity, 235, 279, 414, 560, 561

heart disease and, 391, 392

pregnancy and, 162–64

underweight, 234

see also fat, body

weight training (strength training; resistance training), 525, 531, 537, 542–43, 559

White House Initiative on Women's Health Research, xiii, xxi, 255

Wilkens, Carrie, 464, 478–80

Williams, Serena, xxii

Winsberg, Mimi, 357, 368–70

Winter, Ashley, 109, 113–15

women of color, *see* Black women and people of color

Women's Alzheimer's Movement (WAM), xii–xiii

Women's Comprehensive Health and Research Center, xiii

Women's Health Initiative (WHI), 246, 251–52

World Health Organization, 321, 473

Wright, Vonda, 231, 239–40, 331, 343–44, 352, 353

Y

yeast infection, 87, 125–26, 129, 555

Yu, Christine, 521

Z

Zepbound, 216, 558

zone 2 training, 530

Zoom, 584

zygote, 142